WITHDRAWN FROM LIBRARY

DRUGS & BEHAVIOR

WITHDRAWN FROM LIBRARY

LIBRARY WI

This book is dedicated to the memories of
Rebel Henrikson Montoya
and
Kathryn Lei Kagawa-Webb

WITHDRAWN FROM LIBRARY

MONTGOMERY COLLEGE
ROCKVILLE CAMPUS LIBRARY
ROCKVILLE, MARYLAND

DRUGS & BEHAVIOR

Third Edition

FRED LEAVITT

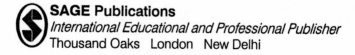

SAGE Publications
International Educational and Professional Publisher
Thousand Oaks   London   New Delhi

289373   APR 3 0 2004

Copyright © 1995 by Sage Publications, Inc.

All rights reserved. No part of this book may be reproduced or utilized in any form or by any means, electronic or mechanical, including photocopying, recording, or by any information storage and retrieval system, without permission in writing from the publisher.

For information address:

SAGE Publications, Inc.
2455 Teller Road
Thousand Oaks, California 91320
E-mail: order@sagepub.com

SAGE Publications Ltd.
6 Bonhill Street
London EC2A 4PU
United Kingdom

SAGE Publications India Pvt. Ltd.
M-32 Market
Greater Kailash I
New Delhi 110 048 India

Printed in the United States of America

Library of Congress Cataloging-in-Publication Data

Leavitt, Fred.
    Drugs and behavior / Fred Leavitt. — 3rd ed.
        p.   cm.
    Includes bibliographical references (pp. 419-504) and index.
    ISBN 0-8039-4783-6 (cloth).   —   ISBN 0-8039-4784-4 (pbk.)
    1. Psychopharmacology. 2. Psychotrophic drugs. I. Title.
RM315.L36   1995
615'.78—dc20   94-35078

96 97 98 99 00 01 10 9 8 7 6 5 4 3 2

Sage Production Editor: Astrid Virding

Brief Table
of Contents

Detailed Table of Contents

5. Variability in Response to Drugs   61

Preface

A reviewer wrote in *The British Journal of Psychiatry* that *Drugs and Behavior* (2nd edition) would become a classic. He was mistaken. Another wrote in *The Journal of the American Medical Association* that *Drugs and Behavior* should be on everyone's reading list of basic texts and standard reference works. That didn't happen either. Still, the book was well-received and I believe that the third edition is better. There are three reasons:

1. Practice in writing doesn't make perfect, but it helps, and I've practiced a lot over the last few years.
2. Computerized bibliographic services have made it much easier to identify and locate the latest and most relevant publications.
3. My editor at Sage, C. Deborah Laughton, is remarkably well-read in psychology and a serious writer herself. Her advice, encouragement, and friendship were invaluable. The rest of the Sage editorial staff helped in many ways.

Thanks to Sheldon Orloff, pediatrician at Oakland's Kaiser Hospital (and star basketball rebounder), for getting me access to Kaiser's excellent library facilities. Melanie Leavitt helped put the references in order. Information specialists at the National Clearinghouse for Alcohol and Drug Information supplied several references, and Terry Smith and Janell Baum at California State University did a great job with the illustrations. Special thanks to Irv Zucker of UC Berkeley, for a variety of reasons.

Introduction

Contents

What Is Psychopharmacology?
Why Study Psychopharmacology?
How This Book Differs From Others

What Is Psychopharmacology?

Psychopharmacology is the science that deals with the effects of drugs on behavior. A *drug* is a chemical that affects living matter. *Behavior,* broadly defined as any observable response, includes measures of perception, mood, thinking, and so forth. Drugs that affect behavior are called **psychoactive.**

Why Study Psychopharmacology?

Works of literature, some labeled fiction and some not so labeled, describe fascinating drug effects. In Greek mythology, travelers through Hades sipped from the River Lethe and became oblivious to all that had gone before. *Time* magazine anticipated in 1966 that memory pills might soon become available for instantly assimilating large bodies of knowledge. Ponce de Leon failed to find a fountain of youth, but physician Brown-Sequard injected himself with an extract of dog testes and became sexually rejuvenated at age 72. (For an explanation of the Brown-Sequard effect, see Chapter 17). The inhabitants of Aldous

1

Huxley's *Brave New World* ingested soma and were content. Kindly Dr. Jekyll swallowed a blood-red potion and was transmogrified into evil Mr. Hyde.

No known drugs produce blissful oblivion or instant knowledge, and the fountain of youth still awaits discovery. Many substances reduce inhibitions, but none transform human to beast. (Some people would disagree.) Drugs are available to make anxieties disappear, but they have undesirable side effects. Nevertheless, newer drugs may someday accomplish most of the above-named ends. That is a major part of the lure of psychopharmacology.

People study psychopharmacology for several reasons. First, they use drugs as tools for discovering the physiological mechanisms underlying particular behaviors. Drugs that reliably induce or suppress sleeping, dreaming, learning, memory, eating, drinking, sex, and aggression have helped researchers identify brain areas that regulate those behaviors.

Second, desirable behaviors are enhanced and undesirable behaviors suppressed by various drugs. Caffeine increases alertness, and chlorpromazine (Thorazine) suppresses many symptoms of schizophrenia. The goal of many psychopharmacologists is to develop drugs that enhance or suppress even more powerfully while producing fewer side effects.

Third, humans are drug-taking animals. Anthropologists have reported drug use in virtually every culture studied. Physicians and unsavory characters on dimly lit street corners are not the only sources of mind-altering substances. Any supermarket will do. Caffeine, nicotine, alcohol, and many vitamins and spices have powerful effects on the brain. Only through careful research will their effects become sufficiently well understood.

Fourth, proper study of the drug field teaches not just about drugs but also about methodology and critical thinking. The facts and skills learned are useful in a variety of occupations, although some require advanced degrees. These include pharmacist (someone who prepares and dispenses drugs), pharmacologist (a scientist who studies the effects and mechanisms of action of drugs), and physician. Pharmaceutical research laboratories hire scientists in many fields including organic, analytic, and biochemistry; molecular and cell biology; biophysics; virology; immunology; toxicology; and pathology.

Clinical psychologists should know about drugs. Jack Wiggins, president of the American Psychological Association, took the controversial position that psychologists should have the right to prescribe (*APA Monitor,* September, 1992). Wiggins wrote that about 20% of all medical prescriptions are for drugs that affect mental processes.

Many jobs available to students right out of college require knowledge of drugs. Drug sales representatives meet with physicians to discuss the advantages of specific products and influence prescribing habits; and marketing representatives probe the needs of health care professionals and their patients. Other jobs in which knowledge of drugs helps include the following: employee assistance counselor, substance abuse counselor, customs inspector, psychology technician, psychiatric technician, high school counselor, social worker, nurse, parole officer, residential counselor/manager, animal trainer, and FBI agent. The opportunities are diverse and considerable.

A fifth reason for studying psychopharmacology is that drug abuse is regarded as among the leading problems facing U.S. citizens (*Bureau of Justice Statistics Sourcebook,* 1992). Yet decisions about drug issues are often based on inadequate or misleading information. The study of psychopharmacology can help people make informed decisions about issues such as the following:

Should drug-testing be allowed (required) in the workplace?

Should pregnant women who use drugs be prosecuted for endangering the lives of their fetuses?

Should patients in institutions have the right to refuse psychiatric drugs?

Should drug-addicted felons be diverted to treatment programs or sent to prison?

Should advertisements for prescription drugs directed at laypeople be allowed?

Should laypeople be allowed to buy prescription drugs without the approval of a physician?

To minimize the spread of AIDS, should drug abusers be allowed to exchange dirty for sterile needles?

Should clinical psychologists, who have no medical training, be allowed to prescribe psychiatric drugs?

Should marijuana be available by prescription for treating glaucoma and the nausea that often follows chemotherapy?

Should people who commit crimes while high on drugs be allowed to plead diminished capacity as a defense?

What rules should govern the use of performance-enhancing drugs by professional athletes?

▩ How This Book Differs From Others

This book differs from most psychopharmacology texts in at least two ways. First, most of the others devote separate chapters to each important drug category. The organization makes it easy for readers to learn all they want about whichever drugs interest them. A disadvantage is that many drugs, both licit and illicit, have short-lived popularity. Thus, knowledge about them becomes obsolete after a few years. Since the last edition of *Drugs and Behavior*, medical barbiturate use declined notably while MDMA (ecstasy), other designer drugs, and crack cocaine became major drugs of abuse. With expiration of the patents on diazepam (Valium) and chlordiazepoxide (Librium), a slew of new antianxiety drugs became available. Fluoxetine (Prozac) and related drugs, unknown 10 years ago, captured a major share of the antidepressant market.

Drugs and Behavior is organized by behavioral categories. Behavioral and methodological principles are not eternal, but their half-lives are considerably longer than those of drugs. Still, the chapters on sleep, sexual behavior, memory, and so forth, all have sections on the effects of popular drugs on those behaviors.

A second advantage of organization by behavior stems from the thorny methodological difficulties that plague most of the fields discussed. For example, few studies on sleep-promoting drugs last longer than 5 weeks; but sleep patterns in research laboratories often do not stabilize in such a short time. Furthermore, the acute and chronic effects of many drugs on sleep differ substantially. Sleep stages during normal, non-drugged sleep and following drug administration may also differ. Discrepancies may appear between objective and subjective measures of quality of sleep. Discussing the problems in one place is more efficient than reintroducing them as they arise for each drug.

The second way in which this book differs from most other texts has been my willingness to tackle controversial issues: Should any or all drugs be legalized? Do pharmaceutical companies develop and promote their products ethically? Does drug therapy cure mental illness? Do programs for preventing and treating drug abuse work? I have tried to explore each issue fairly but have inevitably found myself favoring one side. It seemed important, both pedagogically and morally, to state my views on each issue.

CHAPTER

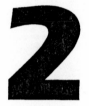

By the time you finish reading this chapter, you should be able to answer the following questions:

What is the functional unit of the central nervous system (CNS)?

How do neurons communicate with each other?

What are receptors?

Two drugs that increase the activity of a given neurotransmitter (NT) to the same extent may have very different actions on behavior. Why?

What criteria must be satisfied to establish a substance as an NT?

Which NTs are released by the autonomic nervous system?

Which NT has been most clearly implicated in development of tolerance?

Which NT is most clearly affected by psychedelic drugs?

Which NT probably mediates the reinforcing effects of cocaine?

Which NT has been most clearly implicated in anxiety disorders?

Neurotransmission

Contents

Psychopharmacologists must know a great deal about the **central nervous system** (CNS), because the CNS is the primary site where psychoactive drugs act. Finding the site of drug action has helped scientists in many different fields. Clinical pharmacologists derived valuable clues for improving psychiatric and other drugs, and they deepened their understanding of disorders treated by the drugs. Neuroscientists identified CNS changes induced by LSD and related drugs, which helped them understand the origins of hallucinations. Others, seeking to unravel the mechanisms of reward, located the brain sites activated by cocaine. The LSD and cocaine research is summarized below, and similar work on sleep, dreams, learning, and memory is discussed in later chapters.

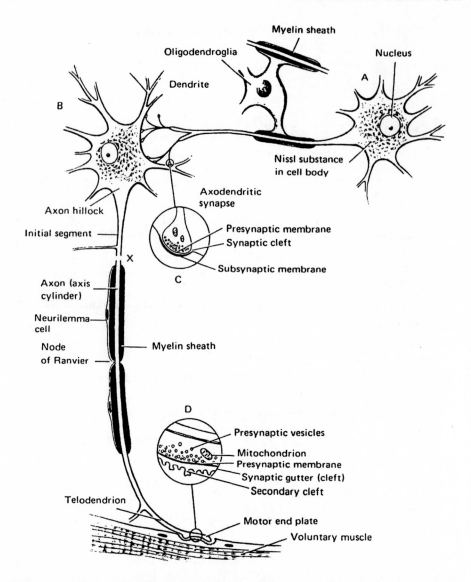

Figure 2.1. Diagram of (A) a neuron located within the CNS and (B) a lower motor neuron located in both the ventral and peripheral nervous systems. The latter synapses with a voluntary muscle cell to form a motor end-plate. Note the similarities, as reconstructed from electron micrographs, between a synapse between two neurons (C) and a motor end-plate (D). The hiatus in the nerve (X) represents the border between the CNS (above the X) and the peripheral nervous system (below the X). Reproduced from *The Nervous System* (3rd ed.), by C. Noback & R. Demarest, 1986, New York: McGraw-Hill. Copyright 1986 by McGraw-Hill. Reproduced with permission of McGraw-Hill.

The functional unit of the CNS is the nerve cell (**neuron**). Although they vary considerably in size and shape, all neurons have three principal parts: a cell body, slender **dendrites** that carry nerve impulses into the cell body (most neurons have a great many dendrites), and one relatively thick **axon** that carries nerve impulses from the cell body (see Figure 2.1). The number of neurons within the human brain has been estimated at 100 billion, and a given neuron may connect with several thousand others. The number of possible combinations of neuronal connections in a single human brain is greater than the total number of atomic particles that make up the known universe (Thompson, 1985).

Neurons float in fluids that contain electrically charged particles called **ions**. Sodium and potassium ions are positively charged, chloride ions negatively charged. Each neuron is covered by a membrane with pores that can open and close. When open, the pores form channels that permit ions to flow through, usually one type per channel. Resting neurons keep most sodium and chloride ions outside the membrane and most potassium ions inside. The result is that resting neurons are negatively charged, with an electric potential of about –70 millivolts.

When a neuron is sufficiently stimulated (by other neurons, light, heat, or pressure), its membrane becomes suddenly and briefly permeable to sodium and other positive ions. They rush inside, and the inside of the neuron becomes positively charged. The change from negative to positive is called an **action potential.**

The action potential lasts for only about a millisecond at a given point along the axon, as sodium channels close behind it and ion pumps restore the membrane to its resting state. But the flow of ions at each point changes the permeability of the membrane at the next point. So the action potential travels as an electrical wave down the axon (see Figure 2.2).

▓ Synaptic Transmission

Whereas transmission within neurons is electrical, transmission between them is primarily chemical. Otto Loewi demonstrated this in a classic series of experiments begun in 1921. Loewi extracted the heart from a frog and bathed it in a special fluid that kept it beating. When he stimulated the vagus nerve leading to the heart, beating slowed as it does following vagal stimulation in normal, healthy frogs. Then Loewi

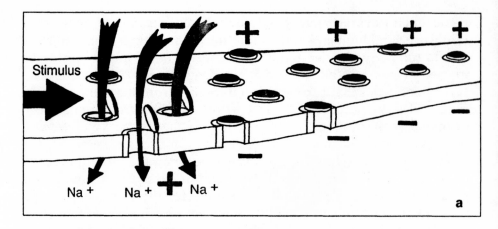

Figure 2.2a. As a neural impulse travels down a neuron, sodium channels open at the point of stimulation and sodium ions rush in.

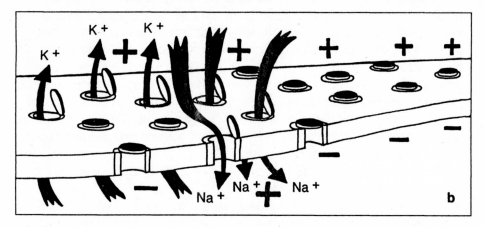

Figure 2.2b. As the neural impulse travels, sodium channels close behind it and potassium channels open. Potassium ions flow outward.

diverted the fluid secreted by the vagus nerve into a vessel containing a second isolated heart. Beating of the second heart slowed. He concluded that the secreted substance, later identified as acetylcholine (ACh), was responsible. Loewi also stimulated the accelerans nerve, which speeds up heart rate in both normal animals and isolated hearts. When exposed to the released fluid, an isolated heart speeded up. The second fluid was norepinephrine (NE). ACh and NE are two of at least 50 compounds called **neurotransmitters** (NTs). Some NTs inhibit activity, as ACh inhibits heart rate. Others stimulate, like NE. Some NTs inhibit at some brain sites and stimulate at others (Erulkar, 1989).

NTs are stored in small sacs called **synaptic vesicles.** The vesicles are located in terminal buttons that branch off the end of neuronal axons. When an action potential reaches the terminal, calcium channels open and positively charged calcium ions rush inside. This triggers the release of one or as many as five or six NTs from the synaptic vesicles. Most neurons release more than one.

The NTs diffuse across the **synaptic cleft** (the gap between neurons) to **receptor** molecules on a second neuron. The first neuron is called **presynaptic** and the second **postsynaptic.** If the released NT is excitatory, it opens channels that let sodium ions flow into the postsynaptic neuron as potassium ions flow out. This increases the likelihood that the postsynaptic neuron will have an action potential. Inhibitory NTs open chloride and/or potassium **ion channels** and reduce the likelihood that the postsynaptic neuron will fire. Box 2.1 describes an extreme consequence of preventing sodium ion flow.

The number of ion channels that open correlates with the amount of NT. The length of time they stay open correlates with the strength of attachment (**affinity**) between the NT and receptors. The affinity determines how long the NT acts on the receptors.

There are two types of synaptic transmission. The type just described, rapid transmission, takes about a millisecond. Slow synaptic transmission occurs over several milliseconds or even minutes. As in fast transmission, an NT activates receptors. This triggers the release of other substances, called **second messengers,** that change the likelihood that the postsynaptic neuron will fire.

Chemical transmission is slower than electrical but more flexible. If a postsynaptic neuron is stimulated excessively, its receptors decrease in number (called **down-regulation**); conversely, the number of receptors increases when levels of stimulation are low (**up-regulation**). Receptor responsiveness is also influenced by neuronal substances called **neuromodulators.**

After an NT acts on the postsynaptic neuron, it must be inactivated. One mechanism is metabolism, which accounts for the rapid inactivation of acetylcholine (ACh). Many insecticides and nerve gases block the enzyme that metabolizes ACh, thus causing continuous, convulsive muscle contractions and eventual death.

Most NTs, although metabolized to some extent, are inactivated primarily by being moved away from the receptors and back into the

Box 2.1
Zombies

The substance tetrodotoxin stops the movement of sodium ions into cells, thus blocking nerve conduction. As a result, tetrodotoxin is at least 500 times more deadly than cyanide. It is found in the ovaries of puffer fish and in certain frogs and newts. The relatively safe puffer fish flesh is regarded as a delicacy in Japan, although chefs must be specially trained and licensed before they are allowed to prepare it. Still, about 100 people die each year after eating the fish.

Harvard ethnobotanist Wade Davis traveled to Haiti to investigate reports of zombies—people who have been drugged, buried alive, and then resurrected. He wrote a fascinating account of his adventures and provided firm evidence that the reports are true. The drug involved is tetrodotoxin. Davis wrote that symptoms of zombification and tetrodotoxin poisoning are remarkably similar. He described the case of a Kyoto man admitted to a hospital in 1977 with puffer fish poisoning. The man eventually stopped breathing. Physicians administered artificial respiration and other treatments, but they didn't help. Twenty-four hours later, he spontaneously began breathing and eventually recovered completely. He said that his senses were unimpaired throughout the ordeal, and he had heard his family weeping over his body, but he was unable to let them know that he was alive.

Davis described how zombies are created. A sorcerer rubs a poison containing tetrodotoxin into the wound of a victim. It slows the victim's metabolism to the point of clinical death. He is pronounced dead and buried alive. In many cases he suffocates in the coffin or dies from the poison. Otherwise, he is dug up from the grave, baptized by the sorcerer with a new name, and given a drug that brings on a state of amnesia and disorientation. The second drug is a species of *Datura,* a powerful anticholinergic. So traumatized, the victim loses volition.

SOURCE: *The Serpent and the Rainbow,* by W. Davis, New York: Warner Books, 1985.

presynaptic terminals. The process, called *reuptake,* conserves the NTs. Many psychoactive drugs affect reuptake. Cocaine, for example, blocks the reuptake of norepinephrine, dopamine, and serotonin, thus augmenting the normal effects of all three NTs. The immediate effect is elevation of mood, but the NTs eventually become depleted and de-

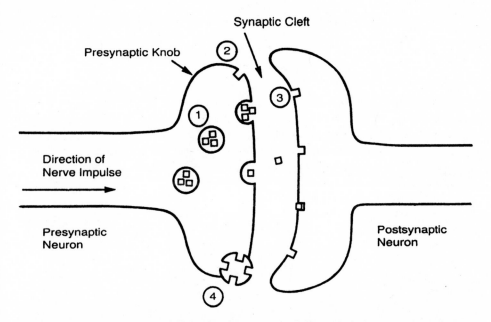

Figure 2.3. 1. Synaptic vesicles (circles) are found in axon terminals, located at the ends of axons. Vesicles contain neurotransmitters (squares).
2. Presynaptic autoreceptors are located on presynaptic neurons.
3. Receptors are located on postsynaptic membranes.
4. Most neurotransmitters are inactivated by a reuptake pump that returns them to presynaptic neurons.
SOURCE: Adapted from Daigle, Clark, & Landry (1988).

pression follows. Figure 2.3 summarizes the typical process of neuro-transmission.

▓ Receptors

All NTs and many drugs bind to one or more receptors. (Substances that bind to receptors are called **ligands.**) Receptor subtypes often differ in their relative affinities for the same ligand and the speed with which they act. The types of receptors on postsynaptic neurons determine how the neurons respond to NTs. Some neurons, for example, are stimulated by ACh and some are inhibited. The diversity of receptors increases the information-handling capacities of the central nervous system (Schofield, Shivers, & Seeburg, 1990).

Agonistic Effects

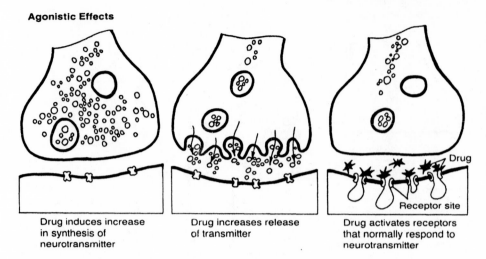

Drug induces increase in synthesis of neurotransmitter

Drug increases release of transmitter

Drug activates receptors that normally respond to neurotransmitter

Figure 2.4. A Drug May Facilitate the Actions of a Neurotransmitter in Any of Several Ways

Determining the location of a drug's receptors is an important step in understanding its mechanism of action. Unwanted effects—side effects—occur when a drug interacts with more than one receptor subtype or with receptors for more than one NT. Cooper, Bloom, and Roth (1991) speculated that drugs of the future will be designed to fit a single receptor, thus minimizing side effects.

⊠ Effects of Psychoactive Drugs on Neurotransmitter Function

Psychoactive drugs influence NT activity. Drugs that potentiate activity are called **agonists,** drugs that interfere are **antagonists.** Leonhard (1992) noted 20 possible sites at which psychoactive drugs affect neurotransmission. Some are listed below and some illustrated in Figures 2.4 and 2.5.

PRESYNAPTIC EFFECTS

Synthesis of NT. NTs are manufactured within the brain from materials called **precursors.** Some drugs change the amount of available precursors. Parkinson's disease is associated with abnormally low levels of dopamine, but peripherally administered dopamine does not enter the

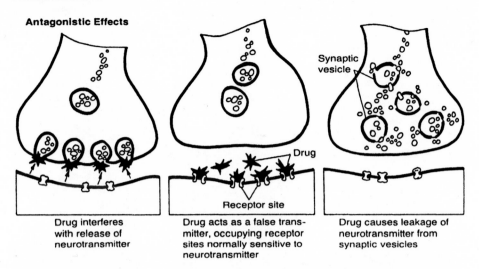

Figure 2.5. A Drug May Antagonize the Actions of a Neurotransmitter in Any of Several Ways

brain. So victims of Parkinson's disease are treated with the dopamine precursor, L-dopa.

Storage of NT. Both cocaine and reserpine inhibit the reuptake of norepinephrine, dopamine, and serotonin; thus, the NTs become vulnerable to metabolism and are depleted. As indicated above, cocaine initially augments NT activity, so it elevates mood in the short term. Reserpine's depleting effects occur more slowly and without an initial augmentation. Prolonged use of either drug causes depression.

Release of NT. Amphetamine promotes release of several NTs, which accounts for its stimulating effects.

Production of False NT. Some drugs replace NTs in synaptic vesicles. The effects range from indistinguishable to highly dissimilar and can be clinically useful. For example, norepinephrine acts at certain postsynaptic sites to increase blood pressure. Drugs that displace stored NE and are less potent than it are used to treat high blood pressure.

POSTSYNAPTIC EFFECTS

Changes in Postsynaptic Receptors. Many scientists believe that schizophrenia is caused by excessive activity of dopamine neurons within the

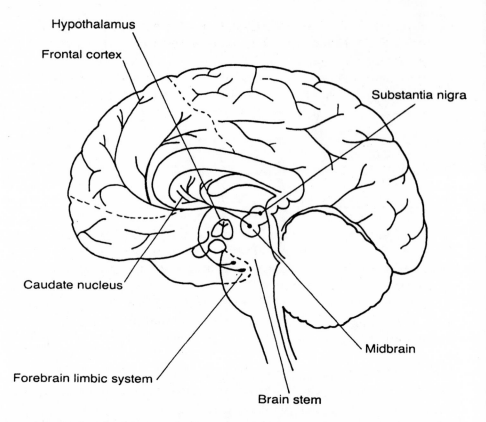

Figure 2.6. The brain has three important dopamine systems: (a) A local circuit on the hypothalamus; (b) A pathway from the substantia nigra to the caudate nucleus; (c) A pathway with cell bodies in the brain stem and midbrain that project to many areas of the cerebral cortex and forebrain limbic system.

brain's **limbic system** (see Figure 2.6). Antipsychotic drugs inhibit activity of limbic dopamine receptors.

Postsynaptic Receptor Adaptation. Chronic administration of antidepressants leads to reduced sensitivity of a set of norepinephrine receptors in the frontal cortex of the rat brain.

INHIBITION OF METABOLIC ENZYMES

The enzyme monoamine oxidase is crucial for metabolizing serotonin, norepinephrine, and dopamine. Some antidepressants, called **mono-**

amine oxidase inhibitors (MAOIs), block the actions of MAO. Thus, activity of the NTs increases and is assumed to be the cause of the antidepressant actions.

A dysfunction of the **cholinergic** system is suspected to cause or contribute to Alzheimer's disease (see Chapter 15). Inhibitors of the enzyme that metabolizes ACh may help Alzheimer's victims.

▓ Difficulties Involved in Assigning Specific Functions to Neurotransmitters

Researchers sometimes administer a drug with known actions on an NT, observe subsequent behavioral changes, and interpret them as evidence that the behaviors are normally controlled by the affected NT. Many examples will be given in the chapters that follow. However, the strategy rarely permits definitive conclusions. The action of a drug on an NT generally triggers a cascade of events that ultimately involves much of the brain. Moreover, drugs have nonspecific effects, both **peripheral** (outside the central nervous system) and central. For example, Satinoff (1988) claimed that all drugs used to study the neuropharmacological substrates of REM sleep alter body temperature, and changes in body temperature profoundly affect sleep.

Few drugs act on just a single NT system. A drug that induces a particular behavior when applied to a specific brain area often produces different effects elsewhere. For example, scopolamine facilitates or impairs learning, depending on whether it is placed in the ventral or dorsal caudate nucleus of rats (Neill & Grossman, 1970).

Many NT manipulations produce species-specific effects. The drug carbachol increases ACh levels. When placed in the lateral hypothalamus of rats, carbachol induces drinking (Grossman, 1960). But carbachol-injected cats sleep and gerbils foot-thump (Block, Vallier, & Glickman, 1974; Hernandez-Peon, 1965).

Mandell, Spooner, and Brunet (1969) tested 25 naturally occurring amino acids on sleep and arousal in young chicks. Six activated, 11 depressed, and only 8 had no effect. Had a researcher tried only one activating and one depressing substance, she might have concluded that she had isolated the crucial NTs.

Compensatory mechanisms, for example, up- or down-regulation of receptors, are usually activated when the concentration of an NT deviates from its normal range. So drug-induced changes are often transient. Moreover, NT systems are interdependent. Gold (1992) cited evidence that levels of circulating glucose affect receptors for serotonin, acetylcholine, GABA, opioid, and excitatory amino acid receptors.

The human brain is enormously complex. Martinez (1986), discussing NT involvement in memory, drew on an analogy from John Garcia to compare the attribute of memory in an organism to the quality of speed in a car. Martinez wrote:

> Speed is the result of most of the parts of the car functioning together. Damage to any number of parts, such as wheels, axles, drive shaft, and so on, will lead to less speed. Similarly, memory results from the simultaneous functioning of many neurotransmitters, and the alteration of functioning of any one will alter learning and memory.

By extension, all single-NT explanations of complex human functions are almost certainly incomplete.

▩ Some Proven and Probable Neurotransmitters

Before a substance is accepted as an NT, it must satisfy several not entirely agreed-upon criteria:

1. The substance must be contained within the presynaptic nerve terminal.
2. It must be released from nerve endings on stimulation of the nerve.
3. Injection of the substance must mimic the synaptic action that normally occurs after NT is released.
4. Some mechanism, enzymatic or otherwise, must exist for terminating its action. The mechanism must fit the time course of NT action.
5. Drugs that interfere with nerve stimulation at the synapse in question must produce similar effects following local application of the substance.

Many substances have been proposed as NTs, but few have been shown to satisfy all the criteria. Several prominent candidates are listed below. Their anatomical distributions, receptor types, and links to specific physiological and psychological functions are indicated.

ACETYLCHOLINE

Functions of Acetylcholine (ACh) Within the Autonomic Nervous System (ANS) and Neuromuscular Junction

The **autonomic nervous system** (ANS) is a motor system that regulates the activities of smooth muscles, cardiac muscles, and glands. Each internal organ receives a double set of fibers, one from the parasympathetic system of the ANS and one from the sympathetic system. The parasympathetic system is most active when an organism is relaxed, and the sympathetic dominates during periods of excitement. The nerves of the ANS consist of two sets of neurons. **Preganglionic neurons** have cell bodies in the brain or spinal cord and axons that terminate in **ganglia** (aggregations of neurons) outside the CNS. Each preganglionic neuron synapses with a **postganglionic neuron** that sends its axons to the effector organs. ACh is released by all preganglionic and all postganglionic parasympathetic neurons. The postganglionic ACh receptors are called **muscarinic.**

A separate motor system, the **somatic** system, controls skeletal muscle movement. Cell bodies within this system arise within the spinal cord and send axons directly to skeletal muscles. ACh is the transmitter released at synapses between CNS and muscle. Receptors at these neuromuscular junctions are called **nicotinic.**

Although ACh acts on both muscarinic and nicotinic receptors, many drugs are specific to one or the other. Ophthalmologists dilate pupils by applying short-acting antimuscarinic drugs. Most antipsychotic and antianxiety drugs, many antidepressants, and all over-the-counter drugs containing scopolamine or an antihistamine, have antimuscarinic effects. These effects include hot, dry skin; dilated pupils; blurred vision; rapid pulse; agitation; confusion; and memory and motor impairment.

Drugs that act at nicotinic synapses affect muscle contractability. They can improve or impair life. The nicotinic drug neostigmine helps victims of myasthenia gravis, a disease characterized by rapid fatigability of skeletal muscle. More powerful nicotinics, when used as key ingredients of insecticides and nerve gases, may kill. Antinicotinics are also used for both helpful and hurtful purposes. Succinylcholine, very

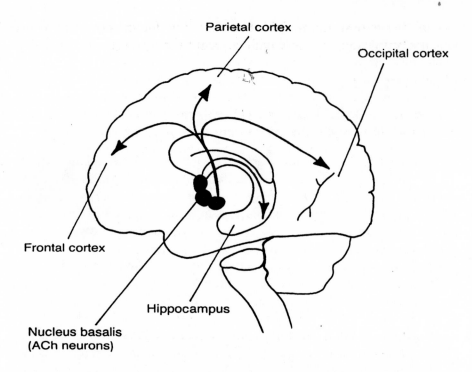

Parietal cortex

Occipital cortex

Frontal cortex

Hippocampus

Nucleus basalis
(ACh neurons)

Figure 2.7. Cell bodies for the ACh system are in the nucleus basalis at the base of the brain. They project throughout the cerebral cortex and hippocampus.

short acting, is valuable when surgical patients must be briefly immobilized. Curare, applied to arrow tips by various South American Indians, immediately paralyzes muscles and causes death from respiratory failure.

Functions of ACh Within the Central Nervous System

ACh is distributed throughout the brain and highly concentrated in the basal ganglia (structures that regulate movement) and motor cortex (see Figure 2.7). ACh is probably involved in regulation of such diverse behaviors as motor activity, food and water intake, sleep and arousal, and learning and memory. Alzheimer's disease is associated with ACh dysfunction (Woolf & Butcher, 1989).

Atropine and related antimuscarinic substances are found in plants of the genus *Datura*. They act both centrally and peripherally to produce a characteristic syndrome: impaired memory and motor ability, slurred speech, drowsiness, confusion, disorientation, feelings of unpleasantness, and visual and auditory hallucinations (Longo & de Carolis, 1968). Some antimuscarinics are used to treat glaucoma. James Joyce suffered from glaucoma, provoking the speculation that his unique writing style, especially in *Finnegan's Wake*, stemmed from the disorienting effects of his medicine. Amazingly, antimuscarinics are taken voluntarily; one species of *Datura* may be the most universally used drug by the Indian tribes of California, Arizona, and New Mexico (*High Times*, 1978).

NOREPINEPHRINE (NE)

Norepinephrine (NE) is one of several compounds called **catecholamines.** They have a common structure: a catechol nucleus (a benzene ring with two hydroxyl groups) and an amine group. Dopamine and epinephrine are two other catecholamine NTs.

Functions of NE Within the Autonomic Nervous System

NE is released by almost all postganglionic sympathetic neurons, so most of its peripheral actions are opposite to those of ACh. Some effects of sympathetic activity are heart rate and blood pressure increases and dilated pupils. Many drugs, including most stimulants, cause sympathetic side effects such as photophobia (extreme sensitivity to light), nausea, headache, and sweating. Most antipsychotic drugs inhibit sympathetic functioning; one result is that users frequently experience dizziness upon arising from a prone position.

Functions of NE Within the Central Nervous System

NE cell bodies cluster heavily in the **locus coeruleus,** a group of about 12,000 large neurons (in humans) on each side of the base of the brain. From there, axons extend upwards and reach almost all brain structures (Cooper et al., 1991) (see Figure 2.8). NE release promotes behavioral arousal and probably affects body temperature, food and water intake, and mood.

Two receptor types, called **alpha** and **beta,** respond to NE. Both have subtypes. Activation of beta$_1$ receptors stimulates the heart and increases blood pressure. Propranolol blocks beta$_1$ receptors and is used to treat hypertension and some types of anxiety.

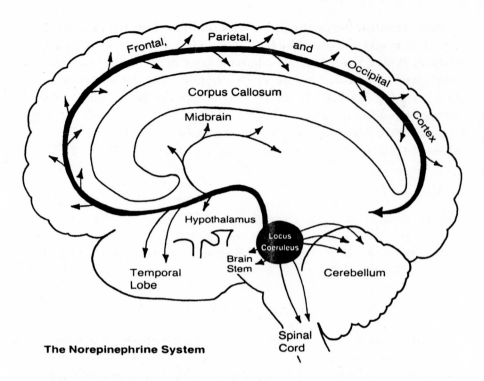

Figure 2.8. Cell bodies of the norepinephrine system cluster in the locus coeroleus and project throughout the cerebral cortex.

EPINEPHRINE

Epinephrine is probably not an important brain neurotransmitter. It is secreted by the adrenal glands in stressful situations.

DOPAMINE (DA)

The brain has three major dopamine (DA) circuits. One connects the hypothalamus and pituitary gland and plays a major role in the manufacture and release of pituitary hormones into the bloodstream. The second, containing about 75% of brain DA, originates in the lower midbrain. This system regulates movement and is deficient in victims of the severe motor disorder, Parkinson's disease. The third DA circuit originates in the midbrain and projects to areas of the cerebral cortex and limbic system. Considerable evidence (see Chapter 14) implicates excess DA within the limbic system to schizophrenia (see Figure 2.6).

Four receptor types have been described for DA. Almost all antipsychotic drugs reduce the activity of limbic system D_2 and D_3 receptors. But clozapine, a highly effective antipsychotic, acts on D_4 receptors. Chronic administration of antipsychotics affects DA receptors controlling motor functions; they may become supersensitive and cause movement disorders (Creese, Burt, & Snyder, 1978).

Cocaine, by binding to receptors that normally carry released DA back to presynaptic neurons, blocks DA reuptake and potentiates its activity. From this and other evidence, Kuhar, Ritz, and Boja (1991) inferred that limbic system DA neurons play a critical role in the reinforcing effects of cocaine and possibly other drugs of abuse. Kuhar et al. offered the following:

- Cocaine administration causes a dose-dependent increase in extracellular DA in limbic areas.
- Blocking postsynaptic DA receptors weakens the reinforcing properties of cocaine.
- DA-like drugs substitute for cocaine.
- The destruction of DA limbic neurons disrupts cocaine self-administration, but destruction of NE or serotonergic neurons does not.
- Many amphetamine actions are similar to those of cocaine, and both nicotine and alcohol also increase extracellular DA in limbic areas. This suggests that limbic neurons are a final common pathway for several drugs of abuse. (Even if the hypothesis is correct, the initial site of action, the receptor, might be located elsewhere.)

SEROTONIN

Serotonin is also called 5-hydroxytryptamine or 5-HT. The cell bodies of serotonin-containing neurons cluster in the **raphe nuclei** of the upper brain stem and project to many areas, including the cerebral cortex, hypothalamus, and limbic system. Serotonin and NE are distributed similarly throughout the brain (see Figures 2.8 and 2.9), but most of their effects are in opposite directions.

Serotonin is found in the pineal gland, smooth muscle, and blood platelets. Most serotonergic drugs administered orally or by injection do not exert specific actions on the brain—they affect the other systems, too. So, central and peripheral effects must be disentangled for proper interpretation of results. Several receptors and subtypes have been identified, but their roles are not clear.

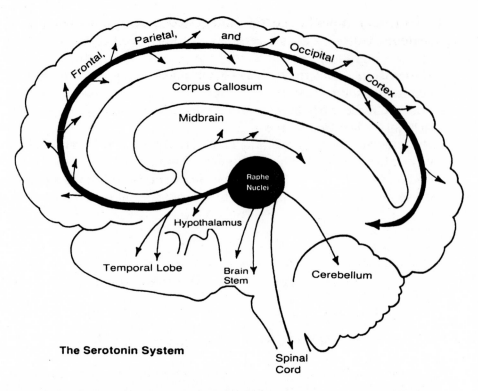

Figure 2.9. Cell bodies of the serotonin system cluster in the raphe nucleus and project throughout the cerebral cortex.

Serotonin plays an important role in the control of sleep. Lesions of the raphe nucleus produce insomnia, and the serotonin precursor L-tryptophan induces sleep. Serotonin affects mood and is implicated in various neuropsychiatric disorders, including anxiety, panic disorder, obsessive-compulsive disorder, depression, schizophrenia, alcoholism, migraine, sexual dysfunction, and Alzheimer's disease (Murphy, 1990). Many antidepressant drugs facilitate serotonergic transmission.

Khanna and his associates (reviewed in Khanna, 1989) showed that brain serotonin plays a role in the development of drug tolerance. Rats given drugs that deplete serotonin levels developed tolerance more slowly and lost it more quickly than did control animals; there were no effects on an already established level of tolerance. Increased serotonin levels led to more rapid development of tolerance. The manipulations worked only when they affected serotonin levels within the median raphe nucleus.

Jacobs (1987) summarized and integrated evidence showing that psychedelic drugs act on a subtype of serotonin receptor:

- The psychedelic LSD works in microgram amounts, suggesting that it acts on specific brain receptors.
- When LSD-like psychedelics are administered to animals, the only reliable changes are in brain serotonin.
- LSD, mescaline, and psilocin are structurally dissimilar but cross-tolerant, which suggests a common site of action.
- LSD suppresses activity of serotonin-containing neurons, which strengthens the hypothesis that it acts on the serotonergic system. But destruction of the neurons enhances LSD's behavioral effects, suggesting that it does not act directly on those neurons. Otherwise, their destruction would remove LSD's site of action and eliminate its effects.
- In rats, even ones with serotonin-depleted brains, many effects of LSD and mescaline mimic those of administered serotonin. That supports the view that the drugs act directly on serotonin receptors.
- Prolonged use of monoamine oxidase inhibitors (MAOIs) reduces the number of brain serotonin receptor sites. Rats, cats, and humans pretreated with MAOIs respond very weakly to LSD.
- Rats can be taught to discriminate between different internal states, for example, by requiring them to press a bar when they have received LSD but not at other times (see p. 93). The rats perceive all the major psychedelics as LSD-like, that is, they press the bar, but they do not bar press for other types of drugs. When LSD was given to rats pretreated with a drug that blocks the actions of serotonin at its receptor sites, the LSD suppressed serotonin neuronal activity as usual. But the rats did not discriminate between LSD and non-LSD-like drugs—further evidence that LSD acts at serotonin receptor sites. The 5-HT$_2$ subtype is most strongly implicated.
- Among 22 drugs drawn from the three different structural groups of human psychedelics, a very high correlation was found between affinity for 5-HT$_2$ receptors and hallucinogenic potency.

HISTAMINE

Histamine-containing neurons have their cell bodies in the hypothalamus and reticular formation and project broadly to the cerebral cortex. This suggests a possible role for histamine in food and water intake, autonomic activity, hormone release, and arousal (Cooper et al., 1991).

Histamine receptors exist in three forms: H_1, acted upon by the common antihistaminic drugs; H_2, on which the common antihistaminics are ineffective; and the recently discovered H_3. Histamine's excitatory actions generally involve interaction with H_1 receptors, its inhibitory actions with H_2.

GAMMA-AMINOBUTYRIC ACID (GABA)

The amino acid gamma-aminobutyric acid (GABA) is probably the major inhibitory neurotransmitter of the cerebral cortex, limbic system, and midbrain. It may play a role in schizophrenia, anxiety states, and epilepsy (low levels of GABA are found in at least one type of epilepsy).

Of the two GABA receptors, $GABA_A$ is much more abundant than $GABA_B$ and linked with receptors for **benzodiazepine** drugs. Benzodiazepines, the most popular antianxiety drugs, potentiate GABA's actions. Gardner (1989) hypothesized that partial activation of benzodiazepine receptors relieves anxiety, and more complete activation produces muscle relaxation and sedation. That suggests a strategy for developing better antianxiety drugs. Of related interest is the observation that the GABA antagonist pentylenetetrazol precipitates anxiety (Hommer, Skolnick, & Paul, 1987).

OTHER AMINO ACIDS

Glycine, the simplest amino acid, is a neurotransmitter in the spinal cord and lower brain stem. Like GABA, it is inhibitory.

Glutamate and aspartate occur in high concentrations in the brain and are powerful neuronal stimulants. Five receptor types have been identified and may be involved in a wide range of processes, including memory acquisition, convulsive disorders, and developmental plasticity.

NEUROPEPTIDES

Peptides are short, connected chains of amino acids. Several dozen are known to affect specific target cells within the brain, and others are being discovered weekly. Neuropeptide research is progressing so rapidly that Cooper et al. (1991) referred to the "peptide parade." At least one neuroactive peptide coexists at neuronal axon terminals with each known NT. Through a variety of mechanisms, they probably modulate the effects of the primary NTs.

Cooper et al. (1991) grouped several peptide families by internal structure: vasopressin and oxytocin, tachykinins, neurotensin, glucagon-related, pancreatic polypeptide-related, and opioid peptides. Only the latter are discussed below, although many other peptides are attracting research attention.

OPIOID PEPTIDES

Many opiates differ only slightly in structure but considerably in their properties. Morphine is a powerful analgesic (pain reliever), codeine a much weaker one. Naloxone is structurally similar to morphine but antagonizes its actions. Several scientists inferred from these observations that specific morphine receptors exist in the brain; naloxone's similarity to morphine allows it to bind to the same receptors and prevent them from responding to morphine. The question then arose, "Why should our brains have receptors for a product of the poppy plant?" The inescapable answer was that our brains produce opiate-like substances. A great search ensued, and the first such compound was isolated in 1975. It was called enkephalin, meaning "in the head." Others were discovered and collectively called endorphins, which is a contraction of "endogenous (produced within the body) morphines."

The four receptor subtypes for opioids are found in high concentration in many limbic structures. Simon and Hiller (1989) stated that the pharmacological effects of opioid peptides are remarkably similar to those of opiate drugs. They probably play a role in regulating blood pressure, stress mechanisms, temperature, feeding, sexual activity, pain perception, the experience of pleasure, tolerance development, physical dependence, and memory.

CONCLUDING COMMENTS

I borrowed heavily from two sources for this very cursory chapter; they offer thorough coverage of mechanisms and discuss additional neurotransmitter candidates. Thompson's small gem (*The Brain*, 1985) includes considerable information on neurotransmission. The Cooper et al. book (*The Biochemical Basis of Neuropharmacology*, 1991), deservedly in its sixth edition, is a classic in the field of neuropharmacology. Both books are lucid and stimulating.

Summary

Neurons communicate with each other chemically, by a process called neurotransmission. The presynaptic neuron releases a chemical, called a neurotransmitter, at the synapse. The NT diffuses across the synaptic cleft and triggers a reaction in the postsynaptic neuron.

Presynaptic receptors modulate the release of NT; postsynaptic receptors increase (decrease) in number if stimulated infrequently (excessively).

Metabolism of ACh terminates its actions. The actions of other NTs are terminated primarily by reuptake.

Each NT binds to one or more receptors, and effects depend on interactions between the NTs and the specific receptors with which they bind. Most psychoactive drugs act by one or more mechanisms on receptors.

Many substances have been identified as probable NTs, but conclusive evidence exists for only a few. ACh and NE are transmitters in both the CNS and autonomic nervous system. Other NTs include dopamine, serotonin, histamine, GABA, and various amino acids and neuropeptides.

Mini-Quiz: Neurotransmission

Name the three principal parts of neurons.

cell body, dendrites, axon

When an action potential reaches the terminal of the axon, ____ ions rush into the terminal and trigger the release of ____.

calcium; one or more NTs

When a neuron fires, NTs diffuse across the ____ to attach to ____ on a second neuron.

synaptic cleft; receptors

When an excitatory NT interacts with a receptor, ____ ion channels open. When the NT is inhibitory, ____ ion channels open.

sodium; chloride and/or potassium

Second messengers act on the ____ cell and change the likelihood that the cell will ____.

postsynaptic; fire in response to the main NT

T/F: Second messengers are associated with fast transmission.

false

If a postsynaptic neuron is stimulated excessively, its receptors ____ in number; the process is called ____.

decrease; down-regulation

The actions of which NT are terminated primarily by metabolism?

ACh

The actions of most NTs are terminated primarily by ____.

reuptake

Substances that bind to receptors are called ____.

ligands

L-DOPA is needed for the _____ of dopamine.

synthesis

Why is L-DOPA rather than dopamine given to Parkinson's victims?

Peripherally administered dopamine doesn't get into the brain.

ACh receptors located on smooth muscles, cardiac muscles, and glands are called _____.

muscarinic

When the autonomic nervous system releases NE, the pupils of the eyes _____.

dilate

The transmitter at neuromuscular junctions is _____.

ACh

Curare, because of its anti_____ actions, causes muscle paralysis.

nicotinic

Three catecholamine NTs are _____.

NE, E, DA

Cocaine stimulates the _____ system of the ANS.

sympathetic

Considerable evidence suggests that the NT _____ is involved in the reward system, and the NT _____ is involved in sleep and development of tolerance.

DA; serotonin

_____ is probably the major inhibitory NT.

GABA

Morphine-like substances produced within the body are collectively called _____.

endorphins

By the time you finish reading this chapter, you should be able to answer the following questions:

What is meant by the site of action of a drug?

Why is it often useful to know the site of action?

What is pharmacokinetics?

What happens to a drug after it is administered? How does it get to the site of action, and what accounts for termination of activity?

What are the different routes of administration and their advantages and disadvantages?

Why is smoking a popular route for drugs of abuse?

Why might two pills with identical amounts of active ingredient have different effects?

What mechanisms often delay or prevent drugs from entering the brain?

How can excretion of acidic (basic) drugs be promoted?

Why do Siberians stand outside bathrooms?

T/F: Some drugs are metabolized into more rather than less active substances.

T/F: The actions of drugs terminate when the drugs are excreted.

Principles
of Drug Action

Contents

▩ Site of Action

Drugs differ in their **sites of action.** Caffeine acts primarily on the brain, digitalis on the heart, and penicillin on infectious bacteria throughout the body. Some drugs affect the site of action directly, others via mediating routes. For example, norepinephrine raises blood pressure by a direct action on small blood vessels. Some drugs cause blood pressure to rise as a secondary effect, by releasing stored norepinephrine; and others do so by inducing pain. Similarly, drugs may lower blood pressure by impairing oxygen transport; promoting an extensive flow of urine or sweat; or acting on blood vessels, the autonomic nervous system, the brain, or the heart. The appropriate treatment for a blood pressure change depends on its cause.

A drug's effects may suggest its site of action. After neuroscientists had shown that an area of the brain called the locus coeruleus plays a vital role in the control of sleep and wakefulness, several investigators studied how drugs that promote or inhibit sleeping affect the locus

33

coeruleus (see Chapter 19). Another clue to site of action is afforded by the unequal distribution of brain neurotransmitters (NTs). For example, the basal ganglia help control movement. Dopamine is heavily concentrated in the basal ganglia, which suggested that it might be helpful in treating victims of movement disorders such as Parkinson's disease. Dopamine did not help—it does not enter the brain after ingestion or injection—but its precursor L-dopa did.

Most drugs act at their site of action upon receptors that normally respond to naturally produced NTs. Drugs that combine with receptors to elicit the normal effects are called agonists. Drugs that interfere with normal physiological processes by blocking the ability of receptors to respond to appropriate stimuli are called antagonists.

As noted above, many drugs act indirectly. To take another example, some drugs cause dry mouth and, as a secondary effect, excessive drinking; the fluid intake lowers body temperature, which in turn affects respiratory rate. These intermediate steps may interfere with an understanding of the relationship between drug and ultimate behavior. So pharmacologists often study simple systems, such as the strength of contractions of guinea pig ileum. Their findings may bore weekend psychopharmacologists but often represent major advances. Exciting research on **endorphins** (naturally produced substances that reduce pain) was stimulated by the report that morphine-like drugs depress contractions of guinea pig ileum.

The higher the dose of drug, the more rapidly it will reach an effective concentration. Other key factors that determine how it acts include extent and rate of **absorption** from the area of administration into the bloodstream; **distribution** throughout the body from the blood; binding or localization in tissues; **metabolic rate** and pathways; and rate of **excretion**. These are discussed in turn.

▧ Pharmacokinetics

Pharmacokinetics refers to the processes of absorption, distribution, metabolism, and excretion of drugs. These affect the onset, duration, and intensity of actions.

ABSORPTION

Neurophysiologists sometimes place drugs directly into the brains of animals, but most drugs gain access to the brain and other parts of the body through the bloodstream. So, drugs that act on the brain must first be absorbed into the bloodstream. Because drugs administered as capsules or other solid forms must dissolve before being absorbed, solubility affects latency of onset. Crushing a tablet or taking it with water speeds up rate of dissolution. (But crushing a sustained-release or buffered tablet defeats its purpose.) Some capsules, even though they dissolve rapidly, are absorbed slowly into the bloodstream from the stomach or intestines. In such cases, and despite television commercials featuring tablets fizzing spectacularly in water glasses, speeding up the rate of dissolution does not affect onset latency.

Almost all solid dosage forms of drugs contain ingredients besides the active agent. Table 3.1 provides an example. Fillers may be used to speed up or slow down absorption, mask unpleasant tastes, increase chemical stability, or add bulk to agents that are active in minute quantities. Because fillers may affect absorption rate, preparations containing identical amounts of active drug but different fillers may have different effects.

Even pills with identical compositions may act differently; four preparations that differed only in size of individual particles produced a sevenfold variation in plasma concentrations after a single dose (Lindenbaum, Mellow, & Blackstone, 1971).

Intravenously injected drugs, put directly into the bloodstream, do not have to be absorbed. Absorption rates from other routes of administration are influenced by blood flow through the tissues at the administration site. Each route has advantages and disadvantages.

Oral

Oral administration is convenient and pain-free. But some orally administered drugs are destroyed by digestive enzymes or metabolized by the liver before reaching the systemic circulation. Patients must be awake and cooperative. Food in the stomach retards absorption, and some drugs irritate the stomach.

Injection

Intravenous injections (injecting directly into a vein) give maximum precision for obtaining a particular blood concentration. But they cause pain. If the needle or injection site isn't sterile, infectious diseases may be transmitted. Germs and additives that are inactivated by stomach

Table 3.1 Contents of a Typical Sugar-Coated Tablet for Oral Administration

Constituent	Content (mg)
Tablet Core	
ABC 789 (active substance)	5.0
Dimethyl silicone oil	0.5
Polyethylene glycol 6000	0.5
Benzensulphonic acid	2.05
Polyvinylpyrrolidone	3.0
Sucrose	3.0
Talc	3.0
Maize starch	6.0
Lactose	26.95
Coating Mass	
Indigotine pigment	0.171
Cetyl alcohol	0.017
Arachis oil hydrogenated	0.017
Stearic acid	0.104
Polyethylene glycol 6000	0.104
Silicic acid	0.174
Polyvinylpyrrolidone	0.174
Cellulose	0.304
Titanium dioxide	0.869
Talc	1.035
Sucrose	7.031
Total Tablet Weight	60.000

SOURCE: From "Formulation and therapeutic efficacy of drugs used in clinical trials" by D. Freestone, 1969, *Lancet*, 2, pp. 98, 99. Copyright 1969 by *Lancet*. Used by permission.

enzymes when swallowed can be dangerous and even fatal when injected. Once a drug is injected, there is no retreat. Intramuscular and **subcutaneous** (under the skin) injections offer similar advantages and disadvantages, and intraperitoneal (into the abdominal cavity) injections are convenient for small laboratory animals.

Inhalation

When drugs are smoked, some portion is changed by the heat and some lost in sidestream smoke. What remains gets to the brain rapidly. Benowitz (1990) estimated that the time from start of a cigarette to delivery of nicotine to the brain is between 9 and 16 seconds in healthy people. In general, the more rapidly a drug reaches the brain, the more intense the effect. Inhalation allows for precise control over dose. The rapid, intense, controlled effects of inhalation make it a popular route for drugs of abuse.

New routes have been developed in recent years. Some drugs are most effective when given as eyedrops (Chiou, 1991). Morphine has been administered in concentrated form through a small inflatable pump; released in a steady stream to the nerves along the spine, the drug provides constant relief to people in severe pain ("Antidepressants Update," 1991). Other exotic methods of administration include tiny biodegradable capsules implanted in arm, thigh, or even brain to release drug slowly over the course of a year or more; nasal sprays that take effect rapidly; and microscopic bubbles of fat filled with anticancer drug and attached to antibodies that distinguish cancer cells from healthy ones. An entire scientific journal, *Advanced Drug Delivery Reviews*, focuses on the development of drug delivery systems.

DISTRIBUTION

The brain is the site of action for most behaviorally active drugs, and that's where they must go. The average human adult has between 12 and 13 pints of blood, and the heart pumps between 12 and 13 pints per minute, so drugs in the bloodstream are distributed throughout the body in about one minute. But two barriers may delay or prevent entirely the entry of a drug into the brain.

Binding to Plasma Proteins

Many drugs combine with proteins within the bloodstream. While bound, they cannot diffuse out. An equilibrium is eventually reached between the unbound drug and the **plasma protein**-drug complex. As the unbound drug is metabolized and excreted, the equilibrium changes and bound drug is released to reestablish it. Drugs that bind tightly to plasma proteins are long-acting. People with impaired kidney or liver function often have reduced levels of plasma proteins, so they bind drugs less completely; they are likely to experience more intense effects and be more susceptible to drug interactions.

Blood-Brain Barrier

The capillary wall in most brain areas differs in structure, function, and permeability characteristics from capillaries elsewhere; and the wall prevents most substances administered outside the CNS from entering the brain. Thus, most acidic dyes injected into laboratory animals will color the internal organs but leave their brains pristine. Even drugs that act on the brain often gain only limited entry. Only 0.002% of intravenously injected mescaline was taken up by the CNS of young rats (cited in Nieforth, 1971).

Drugs with structures least like the water molecule are most soluble in lipids, and lipid-soluble substances enter the brain most easily. They also dissolve readily in neutral fat deposits and are often stored there. Dewhurst (1970) described a method for measuring lipid solubility: The drug is added to a mixture of equal parts of olive oil and water and shaken well; then the two phases are separated and the amount of drug in the oil fraction is divided by the amount in water. (With proper attention to materials, this method yields magnificent salads.)

Lipid solubility is reduced by addition of an OH group to a molecule. When an OH group is added to the powerful psychoactive drug tryptamine, the new compound 5-hydroxytryptamine (serotonin) is not active unless injected directly into the brain. Serotonin is a neurotransmitter that, like other NTs, does not get through the **blood-brain barrier**. The barrier is, however, permeable to the precursors from which the NTs are synthesized. Oldendorf (1978) speculated that the selective impermeability serves to conserve NTs, as they cannot be removed from the brain by the blood. Moreover, they are prevented from diffusing throughout the brain and altering its activity. The barrier also blocks entry into the brain of transmitters that act elsewhere in the body, such as norepinephrine within the autonomic nervous system.

Increasing lipid solubility is not the only way to improve delivery of therapeutic drugs to the brain (Madrid, Feigenbaum, Brem, & Langer, 1991). Administration of certain drugs increases blood-brain barrier permeability to others. The barrier can be circumvented by injecting the drug directly into the brain. Some drugs can be sent to the brain by indirect routes, for example, via the cerebrospinal fluid; and to some parts of the brain that lie outside the blood-brain barrier (Martinez, Schulteis, & Weinberger, 1991).

The entry of molecules into the brain is affected by their size and degree of ionization. Small, un-ionized molecules penetrate best and are also absorbed more rapidly from the alimentary tract. Paton (1960) concluded that all drugs that act on the CNS can be taken orally, and Benowitz (1990) claimed that all common drugs of abuse are un-ionized and lipid soluble.

Lorenzo, Fernandez, and Roth (1965) injected sodium sulfate into cats and then exposed the animals to either rapid flashes of light or various tones. The animals were then killed and their brains assayed. Sulfate penetration into two important stations in the visual pathway was greater in those cats that had received visual stimulation; and penetration was greater in the auditory pathway for cats that had been exposed to tones. Interestingly, music festivals with light shows as accompaniment are common settings for use of illicit drugs.

METABOLISM

Blood leaving the brain carries drugs out and lessens their effects. The primary mechanisms for terminating effects are metabolism, which occurs in several organs but especially the liver, and excretion, mainly by the kidneys. The liver is the primary site for metabolism, although some metabolic reactions occur in plasma, kidneys, and other tissues. Considering the enormous diversity of drug types, just a few biochemical transformations are used. The main effect of metabolism is to convert lipid- into water-soluble substances, which the kidneys process more readily. Rapidly metabolized drugs generally have smaller effects than more slowly metabolized ones.

Some drugs are metabolized into more rather than less active substances. About 10% of administered codeine is metabolized to the much more powerful morphine. About 80 metabolites of marijuana have been identified (Chiang & Rapaka, 1987), and at least one is more potent than the parent compound (Martin, Dewey, & Harris, 1984).

Laboratory animals generally metabolize drugs more rapidly than humans do, and often by different metabolic pathways (Vocci, 1989). The differences should not be ignored. For example, tilidine is a potential drug of abuse because of its morphine-like effects on people. Yet tilidine has mild or no effects on rats and monkeys; they, unlike humans, do not metabolize it to an active substance.

EXCRETION

Drugs can be excreted in urine, feces, expired air, sweat, and the milk of a nursing mother. The primary excretory pathway is via the kidneys. Some drugs, such as nitrous oxide and the hallucinogenic mushroom *Amanita muscaria*, are excreted unchanged. *Amanita* users in Siberia frequently collected the urine of people who had recently eaten some, so they could use it in turn. Reindeer also like the mushroom, and with their keen sense of smell can detect human urine—so much so that Wasson (1968) wrote, "It is likely to make it dangerous to relieve oneself in the open when there are reindeer around." (This book is full of practical information.)

The rate of excretion is pH-dependent. Basic drugs are excreted most rapidly when the urine is acidic, acidic drugs when the urine is alkaline. These factors can be critically important in the event of poisoning. A weak base such as sodium bicarbonate has saved overdose victims of weakly acidic drugs such as phenobarbital; and ascorbic acid has been used to treat overdose with the weakly basic amphetamine. (Some amphetamine users prolong its effects by first ingesting sodium bicarbonate.)

Nicotine is basic, so excreted more slowly in alkaline urine. Schachter et al. (1977) gave daily doses of vitamin C, sodium bicarbonate, or placebo to heavy smokers and asked them to keep careful records of number of cigarettes smoked. The vitamin C group smoked most, the bicarbonate group least. Schachter et al. noted that many smokers routinely light up after meals, when the urine is most acidic. Fox (cited in Garfield, 1979) designed a smoking-cessation clinic around Schachter's procedures. He too used a sodium bicarbonate, a vitamin C, and a placebo group. After 5 weeks the average daily cigarette consumption was 7.8 in the latter two groups and only 0.14 in the bicarbonate group.

RESIDUAL EFFECTS

During withdrawal from drugs, physiological and behavioral systems often respond in the opposite direction from how they did initially. Cocaine-induced euphoria is often a prelude to severe depression. Withdrawal from chronic high doses of CNS depressants such as barbiturates can precipitate severe, even life-threatening, seizures.

Heroin reduces sex drive, and withdrawing male addicts have reported ejaculating merely upon brushing against a woman. Many drugs suppress both the frequency and vividness of dreams; both increase during withdrawal and may account in part for the development of drug addiction: A person suffering from rebound depression or nightmares can relieve the symptoms by taking more drugs.

Spencer and Boren (1990) edited a recent symposium on the **residual effects** of abused drugs on behavior. Effects may even persist into the next generation. Friedler and Cochin (1972) injected morphine into female rats 5 days before the rats conceived; their offspring differed from uninjected controls in both physical development and response to morphine. Gauron and Rowley (1969) injected 5-day-old rats daily for 50 days with either saline or one of three antipsychotic drugs. Then the rats were put aside until tested at age 75 days in an avoidance conditioning apparatus; saline-treated rats made the fewest errors. At 120 days, all the females were bred with males that had never received drugs. Females that had been treated with drugs were the poorest breeders. No offspring were exposed directly to drugs; nevertheless, when tested in the conditioning apparatus at 75 days, offspring of drug-treated mothers did not learn as well as the others.

McLellan, Woody, and O'Brien (1979) grouped hospitalized drug abusers into three categories according to their primary drugs: stimulants, depressants, and opioids. The patients, all at an early stage in their drug-taking careers, must have already differed or they would have had the same drugs of choice. But the differences were subtle and not detected by the Minnesota Multiphasic Personality Inventory (MMPI; given long enough after hospitalization that most acute drug effects had disappeared). The groups were also similar in demographic variables. Some patients became frequent repeat offenders over the next 6 years, giving McLellan and colleagues an opportunity to study residual effects of drugs. They gave the patients repeated psychiatric evaluations, always at least 2 weeks after hospitalization so that acute drug effects and withdrawal symptoms were minimized. Over time, the stimulant abusers increased in schizophrenia-like symptoms, especially paranoia. The depressant group increased in depressive symptoms, cognitive impairment, and anxiety. The opioid abusers did not increase in psychiatric symptoms.

Summary

To produce an effect, a drug must achieve an adequate concentration at its site of action. This typically involves several steps, collectively called pharmacokinetics:

1. Absorption: The rate of absorption of a drug into the bloodstream is influenced by blood flow through the tissues at the site of administration. Absorption rates differ for oral, injection, and inhalation routes of administration.
2. Distribution: Two factors retard distribution of drugs to the brain. (a) Drugs in the bloodstream cannot diffuse out while bound to plasma proteins. (b) The blood-brain barrier prevents entry of many drugs into the brain.
3. Metabolism: Most but not all drugs are metabolized to less active products. The liver is the main organ of metabolism.
4. Excretion: Some drugs are excreted unchanged. The kidneys are the primary excretory organs.

Even after a drug has been metabolized and excreted, it may continue to exert residual effects.

Mini-Quiz: Principles of Drug Action

Most drugs act at their _____ upon _____ that normally respond to naturally produced _____.

site of action; receptors; NTs

Drugs that combine with receptors to elicit the normal effects are called _____.

agonists

The processes of absorption, distribution, metabolism, and excretion are collectively called _____.

pharmacokinetics

Which aspect of pharmacokinetics is affected most by a drug's solubility?

absorption

Which common route of administration bypasses absorption?

intravenous injection

Which common route of administration is most affected by food in the stomach?

absorption

Which route of administration gives most precision?

intravenous injection

T/F: In general, the more rapidly a drug reaches the brain the weaker the effect.

false

What two barriers delay entry of drugs into the brain?

binding to plasma proteins; blood-brain barrier

Drugs soluble in _____ enter the brain most readily.

lipids

The drug tilidine has morphine-like effects on people but mild effects on rats. What accounts for the difference?

tilidine is metabolized to an active substance by people, not by rats

Name two drugs that are excreted unchanged.

nitrous oxide; *Amanita muscaria* mushroom

Basic drugs are excreted more rapidly when the urine is _____.

acidic

T/F: The effects of some drugs persist long after drug use is discontinued.

true

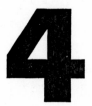

By the time you finish reading this chapter, you should be able to answer the following questions:

What is the purpose of classifying drugs?

Why is classification by molecular structure not necessarily best for psychopharmacologists?

Why are all classification systems inevitably oversimplifications?

Why should drugs be prescribed by official rather than brand name?

What are the main categories of drugs used clinically?

Classification

Contents

Although no two drugs are identical in all respects, many are qualitatively similar. For example, all the more than 2,500 barbiturates are central nervous system depressants. They inhibit convulsions, depress respiration, and have characteristic effects on the liver, kidneys, gastrointestinal tract, and cardiovascular system. Calling a drug a barbiturate conveys a great deal of information.

The purpose of classifying is to provide a framework around which to organize facts and thinking. Hence, the system chosen should reflect the classifier's interests; none is universally best. The Federal government, law enforcement agencies, judges, and lawyers sort by legal status, whereas some users classify all drugs as uppers or downers. Box 4.1 gives the government schedules of controlled substances. Serious scientists need more elaborate categories. Both chemists and pharmacologists classify according to molecular structure, which helps chemists plan syntheses of new compounds and pharmacologists uncover relationships between structure and effects. Structural similarity does not guarantee pharmacological similarity, however. The powerful psychedelic LSD has a close relative, 2-bromo-LSD, which is only weakly active.

The reason is that 2-bromo-LSD does not reach the brain after ingestion (Cerletti & Rothlin, 1955).

Box 4.1
Schedules of Controlled Substances

The Federal government classifies drugs for legal purposes. Controlled drugs are put into one of five classes:

Schedule I: No currently accepted medical use and high abuse potential. Not obtainable by prescription. Examples—heroin, LSD, marijuana, mescaline.

Schedule II: Some currently accepted medical use and high abuse potential. Prescription required. Examples—cocaine, methadone, morphine, amphetamine.

Schedule III: Some currently accepted medical use and moderate abuse potential. Prescription required. Examples—glutethimide, nalorphine, certain stimulants and depressants not listed in Schedules I or II.

Schedule IV: Some currently accepted medical use and lower abuse potential than Schedule III drugs. Prescription required. Examples—alprazolam, chlordiazepoxide, diazepam.

Schedule V: Some currently accepted medical use and low abuse potential. No prescription required but certain conditions must be met, for example, the drug must be sold by a pharmacist, the purchaser must be at least 18, and the pharmacist must keep an official record of the sale. Examples—buprenorphine, preparations containing limited amounts of certain opioids.

The classification system below is provided partly as a preview of what's to come and partly for quick reference. No more arbitrary than any other, it arranges drugs according to both clinical and nonclinical use. The drugs used clinically are available only by prescription. Two points must be noted: First, all drugs have many actions. Chlorpromazine, classified as an **antipsychotic drug,** affects the heart, kidneys, eyes, endocrine system, autonomic nervous system, dreaming, learning, motor activity, and proneness to seizures. Second, drug actions are influenced by many factors. For example, 75% of U.S. respondents answered that they enjoyed food more and ate increased amounts after smoking marijuana (Tart, 1971); yet 60% of Jamaican users reported that marijuana reduces hunger (Rubin & Comitas, 1976).

When a new drug is developed, it is given a **chemical name** that indicates its structural formula and enables chemists around the world to reproduce it. Upon approval for manufacture, a special committee gives the drug an **official name.** The drug's manufacturer gives it a proprietary (brand) name. Chemical names are formidable: the chemical name of one widely used antianxiety drug is 7-chloro-2-methylamino-5-phenyl-3H-1, 4 benzodiazepine-4-oxide. Chlordiazepoxide is its official name and Librium the brand name.

Prescribing by official rather than brand name may save patients money. It also eliminates a source of potential confusion, as each drug has only one official name but may have many brand names. Pyrilamine maleate has had more than 40 and thalidomide more than 50. Should a drug prove hazardous, multiple names increase the difficulty of notifying the public and removing it from the market.

▓ Drugs Used Clinically

Mental health professionals have not reached consensus on the best method for classifying mental disorders, but they generally agree on the major categories. The most widely used system, *The Diagnostic and Statistical Manual of Mental Disorders* (DSM), is published by the American Psychiatric Association and periodically revised. The 1994 revision, *DSM-IV,* lists more than 400 different disorders. Conditions listed in the *DSM-IV* that afflict large numbers of people and are frequently treated with drugs form the basis of the drug classification system below. Only a few drugs are listed for each category, with a common brand name for each in parentheses.

ANXIETY DISORDERS

People who suffer from generalized anxiety disorder experience unfocused anxiety, tension, and agitation. They don't worry about any one specific thing, but they spend much of their lives worrying. **Antianxiety drugs** help calm them. The common antianxiety drugs resemble each other in molecular structure. Most are derivatives of the compound **benzodiazepine.** They differ among themselves primarily in latency of onset (time to take effect) and duration of action. High

Table 4.1 Drugs Used to Treat the Anxiety Disorders

Generalized Anxiety Disorder	Panic Disorder	Obsessive- Compulsive Disorder
Benzodiazepines		
alprazolam (Xanax)	alprazolam (Xanax)	clomipramine
chlordiazepoxide (Librium)		
diazepam (Valium)		
triazolam (Halcion)		
Nonbenzodiazepine		
buspirone (BuSpar)		

doses of benzodiazepines relax muscles and induce sleep, so they are widely prescribed for people with sleeping problems. Although they may help in the short run, they are not a good long-term solution. They have serious abuse potential and, in one study, nearly a third of abusers had received their first prescription for insomnia (Ladewig, 1983). Representative benzodiazepines are alprazolam (Xanax), chlordiazepoxide (Librium), diazepam (Valium), and triazolam (Halcion). Buspirone (BuSpar) is an important nonbenzodiazepine antianxiety drug.

Two other types of anxiety disorders are **panic disorder** and **obsessive-compulsive disorder.** Panic disorder is often treated with antianxiety drugs, especially alprazolam, and with antidepressants. The drug of choice for obsessive-compulsive disorder is clomipramine. Alternative treatments include several drugs that increase brain levels of the neurotransmitter serotonin. (Recall from Chapter 2 that NTs are chemicals produced within the brain that allow for communication between nerve cells.) Table 4.1 lists the antianxiety drugs mentioned above.

DEPRESSION

Depression is a mental state characterized by sustained and extreme sadness. Depressed people become demoralized and lose interest in life's normal activities. Antidepressant drugs play a major role in treating them. Two alternatives are psychotherapy and, in severe cases, electroconvulsive shock.

Table 4.2 Drugs Used to Treat Mood Disorders

Tricyclics (TCAs)	Selective Serotonin Reuptake Inhibitors (SSRIs)	Monoamine Oxidase Inhibitors (MAOIs)
imipramine (Tofranil)	fluoxetine (Prozac)	moclobemide (Aurorix)
amitriptyline (Elavil)	sertraline (Zoloft)	brofaromine (Consonar)
nortriptyline (Pamelor)	paroxetine (Paxil)	
doxepin (Sinequan)	fluvoxamine (Luvox)	
Miscellaneous Drugs		
trazodone (Desyrel)		
bupropion (Wellbutrin)		
lithium (Eskalith)		

The antidepressants are subdivided according to chemical structure and mechanism of action. There are three main types:

Tricyclic antidepressants (TCAs) increase brain activity of the NTs norepinephrine and serotonin. They include imipramine (Tofranil), amitriptyline (Elavil), nortriptyline (Pamelor), and doxepin (Sinequan).

The **serotonin selective reuptake inhibitors** (SSRIs) are structurally diverse. All, however, increase serotonin activity. Four drugs in this class are fluoxetine (Prozac), sertraline (Zoloft), paroxetine (Paxil), and fluvoxamine (Luvox).

Monoamine oxidase inhibitors (MAOIs) enhance the activity of epinephrine, norepinephrine, dopamine, and serotonin. MAOIs act by blocking the enzyme that metabolizes the NTs. The first-generation MAOIs fell out of favor, because they interact with many other drugs and common foods to produce dangerous increases in blood pressure. Several newly developed MAOIs, including moclobemide (Aurorix) and brofaromine (Consonar), have much briefer actions and as a result are safer.

Trazodone (Desyrel) is an antidepressant that increases serotonin levels by a mechanism different from that of the SSRIs. Bupropion (Wellbutrin) increases dopamine activity.

Depressed people given lithium (Eskalith) can often reduce their dose levels of traditional antidepressants. Some improve on lithium after failing to respond to other drugs. Table 4.2 lists the antidepressants mentioned above.

BIPOLAR DISORDER

Manic people are full of energy and enthusiasm. They don't need much sleep and enjoy taking on difficult, speculative projects. But they are easily distracted, often failing to finish what they start. Most manics alternate between periods of mania and depression, so the condition was once called manic-depression. The current term is bipolar disorder. Lithium is used to treat and prevent both mania and recurrent manic-depressive episodes. Carbamazepine (Tegretol) and sodium valproate (Depakene) are alternatives.

SCHIZOPHRENIA

Antipsychotic drugs are used to treat schizophrenia. Although all antipsychotics are similar in effectiveness, they produce different patterns of side effects. Some, such as haloperidol (Haldol), are prescribed in relatively low doses, have weak sedative actions, and frequently cause movement disorders. Others, such as chlorpromazine (Thorazine) and thioridazine (Mellaril), require high doses, sedate, and are relatively free of motor side effects. Many patients respond favorably to clozapine, but some develop a potentially fatal blood disorder. See Chapter 14 for further discussion.

ATTENTION-DEFICIT DISORDER

Attention-deficit disorder is a group of symptoms that usually includes hyperactivity and difficulty in concentrating. It is treated with psychomotor stimulants, which increase alertness and decrease drowsiness. Representative psychomotor stimulants are d-amphetamine (Dexedrine), methylphenidate (Ritalin), and pemoline (Cylert).

DRUG ABUSE

Several antidepressant and antianxiety drugs ease symptoms of drug withdrawal.

Abuse of Alcohol

Disulfiram (Antabuse) interferes with the metabolism of alcohol. People pretreated with disulfiram experience a variety of unpleasant reactions if they drink within several days. Other drugs, including lithium and the experimental drug RO15-4513, reduce the intoxicating effects of alcohol. (But RO15-4513 has little clinical potential because it doesn't reduce alcohol toxicity; people pretreated with RO15-4513 might try to overcome its effects by drinking much more than usual; they might die.)

Abuse of Cocaine

Bromocriptine (Parlodel) and desipramine (Pertofran) reduce craving for cocaine.

Abuse of Nicotine

Nicotine chewing gum and nicotine patches (both available by prescription only) pose fewer health risks than cigarettes.

Abuse of Opioids

Opiate antagonists like naltrexone (Trexan) reverse the effects of opium, heroin, and other narcotics, so they are used to treat both overdose and dependency. Methadone (Dolophine), pharmacologically similar to heroin but longer acting and effective orally, eases the pain of withdrawal and substitutes for heroin in treatment programs.

▓ Drugs Commonly Used Nonmedically for Recreational Purposes

Jaffe (1990) used eight categories to classify drugs (excluding caffeine) taken recreationally: (1) opioids, (2) central nervous system depressants, (3) psychostimulants, (4) nicotine and tobacco, (5) cannabinoids, (6) psychedelics (hallucinogens, psychotomimetics), (7) arylcyclohexylamines, and (8) inhalants. He added a miscellaneous group and noted that the drugs are rarely used alone. "Opioid abusers commonly smoke cigarettes and use and abuse alcohol, cannabis, sedatives, stimulants, and cocaine. Similarly, alcoholics smoke heavily and typically use and abuse anxiolytics."

OPIOIDS

Opiates are extracts of opium. Opiates, opiate derivatives, and synthetic opiate-like drugs are collectively called opioids and include opium, heroin, morphine, methadone, and codeine. The terms *opioid* and *opiate* are often used interchangeably. The drugs are also called narcotics. All are analgesic (pain-relieving) and induce a euphoric (highly pleasurable) state. The first experience, however, often ends in nausea and vomiting.

CENTRAL NERVOUS SYSTEM DEPRESSANTS

Barbiturates, benzodiazepines, methaqualone (Quaalude), and related drugs are used extensively and illegally outside of medical practice. In fact, their nonmedical use exceeds that of the opioids (Jaffe, 1990). On the street, they are called downers. Many people enjoy their disinhibiting, antianxiety, and sleep-promoting effects. Alcohol (more properly, ethyl alcohol or ethanol) shares many properties with barbiturates and benzodiazepines.

PSYCHOMOTOR STIMULANTS

Amphetamine and methylphenidate are used recreationally as well as clinically. On the street, they are called uppers. Other slang names include speed, crystal, and meth. They and cocaine enhance self-confidence and sense of well-being. Nicotine and caffeine have much in common with drugs in this category.

NICOTINE AND TOBACCO

Nicotine, among the most popular drugs in the world, is a major ingredient of tobacco. Nicotine stimulates, improves mood, facilitates learning and memory, and promotes weight loss. Offsetting the beneficial effects, however, are several major adverse consequences that are discussed in Chapter 7.

CANNABINOIDS

The hemp plant synthesizes at least 400 chemicals. More than 60, including delta-9-tetrahydrocannabinol, are cannabinoids. The cannabinoid delta-9-tetrahydrocannabinol is responsible for most of the psychological effects of marijuana, a drug used socially to facilitate interactions, relieve stress, and induce a relaxed, pleasant state. Slang names include pot, weed, and Mary Jane.

PSYCHEDELICS

These drugs, also called psychotomimetics and hallucinogens, distort cognition and perception. They heighten awareness of sensory stimuli while reducing ability to control what is experienced. They promote introspection and feelings of profundity. The **psychedelics** include LSD (acid), peyote, mescaline, psilocybin, and MDMA (ecstasy). Although MDMA is illegal, many psychiatrists endorse it as a means to enhance openness, empathy, and compassion.

ARYLCYCLOHEXYLAMINES (PSYCHEDELIC ANESTHETICS)

Phencyclidine (PCP, angel dust) is a once-popular veterinary anesthetic, and ketamine is still used in animal surgery. Both drugs are hallucinogenic and cause users to feel dissociated from themselves and their environments. Some people enjoy the experience.

INHALANTS

The intoxicating effects of nitrous oxide and ethyl ether have attracted users for more than 100 years. Other often-abused inhalants include antifreeze, paint thinner, and industrial solvents such as toluene. All cause many harmful effects such as memory loss and irreversible neurological damage. Both butyl nitrite and amyl nitrite (poppers) dilate blood vessels; some people inhale one or the other to intensify and prolong sexual orgasm.

MISCELLANEOUS DRUGS

About 80% of the world's population uses caffeine, a stimulant that increases alertness and induces a sense of well-being. Caffeine is in a chemical family, the methylated xanthines, that includes theophylline (a key ingredient of tea) and theobromine (found in cocoa).

Mescaline and about 60 other substances contribute to the powerful visual effects of the peyote cactus. The drug kava, which initially stimulates and then induces a pleasant sleep-like state, and the powerful psychedelic *Amanita muscaria* (the fly agaric mushroom) are used in many parts of the world. Prisoners unable to get marijuana often use the common household spice nutmeg as a substitute. Nutmeg, however, has a much smaller margin of safety between intoxicating and toxic doses.

Summary

The purpose of classifying is to provide a framework for organizing facts and thinking. Because different users have different needs, no system is universally best.

Chemists who work on synthesizing new drugs find classification by molecular structure helpful. But drugs with similar molecular structures may affect organisms in vastly different ways. Scientists interested in behavioral endpoints often classify according to clinical and recreational use.

Regardless of the classification scheme, two points should be kept in mind: (a) All drugs have many effects. (b) The actions of drugs are influenced by many factors.

The chemical name of a drug indicates its structural formula. Upon approval for manufacture, the drug is given an official name. The drug's manufacturer gives it a proprietary (brand) name.

Important categories of clinical drugs include the following: antianxiety drugs, which in high doses induce sleep; antidepressants; drugs for treating mania and bipolar disorder; antipsychotics; drugs for treating attention-deficit disorder; and drugs for treating drug abuse.

Drugs used recreationally can be categorized as follows: (a) opioids; (b) central nervous system depressants; (c) psychostimulants; (d) nicotine and tobacco; (e) cannabinoids; (f) psychedelics (hallucinogens, psychotomimetics); (g) arylcyclohexylamines; (h) inhalants; and miscellaneous drugs, including caffeine.

Mini-Quiz: Classification

Most pharmacologists classify drugs according to _____.

molecular structure

2-bromo-LSD has weak effects on the central nervous system because _____.

it doesn't get into the CNS

Drugs that change cognitions, perceptions, and moods are called _____.

psychoactive

Chlorpromazine is classified as an _____ drug.

antipsychotic

Give an example from the text of a cultural difference in response to a drug.

Marijuana users in the United States say that the drug increases appetite whereas users in Jamaica say it depresses appetite.

Match the drug with the condition for which it is most frequently prescribed.

1. chlordiazepoxide
2. phenelzine
3. buspirone
4. lithium
5. moclobemide
6. fluoxetine
7. alprazolam
8. clozapine
9. clomipramine
10. methylphenidate

a. schizophrenia
b. anxiety
c. depression
d. attention-deficit disorder
e. bipolar disorder
f. obsessive compulsive disorder

1a; 2c; 3b; 4c & e; 5c; 6c; 7b; 8a; 9f; 10d

Disulfiram interferes with the metabolism of _____.

alcohol

Bromocriptine reduces craving for _____.

cocaine

Match the drug with its class.

1. amphetamine	a. opioids
2. LSD	b. CNS depressants
3. heroin	c. psychostimulants
4. marijuana	d. cannabinoids
5. phencyclidine (PCP)	e. psychedelics
6. MDMA (ecstasy)	f. arylcyclohexylamines
7. amyl nitrite	g. inhalants
8. alcohol	

1c; 2e; 3a; 4d; 5f; 6e; 7g; 8b

By the time you finish reading this chapter, you should be able to answer the following questions:

Why do many patients receive suboptimal doses of therapeutic drugs?

What types of factors affect responsiveness to drugs?

Why are elderly people often more sensitive than others to the effects of drugs?

How is dose calculated to adjust for body weight?

How do pharmacological and behavioral tolerance differ?

What is polypharmacy and why is it generally inadvisable?

T/F: Placebos affect subjective but not objective measures.

Variability in Response to Drugs

Contents

The *Physicians' Desk Reference* (*PDR*) is a valuable handbook for pharmacology students and practitioners. The *PDR* lists drugs by class and includes information on dosages and contraindications. But reliance on the *PDR* should be tempered by certain considerations: The information is supplied by the pharmaceutical houses that developed each drug and, as indicated in Chapter 6, the houses often suggest uses that cannot be justified on scientific or medical grounds; in addition, reports of adverse effects do not always find their way into the *PDR* (Lowinger, 1975). In any event, physicians should use the listed dosage ranges only as starting points; they should make adjustments according to the needs of individual patients.

Reactions to drugs are influenced by many factors, and people respond variably. To protect against unpredictable adverse effects to normal therapeutic doses, many physicians prescribe conservatively and their patients receive less than optimal doses. Fortunately, even suboptimal doses are usually beneficial. A second consequence of variability is that knowledge of a drug's classification may not be enough for accurately predicting how the drug will act in a particular situation. Stimulants sometimes sedate, depressants stimulate, euphoriants cause anguish, and placebos duplicate virtually any action of any drug. Atropine accelerates heart rate to varying degree in almost all recipients—yet slows it in some (Smith & Rawlins, 1973).

Jones (1990) had 10 volunteers smoke cocaine base under controlled conditions. Their peak plasma levels varied about fivefold each time. On a different day, he observed similar variability after injecting them with precise amounts of cocaine. Perez-Reyes (1990) found wide variations in peak plasma concentrations of delta-9-tetrahydrocannabinol (the major active ingredient of marijuana).

Even if pharmacokinetics were identical in different people, responsiveness to a prescribed drug regimen would vary. First, people who differ in degree of severity of an illness are likely to respond differently to treatment. Second, a single diagnostic label may cover several diseases. For example, depression may or may not be associated with a well-defined precipitating event; some depressives show decreased levels of serotonin, some of norepinephrine; some but not all lose weight, are constipated, and experience sleeping difficulties. The symptoms differ in young and old. Third, patients comply in varying degree with physicians' instructions. As many as 20% of inpatient and 50% of outpatient schizophrenics do not follow their prescribed regimens (Hare & Willcox, 1967; Willcox, Gillan, & Hare, 1965). In this respect, schizophrenics are perfectly normal—between 25% and 80% of patients of diverse types are noncompliant (Sackett, 1976, 1980). A fourth problem is that people who prescribe and fill drug orders make errors. Lesar et al. (1990) had pharmacists in a teaching hospital evaluate the appropriateness of each prescription written by hospital physicians during a one-year period. Of 289,411 orders by 840 physicians, 905 errors (none of which were implemented) were identified—58 were considered potentially serious, severe, or fatal.

▩ Responsiveness to Drugs: Four Important Influences

The influences on drug response may be grouped under four somewhat arbitrary and overlapping headings: organismic variables, drug variables, environmental variables, and situational variables.

ORGANISMIC VARIABLES

Age

Children's metabolic enzyme systems and blood-brain barriers are incompletely developed and, until they reach age 3, their gastric fluids are less acidic than those of adults. Children have a higher percentage of body fluid, a lower percentage of body fat, and fewer plasma proteins. Thus, children react differently than adults to many drugs. Pediatric pharmacology has become an important specialty (cf. Campbell & Spencer, 1988; Levin, 1987).

Glantz, Petersen, and Whittington (1983) edited a volume that summarizes a great deal of research on drugs and the elderly. Elderly people are likely to take drugs for chronic illnesses, and each new drug increases the risk of interactions. Metabolic and excretory systems become less efficient, plasma protein levels decrease, and the blood-brain barrier becomes more permeable with age. All these factors increase the likelihood of prolonged drug effects and the risk of an adverse reaction.

Weight

In animal work, dosages are usually calculated in milligrams of drug per kilogram of body weight (mg/kg). Clinical practitioners often require greater precision, so they consider proportion of body fat to muscle. (Many drugs are stored in fat and remain active longer in overweight people than more muscular people of the same weight.) To calculate how much drug to administer, with no adjustment for body fat:

1. Determine the suggested dosage, in mg/kg.
2. Weigh the recipient and express the weight in kg (1 kg = about 2.2 pounds).
3. From the above, calculate the mg dose.
4. If the drug is in pill form, the number of mg per tablet should be known.
5. For drugs in solution, read the concentration in mg/cc. Divide the quantity obtained in (3) by the number of mg/cc.

Suppose the recommended dosage is 0.05 mg/kg, and the drug is supplied in 1-cc vials containing 20 mg. A man weighing 70 kg should receive $0.05 \times 70 = 3.5$ mg; $3.5/20 = 0.175$ cc. Give 0.175 cc of solution.

First-time experimenters are often surprised by the minute amounts of drugs needed to produce powerful effects. To anesthetize a 20-gm mouse with pentobarbital, which is available in concentrations of 50 mg/cc, the recommended dose is 60 mg/kg when given intraperitoneally. The amount administered would be $(60 \times 0.02)/50 = 0.024$ cc.

Biological Rhythms

Physiological systems as simple as single cells and as complex as humans are rhythmically active, and rhythmicity affects responsiveness to many drugs. For example, the mortality rate was 80% in mice injected during early evening with a toxin, and only 15% in similar mice injected 8 hours later (Halberg, 1960). In people, daily, hourly, and seasonal sensitivity changes to drugs have been reported (Reinberg & Smolensky, 1983). Drugs whose actions are affected in important ways by time of administration include several over-the-counter analgesics; drugs for heart problems; anticancer and antibacterial drugs; and drugs used in neurology and psychiatry (Reinberg & Smolensky, 1983).

Reactions to alcohol, lithium, diazepam, and propranolol vary throughout the menstrual cycle (Jones & Jones, 1976; Kahn, 1991). (Note: Women, because of those "terrible monthly rhythms," must of course be "precluded from serious consideration for high government office"; not well publicized is that men have similar rhythms. Hersey [1931] found that male industrial workers experienced 4- to 6-week cycles of emotional changes; and Doering, Kraemer, Keith, Brodie, & Hamburg [1975] reported cycles of testosterone levels that clustered at periods of 3 weeks.)

Reinberg (1991) discussed several findings and implications of **chronopharmacology** (the study of drug effects as a function of body time and upon the body's time structure):

- Even if administered in sustained-release form, a drug may not achieve steady plasma levels.
- Pharmacokinetic characteristics such as maximum concentration and half-life, as well as effectiveness, may change rhythmically.
- Target systems may change rhythmically in susceptibility or sensitivity.
- Rhythmic changes may differ in males and females.

To the above may be added Langevin's (1991) comment that drug prescriptions should read not only how much and how often but at what time. It should also be noted that drugs are more likely to be prescribed in error at certain times. When pharmacists evaluated the appropriateness of physicians' written prescriptions, both total errors and significant errors were greatest on orders written between noon and 3:59 p.m. (Lesar et al., 1990).

Personality

Personality variables affect both proneness to drug use and responsiveness. Eysenck (1963, 1983) showed in an extensive series of experiments that the personalities of drug recipients influence how drugs affect them. In considering the examples below, keep in mind Wilder's *"Law of Initial Value"*:

> Not only the intensity but also the direction of a response of a body function to any agent depends to a large degree upon the initial level of that function at the start of the experiment. The higher this "initial level," the smaller is the response to function-raising, the greater is the response to function-depressing agents. At more extreme initial levels there is a progressive tendency to "no response" and to "paradoxical reactions," i.e., a reversal of the usual direction of response. (Wilder, 1957)

1. Small doses of morphine given to people suffering physical or mental pain produce euphoria; given to happy, pain-free people, similar doses often precipitate mild anxiety and fear (Innes & Nickerson, 1965).
2. Amphetamine-like drugs amplify existing mood: Anxious people become more anxious, mild depression becomes pronounced, and euphorics attain even greater heights (Lehmann, 1966).
3. The more variable people were on perceptual tasks prior to taking psilocybin, the smaller were their reactions to the drug (Fischer, Hill, & Warshay, 1969). Both threshold and intensity of response to one drug predicted responses to others (Kornetsky, 1960; Shagass, 1960). Perhaps simple behavioral pre-tests can be developed to improve dosing accuracy.
4. Employed and/or married opiate addicts responded most favorably to treatment with the narcotic antagonist naltrexone (Greenstein et al., 1983).
5. Even rats have personalities. Rats that increase activity most in new environments are most likely to self-administer and respond to amphetamine (Piazza, Deminiere, LeMoel, & Simon, 1989).

Physiological State

Kidney and liver function affect responsiveness to drugs. So do other physiological conditions. For example:

1. Aspirin lowers body temperature but only in people with fever.
2. Pain interferes with morphine-induced respiratory depression; in fact, people often treat overdose victims by deliberately inflicting pain (Jaffe, 1965).
3. Cutler, Sramek, Murphy, and Nash (1992) administered a drug to elderly men, some healthy and some suffering from Alzheimer's disease. The healthy men had few side effects, the Alzheimer's victims many.
4. Food intake can enhance, impair, or leave unchanged absorption and distribution of various drugs (cf. Melander [1978] for review). Foods such as cabbage, brussels sprouts, and charcoal-broiled beef can affect drug metabolism. So can vitamin deficiency or excess (cf. Anderson [1988] for review). Stewart (1992) reported three cases in which a high-fiber diet inhibited absorption of antidepressants.
5. Chronic drinkers become tolerant to alcohol's effects, because the enzymes that metabolize alcohol become more numerous. The drinkers then show tolerance to many other drugs metabolized by the same enzymes (Shoaf & Linnoila, 1991). Cigarette smokers metabolize caffeine more rapidly than do nonsmokers. If they stop smoking, caffeine plasma levels may become very high and cause nervousness, and that may cause them to start smoking again (Benowitz, 1990).

Genetics

Inherited characteristics influence responsiveness to drugs (cf. Spielberg, 1984; Thompson & Thompson, 1986; Vesell, 1979; Weinshilboum, 1984). Thompson and Olian (1961) injected pregnant mice of three different strains with epinephrine, then compared the offspring with offspring born to untreated mothers of the same strains. Activity was elevated above control levels in one strain, depressed in another, and not significantly changed in the third. (The changes followed the predictions of the Law of Initial Value.) The results have important implications for anyone interested in deriving general laws about behavior.

Monoamine oxidase inhibitors and structurally similar drugs are metabolized rapidly by about 50% of African Americans and Caucasians, much more slowly by the other 50%. The proportion of fast and slow MAOI metabolizers varies considerably in other racial groups. Slow metabolizers respond better to antidepressant therapy with MAOIs (Johnstone & Meersch, 1973). As seen in Table 5.1, the enzyme glucose-6-phosphate dehydrogenase is distributed unevenly in different racial groups. People deficient in the enzyme are susceptible to

Table 5.1 Incidence of Glucose-6-Phosphate Dehydrogenase Deficiency in Men

Nigerian Negroes	20
American Negroes	10-15
American Caucasians	1
Kurdish Jews	58
Ashkenazi Jews	0.4
Sardinians	4-30
Iranians	8.5
Arabs	4-5
Greeks	1-3
American Indians	
Oyana	16
Carib	2

SOURCE: From "The genetics of drug susceptibility" by I. Porter, 1966, *Diseases of the Nervous System, 27*, pp. 25-36.
NOTE: Amounts given are percentages.

anemia after being treated with a variety of drugs including aspirin, antimalarials, and sulfa drugs. Some otherwise normal people have a genetic defect that causes them to respond unusually to the antihypertensive drug debrisoquine. If they smoke, they are less likely to develop lung cancer than people without the defect (Caporaso et al., 1989).

When men and women with a history of sedative abuse were allowed to self-administer pentobarbital, their daily intakes varied more than tenfold. Intake was higher for people with faster metabolic rates (Pickens & Heston, 1981).

Propranolol, used for a variety of purposes including the prevention of migraine headaches, induces significantly larger blood pressure and heart rate reductions in Chinese men than U.S. white men (Zhou, Koshakji, Silberstein, Wilkinson, & Wood, 1989). Lin et al. (1989) treated Asian and Caucasian schizophrenics with the **antipsychotic** drug haloperidol. For a given dosage, Asians on average had higher serum concentrations and more side effects. Haring et al. (1990) found that age, gender, weight, and smoking habits all affected plasma concentration of the antipsychotic drug clozapine.

Male mammals have an X and a Y chromosome whereas females have two Xs. The genetic difference mediates many gender differences, such as those listed below (from Yonkers, Kando, Cole, & Blumenthal, 1992).

- Absorption differs, because women secrete less gastric acid than men.
- Women have a lower ratio of lean body mass to **adipose tissue,** which
  results in lower initial serum concentrations of many drugs. But drugs stored
  in adipose tissue have longer half-lives in women.
- Women and men differ in metabolic enzymes. Women have less **alcohol
  dehydrogenase,** the enzyme that breaks down alcohol before it enters the
  bloodstream, so women absorb about 30% more alcohol than men of equal
  weight who drink the same amount (Frezza et al., 1990).
- Women require smaller doses per body weight of antipsychotics.
- Following antipsychotic drug treatment, both incidence and severity of
  the side effect tardive dyskinesia are greatest in elderly women.
- Certain **antianxiety** and **hypnotic** drugs are eliminated more slowly in
  women than men.
- Female victims of depressive illness with panic attacks respond better to
  monoamine oxidase inhibitors, male victims to tricyclic antidepressants.
- Women experience more adverse reactions to lithium.

Kalow (1967) described a tragic case resulting from a physician's
failure to recognize that many untoward drug reactions have a genetic
basis. A young boy died following general anesthesia. Some time later,
his sister required an operation and her troubled parents consulted their
anesthesiologist. He assured them that the boy's death had been an
extremely rare occurrence and no special precautions were needed. The
girl died under the same circumstances. One of the goals of **pharmacogenetics** is to develop techniques for anticipating such **idiosyncratic**
responses.

Handedness

The relative contributions of genetic and environment factors to
handedness are in dispute, but there is clear evidence that left- and
right-handers respond differently to drugs. Irwin (1985) found that EEG
changes in left-handers were greater to a variety of drugs.

DRUG VARIABLES

The Dose-Response Curve

Small quantities of alcohol promote sociability and liveliness, larger
amounts cause stupor. Strychnine in very small doses facilitates learning

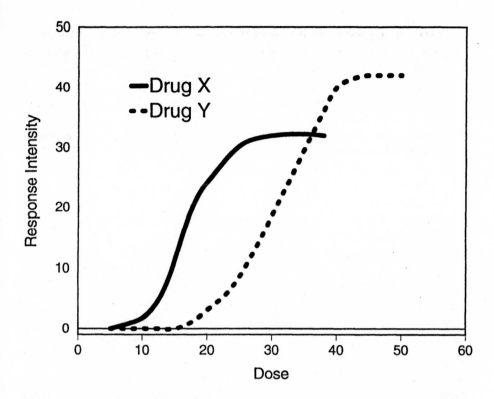

Figure 5.1a. Typical Dose Response Curves
NOTE: Drug X is more potent than drug Y: A smaller dose of X than Y is required to produce a given response.
Drug Y has greater maximum efficacy: The maximum response it produces is greater than that of drug X.

and memory, but larger doses kill. More generally, the magnitude and type of response to a drug depend greatly on the dose administered. The graphic display of effects as a function of dosage is called the dose-effect or dose-response curve. It is often but not always S-shaped (see Figure 5.1a). A given drug may yield different dose-response curves for each response measured.

The highest point on the curve represents the maximum efficacy of the drug. (More correctly, maximum efficacy is the strongest effect not accompanied by undesirable side effects.) Potency refers to the amount of drug needed to be effective. One drug may be more potent than another but with a smaller maximum efficacy; the latter is the more important characteristic. Television pitchmen who exhort viewers to buy their brand of aspirin sometimes try to exploit differences in potency, that is, they say that one tablet of their brand is as powerful as two of brand X. But if two brand X tablets are cheaper, safer, and more effective, then brand X is the better buy.

Consider the following problem:

> Drugs X and Y both relieve headache pain. However, 50% of people given 5 mg/kg of drug X complain of nausea. Drug Y does not produce undesirable side effects in 50% of users until doses of 1,000 mg/kg are given. Which drug is safer?

The question cannot be answered without first knowing the dose of each drug that relieves headache. Suppose a 0.005 mg/kg dose of drug X relieves pain in 50% of people, and the corresponding Y dose is 500 mg/kg. Drug X would have a much greater margin of safety between therapeutic and toxic doses. In general, the steeper the slope of a dose-response curve, the greater the likelihood that an effective dose will produce unwanted side effects.

Referring to dose in terms of effects on 50% of subjects emphasizes the point of this chapter: A given dose affects different people differently. The dose that produces a specified intensity of effect in 50% of subjects is called the median effective dose (ED50). The TD50 and LD50 refer, respectively, to the dose that produces any type of toxic effect, and the lethal dose, in 50% of subjects. A drug's therapeutic index is the ratio between its TD50 and ED50, although other proportions are sometimes used. (The ratio TD25/ED90 would refer to the dose that produces toxic effects in 25% of recipients and is effective in 90%.) The greater the value TD50/ED50, the safer the drug. But there are no hard-and-fast rules. A low therapeutic index might be acceptable for terminal cancer patients but not headache sufferers.

In contrast to the typical S-shaped dose-response curves for single individuals, curves showing the number of individuals who respond to a given dose with a specified effect are usually normally distributed (see Figure 5.1b).

Repeated Administrations of the Same Drug

Tolerance to a drug occurs when a given dose produces a smaller effect than it did initially. In a survey, Anthony and Trinkoff (1989) asked users of illegal drugs, "Did you find that you needed larger amounts of these drugs to get an effect—or that you could no longer get high on

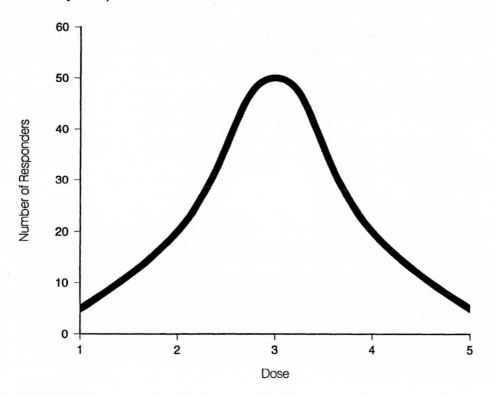

Figure 5.1b.

the amount you used to use?" Approximately two thirds of daily heroin users, 43% of daily cocaine users, and 21% of daily marijuana users answered, "Yes." The degree of tolerance is sometimes striking: The usual therapeutic dose of amphetamine is about 10 mg, but addicts have taken doses as high as 1,700 mg without ill effect (Innes & Nickerson, 1965). Tolerance is most likely to develop with frequent dosing of drugs that have a long half-life (the time needed for half the dose to be removed), whereas short half-lives are associated with earlier and more severe withdrawal (Sellers, Busto, & Kaplan, 1989). Jones (1990) noted that tolerance for many psychoactive drugs begins to occur within seconds or minutes. When a drug is eaten rather than inhaled or injected, the rapid onset of tolerance counteracts the slowly arising effects and reduces their intensity.

Tolerance is called **pharmacological** when changes in response to a drug result from such factors as decreased absorption, more rapid metabolism and excretion, and decreased receptor affinity. Some tolerance develops as recipients begin compensating for drug actions. Siegel (1988) reasoned that principles of learning account for this **behavioral tolerance.** Thus, if a drug elicits responses when administered repeatedly under standardized conditions, environmental cues associated with administration of the drug often elicit anticipatory responses in the opposite direction. The anticipatory responses partially cancel the drug effect. For example, alcohol produces **hypothermia.** Rats given alcohol repeatedly and then a placebo under identical conditions, become briefly hyperthermic.

Behavioral tolerance accounts for many drug phenomena. Siegel (1988) noted that morphine's analgesic effects become weakened over time but can be reinstated by changing the circumstances of administration. And people who self-administer drugs, if they abruptly vary their routine, risk overdose.

Tolerance does not develop equally to all aspects of drug action, so repeated administrations can change therapeutic effectiveness. Chronic users of alcohol and other sedating, antianxiety drugs become resistant to the sedative and intoxicating effects but not to the lethal dose (Okamoto, Boisse, Rosenberg, & Rosen, 1978). The constipating effects of heroin persist long after the same dose no longer produces euphoria.

A drug given repeatedly over a short time period may promote very rapid tolerance, called **tachyphylaxis.** For example, for a given blood alcohol level, cognitive performance and memory are impaired more while people drink and the level is increasing than when they have stopped and it is falling (Jones, 1973). Reverse tolerance, in which responsiveness to a drug increases with repeated administration, has been demonstrated under certain circumstances for marijuana, phencyclidine, cocaine, and others (French, 1988; Snyder, 1971; Stripling & Hendricks, 1981). **Cross tolerance** may develop among related drugs (mescaline and LSD, heroin and morphine, alcohol and many different CNS depressants) and to similar effects produced by unrelated drugs. For example, both alcohol and morphine produce hypothermia, and cross tolerance develops to the hypothermic effect (Khanna, Le, Kalant, & LeBlanc, 1979).

Porchet, Benowitz, and Sheiner (1988) gave subjects two intravenous infusions of nicotine. When the second was given within 120 minutes of the first, blood concentrations rose but heart rate acceleration and subjective effects were smaller than after the first. At 240 minutes, the initial response was fully restored. Benowitz (1990) explained a typical daily smoking cycle in terms of this rapid development and regression of tolerance. The morning cigarette is strongly arousing and starts the day's development of tolerance. As smoking continues throughout the day, nicotine accumulates; this results in more tolerance, withdrawal symptoms between smokes, and weaker positive effects of individual cigarettes. The effects are restored after a night's abstinence. Because of the dose-response and dose-tolerance characteristics, habitual smokers must smoke at least 15 cigarettes per day to achieve the positive effects and minimize withdrawal discomfort.

Method of Administration

Even for a single route of administration, differences in technique may affect response. Patients injected with diazepam by nurses had plasma levels only about one third as high as patients injected by physicians (Dundee, Gamble, & Assaf, 1974). The nurses were neither hitting the right spot nor injecting the drug deeply enough into the buttocks. Doctors stuck it more efficiently to patients.

Dosage Regimen

If a drug's level within blood plasma is too low, the drug will be ineffective; too high, and there may be toxicity. To maintain steady state levels, drugs should be given at uniform intervals equal to the drug's half-life. Thus, a drug with a half-life of 8 hours should be given at 8-hour intervals. Niebergall, Sugita, and Schnaare (1974) showed that the standard intervals prescribed for many drugs result in plasma levels outside the therapeutic range for much of the day. Dosage regimen is sometimes more important than the total amount administered. Baker and Alcock (cited in Worden, 1974) reported no cataracts in rats given a particular drug 5 days per week in 250-mg doses (total dose of 1,250 mg per week); but 22% developed cataracts when given 100 mg per day (700 mg per week).

Drug Interactions

The pharmacokinetics of one drug—the rate or pattern at which it is absorbed, the extent to which it is bound to plasma proteins, or the rate or pattern of its metabolism or excretion—may be affected by the presence of another. Drugs may interact in several other ways as well. An antagonist of a drug prevents receptors from reacting fully to that drug, whereas an agonist combines with receptors to mimic the activity of the drug or a naturally occurring substance. Following are a few examples of **interactions:**

1. Many drugs interfere with the positively reinforcing effects of other drugs, so have been used to treat addiction. A person who takes disulfiram and then alcohol within 5 days will have a violently unpleasant reaction (Fox, 1967). Monkeys suppress their self-administration of cocaine when pretreated with buprenorphine, presumably because positive reinforcement is blocked (Mello, Mendelson, Bree, & Lukas, 1989).

2. Rats pretreated with caffeine self-administer twice as much cocaine as do rats pretreated with water, indicating that caffeine increases the positive effects of cocaine (Schenk, Horger, & Snow, 1989-1990).

3. Both cocaine and marijuana increase heart rate in men. Taken together, the heart rate increase is comparable to that following marijuana alone (Foltin & Fischman, 1989a).

4. Hearn et al. (1991) identified a metabolite, cocaethylene, that is produced within the body by the combination of cocaine and alcohol. Cocaethylene intensifies the euphoric effects of cocaine while increasing the risk of sudden death.

5. Monoamine oxidase inhibitors are safe antidepressants if used properly but may cause a **hypertensive** crisis if combined with caffeine, chianti wine, or a variety of foods.

6. Garza-Trevino et al. (1989) administered the sedative-hypnotic drug lorazepam in combination with the antipsychotic drug haloperidol to agitated hospital patients. The combination achieved quicker, longer-lasting sedation at lower doses than did either alone.

7. Figure 5.2, from Kreek (1991), gives frequent combinations of drugs and their desired effects.

Given that interactions can occur in so many different ways, it is clear that drug combinations should be administered rarely—and then only when the interactions are fully understood. McCarthy (1974), however, used simple mathematics to show that the latter condition cannot often be met. If there were a pool of only 20 drugs, 190 different pairs and 1,140 triplets would be possible. Twenty-four drugs mixed 2, 3, or 4 at a time yield 11,000 possible combinations. Yet **polypharmacy** is common even though industrialized countries regularly use about 5,000 drugs (Albert, 1987; there seem more because of the abundance of trade names). Ayd (1974) reported that most psychiatric patients take at least six drugs daily. James (1976) found that 18.8% of hospitalized patients who

Combination	Desired Effect
1. Heroin plus alcohol	Enhance heroin "high" or euphoria
2. Heroin followed by alcohol	Self-medicate narcotic withdrawal symptoms
3. Heroin followed by cocaine	Self-medicate narcotic withdrawal symptoms
4. Cocaine plus alcohol	Enhance cocaine "high" or euphoria
5. Cocaine followed by alcohol	Self-medicate anxiety, nervousness, and overstimulation ("crash") followed by cocaine use
6. Cocaine plus heroin	Enhance or alter cocaine "high" or euphoria
7. Cocaine followed by heroin	Self-medicate anxiety, nervousness, and overstimulation ("crash") followed by cocaine use

Figure 5.2. Patterns of Heroin, Cocaine, and Alcohol Use in Combination
SOURCE: From Kreek (1991).

received five or fewer prescribed drugs had adverse drug reactions; for those taking more than five, it was 81.4%. Mason, Nerviano, and DeBurger (1977), commenting on the problem, wrote:

> Even though there is no basis in fact for the existence of polypharmacy as a treatment method, it continues to be a prominent aberrant form of drug therapy. The situation seems to be indicative of a serious gap in the fundamental knowledge of antipsychotic drugs and their clinical use.

Polypharmacy is common among drug abusers. Senay (1989) paid users on the street who were not in treatment for urine samples. Many tested positive for more than nine common substances of abuse not counting nicotine. Though probably honest with him, they did not acknowledge taking many drugs for which they tested positive; he concluded that they did not know what they were taking. Sellers et al. (1989) found that 86% of patients classified as benzodiazepine abusers abused at least one other drug not counting nicotine or caffeine.

Drugs are most rewarding when they reach the brain rapidly; so anything, including other drugs, that increases rate of absorption or decreases metabolism may intensify effects. Sellers et al. (1989) gave examples.

1. Diazepam blood plasma concentration is 100% greater 15 minutes after administration when taken with alcohol than alone.
2. Alcohol greatly increases blood plasma concentrations of amitriptyline.
3. The half-life of caffeine is 10.4 hours in women on oral contraceptives, 4 hours in women not on contraceptives.

ENVIRONMENTAL VARIABLES

Many environmental factors affect responsiveness to drugs. Chlorpromazine injected into rats and mice in a cold room induced neurological depression; at higher temperatures, the same dose caused hyperexcitability (Quadbeck, 1962). High temperatures weakened the convulsant effects of both pentylenetetrazol and strychnine (Hall, Nelson, & Edlin, 1967). Other variations that had significant effects include level of illumination (Watzman, Barry, Kinnard, & Buckley, 1968), whether subjects were tested singly or in groups (Chance, 1946), noise level (Chance, 1947), and whether the cages in which subjects were housed had ground corncob or red cedar chip bedding (Ferguson, 1966). In people, skin eruptions may occur if they take any of a variety of drugs, including antihistamines, antibiotics, antianxiety drugs, and birth control pills, and are then exposed to direct sunlight (Chambers, 1987).

Vesell et al. (1973) allowed urine and feces to accumulate under the wire mesh cages of one group of rats, and they cleaned cages daily for a second group. Liver enzyme activity was inhibited in the rats in the dirty cages. The results may explain some large discrepancies among laboratories studying drug metabolism. Another implication is that unwashed drug users may have known what they were doing. And, for maximum drug effects, it might be wise to move to New York or Los Angeles.

In people, alcohol produces a great variety of behavioral changes. Recognizable stereotypes exist for belligerent, loquacious, maudlin, uninhibited, and sleepy drunks. The range of anticipated behaviors is much less for other drugs, probably because alcohol has greater legal and cultural acceptance; consequently, it is used by a broader sample of people and in more diverse settings.

Pliner and Cappell (1974) studied volunteer subjects who drank alcohol, then worked on a task either alone or in a three-person group. The isolated subjects reported that alcohol made them less clear-thinking, dizzier, and sleepier; the grouped ones felt less bored and happier.

SITUATIONAL VARIABLES

Expectations

The Placebo Effect. An enterprising friend once wanted to market a new substance that he intended to call PLEEZBO. He was going to claim that PLEEZBO offered significant relief from cough, headache, postoperative pain, seasickness, anxiety, tension, pain from angina pectoris, and virtually every other human ailment. Amazingly, he would have been telling the truth. But he was deprived of an opportunity to make a fortune when the Food and Drug Administration passed a law requiring listing of active ingredients. His substance, the **placebo,** has no active ingredients.

Placebos, narrowly conceived as inactive *drugs,* are important in medical practice. Viewed more broadly, as any form of therapy without specific activity for the condition being treated, their role expands considerably. Beecher (1961) found that the substantial improvements following a once-popular surgical procedure for angina pectoris were no greater than those following skin incision alone. Sox, Margulies, and Sox (1981) reported that patients complaining of chest pain who received diagnostic tests were less likely to claim short-term disability than those not receiving the tests. And Yoken and Berman (1984) found that clients who paid for psychotherapy had better outcomes than those who didn't. Shapiro and Morris (1978) wrote,

> The placebo effect may have greater implications for psychotherapy than any other form of treatment because both psychotherapy and the placebo effect function primarily through psychological mechanisms. . . . [It] is an important component and perhaps the entire basis for the existence, popularity, and effectiveness of numerous methods of psychotherapy. . . . Much can be learned about psychotherapy from study of the placebo effect.

Placebos influence both subjective measures like mood and objective measures like reaction time. Physiological systems respond—for example, Beecher (1955) cited a study in which injection of isotonic saline produced several reliable changes in the composition of the blood of severely anxious patients; and another in which 7 of 15 subjects given a placebo they thought to be morphine responded with constricted pupils. Cousins (1977) cited a report from the National Institute of Geriatrics in Romania. A new drug, believed to have rejuvenative powers, was given to 60-year-old subjects. Their **morbidity** and mortality rates were substantially lower than control subjects who received nothing; but a third group, given placebos, stayed as healthy and lived as long as the drug recipients.

Nisbett and Schachter (1966) gave placebos to two groups of people. Group 1 was told to expect symptoms such as hand tremor, breathing rate changes, and a sinking feeling in the pit of the stomach; these normally occur in fearful situations. Group 2 received descriptions unrelated to fear: itching and numb feet. Both groups then self-administered shocks from a machine with an adjustable dial, increasing intensity until the pain became unbearable. Subjects in the first group withstood considerably greater intensities. The authors reasoned that pain from shock is normally augmented by symptoms of fear, and subjects told to expect such symptoms attributed them to the drug rather than the shock.

Placebo actions, mediated by expectations, are influenced by many factors. As with active drugs, their effects are sometimes influenced by biological rhythms (Pollman, reported in Reinberg & Smolensky, 1983). Leslie (1954) found that red, yellow, and brown pills are more effective than blue or green; and that unusual sizes (tiny or huge), dosages (9 or 11, but not 10, drops), and tastes yield best results. Because expectations depend on the recipient's prior history and presenting problem, probably no specific color or size is universally best.

Whether deliberate or otherwise, whoever administers a placebo influences recipients' expectations. A nurse with an openly negative attitude reduced placebo effectiveness from 70% to 25% (Broadhurst, 1977). Wolf (1962) reported that one of two physicians who administered placebos increased his patients' gastric acid secretions consistently; the second consistently decreased secretions.

Drugs that produce discernible effects, but not on the condition being treated, are called **active placebos.** For example, atropine causes dry mouth and has been used as an active placebo in studies of antidepressants. Researchers are more likely to conclude that an antidepressant works if they've used an inert rather than active placebo control group (Thomson, 1982). Also, an active placebo given with an active drug can modify the actions of the latter (Lipman, Park, & Rickels, 1966). The significance of these findings is discussed in Chapter 13.

Benson and Epstein (1975) contended that physician cures until the 20th century were due primarily to placebo effects. Yet physicians cured many people, as witch doctors do today. Cousins (1977) quoted Albert Schweitzer:

> The witch doctor succeeds for the same reason all the rest of us succeed. Each patient carries his own doctor inside him. They come to us not knowing that truth. We are at our best when we give the doctor who resides within each patient a chance to go to work.

Cousins concluded that, "the placebo is the doctor who resides within."

Double-blind placebo controlled studies yield relatively weak non-specific effects. For one thing, both doctors and patients know that some patients will receive an ineffective drug. Second, they sometimes figure out who has received what. Roberts, Kewman, Mercier, and Hovell (1993) sought conditions under which the effects would be maximized. They reviewed the literature on five medical and surgical procedures[1] that were thought effective at the time they were administered. Physicians had used them to cure, not as part of an experiment. Subsequent research showed that the procedures were no more effective than placebo. Nevertheless, of 6,931 patients treated, 40% were reported to have had excellent outcomes, 30% good outcomes, and 30% poor outcomes.

The Effects of Expectations on Active Drugs. The effects of active drugs are the result of pharmacology and nonspecific variables (cf. Rickels, 1968). Wolf (1950) administered ipecac to a pregnant woman suffering from intense nausea and vomiting—symptoms normally *caused* by ipecac. She was cured within 20 minutes. Wolf gave atropine, a gastric secretion inhibitor, to a patient who believed he was receiving a drug that had previously caused him to hypersecrete. He hypersecreted.

Patients improved more on placebos than tranquilizers when the substances were administered by nurses who opposed drug therapy for those patients (Baker & Thorpe, 1957). In another study, outcome depended considerably on whether or not drug administrator and recipient were of the same gender (Kerekjarto, 1968). Fisher et al. (1964) asked physicians to act either enthusiastically or with scientific skepticism while they administered either the antianxiety drug meprobamate or placebo. When physicians were enthusiastic, patients improved much more with meprobamate than placebo. With skeptical physicians, they did not. The demonstration may explain why many enthusiastic clinician claims fail to be substantiated within the sterile confines of laboratories. It is not a good argument against laboratory testing; both laboratory scientists and clinicians should treat all patients with enthusiasm and encouragement. Along those lines, Wheatley (1968) reported more favorable outcomes from patients with optimistic compared with pessimistic physicians.

Rickels (1968) edited a volume that documents a wide variety of nonspecific effects on drug response. These include characteristics such as color, size, and shape. For example, Schapira, McClelland, Griffiths, and Newell (1970) found that phobic patients treated with the drug oxazepam improved most when the pills were green and least when they were red. Unfortunately, little research goes on in this area; I wrote or called 15 of the largest pharmaceutical companies in the United States—none of the respondents knew of any work in progress on the relationship between a drug's appearance and effectiveness.

Many new medical treatments owe their effectiveness to the enthusiasm of advocates. An initial pattern of improvement of 70% to 90% declines to 30% to 40% as skeptical investigators are attracted and test the treatment under circumstances that minimize the placebo effect. The treatment is then abandoned. Benson and McCallie (1979) quoted the 19th-century physician Trousseau: "You should treat as many patients as possible with the new drugs while they still have the power to heal."

Task Variables

In 1955, Dews published the first of an extensive series of experiments demonstrating that drug actions are influenced considerably by what the recipient is doing. He deprived pigeons of food and required them to peck at a recessed disc of transparent plastic, called a key, for food reward. Some birds were required to peck 50 times for a single brief access to food. This is called a fixed ratio schedule. Other birds had to wait 15 minutes between rewards. (Pecks made before 15 minutes had elapsed were not rewarded; this is a fixed interval schedule.) Pentobarbital, in keeping with its classification as a CNS depressant, reduced responding of pigeons on the fixed interval schedule. But pigeons on the fixed ratio schedule responded more rapidly.

Barrett (1981) summarized the results of several experiments to show the complexity of drug/task interactions:

1. Morphine and methadone decreased responding of animals on fixed interval schedules for food reward.
2. Morphine and methadone increased responding of animals that received electric shock when they responded.
3. Amphetamine and cocaine increased responding of animals in both situations.
4. Pentobarbital, alcohol, and chlordiazepoxide increased responding of animals on fixed interval schedules for food reward.
5. Pentobarbital, alcohol, and chlordiazepoxide decreased responding of animals that received electric shock when they responded.

Steele and Josephs (1990) raised anxiety in both intoxicated and sober volunteer subjects by telling them they would have to give a speech in 15 minutes, to be evaluated by psychology graduate students, on "What I dislike most about my body and physical appearance." One half of the intoxicated and sober subjects spent the next 7 minutes in the distracting activity of rating esthetic features of art slides, and the other half sat quietly. Sober subjects were unaffected by the interim activities; but anxiety was reduced in intoxicated subjects who rated slides and worsened in those who sat quietly.

Summary

Reactions to drugs are influenced by many variables, grouped under four broad headings: organismic, drug, environmental, and situational. Because so many factors are involved, there is enormous variability in response to drugs.

Organismic variables include age, weight, biological rhythms, personality, physiological state, and genetics.

Drug variables include dose, frequency and method of administration, dosage regimen, and coadministration of other drugs.

Environmental variables include temperature, degree of crowding, lighting, noise level, and cleanliness.

Situational variables include expectations and task variables.

▨ **Note**

1. The treatments were: removal of the carotid body to treat bronchial asthma; the drug levamisole for herpes simplex virus; photodynamic inactivation for herpes simplex virus; topical application of organic solvents for herpes simplex virus; and gastric freezing for duodenal ulcer.

Mini-Quiz: Variability in Response to Drugs

The _____ is a reference book that lists drugs by class and includes information on dosages and contraindications.

Physician's Desk Reference

The text groups influences on drug response under four headings. Name them.

organismic, drug, environmental, and situational variables

The field that studies drug effects as a function of body time is _____.

chronopharmacology

T/F: Atropine normally increases heart rate. According to the Law of Initial Value, atropine will probably have a greater effect on someone whose initial heart rate is 80/min rather than 60/min.

false

Strychnine is a powerful poison but has been used to improve learning. The two different effects show the importance of _____.

dose

When, after repeated administrations of a drug, a given dose produces a smaller effect than it did initially, we say that _____ has occurred.

tolerance

Morphine's analgesic effects weaken over time but can be reinstated by administering it under different circumstances. The weakened effects are attributed to _____.

behavioral tolerance

Very rapid development of tolerance is called _____.

tachyphylaxis

Mescaline and LSD are _____ tolerant.

cross

MAOIs may _____ with various foods to cause a hypertensive crisis.

interact

Taking more than one drug at a time is called _____.

polypharmacy

T/F: Placebos influence both subjective and objective measures.

true

Atropine causes dry mouth. When given to control subjects in a study of antidepressants, atropine is a(n) _____.

active placebo

T/F: Expectations affect response to placebo but not to active drug.

false

_____

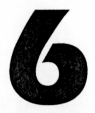

By the time you finish reading this chapter, you should be able to answer the following questions:

What are the different strategies used by pharmaceutical companies for developing new drugs?

Into which two structural groups can about 200 known psychedelics be classified?

What are the advantages and disadvantages of in vitro screening tests?

Why should drugs be tested on more than one animal species?

What are teratogens?

Why are animals given the opportunity to work for continuous access to drugs?

Are screening tests accurate?

At what point is an investigational drug (a) tested on humans? (b) released for general use?

Do informed consent forms offer sufficient protection for research subjects?

What are the arguments for assigning patients randomly to groups, so that some fail to receive the proper dose of a medicine likely to help them?

What types of questionable strategies have drug companies used to increase their profits?

T/F: Both men and women and people of various ethnic groups should be represented in trials of new drugs.

ugs

)ment,
), and Promotion

Contents

For every chemical that reaches U.S. pharmacy shelves, scientists reject between 2,000 and 10,000 others as either ineffective or unsafe (*FDA Consumer* Staff, 1990). But with approximately 5,000 drugs in regular use and 1.6 billion prescriptions filled each year, pharmaceutical manufacturers have ample incentive for seeking competitive products. Several developmental strategies are used.

1. Scientists study the cellular and molecular events that occur during health and disease. Then, often with the help of computers, they try to tailor compounds to act or block activity at relevant biochemical pathways. For example, the naturally occurring substance hypoxanthine is oxidized to uric acid and leads to kidney stones or gout in

85

susceptible people. Allopurinol, which interferes with the oxidation of hypoxanthine, blocks the production of uric acid and is thus valuable for treating gout (Burger, 1982).

2. Some drugs serve as leads to new and better ones. The antimalarial activity of chlorguanide is due to one of its metabolites. Although not itself a good antimalarial, the metabolite served as a starting point for molecular modification that led to the useful drug amodiaquine (Burger, 1982).

3. **Ethnobotanists** study how people in preindustrial societies use plants. Schultes (1963) urged scientists to consider the 800,000 species in the plant kingdom as potential drug sources. He advised ethnobotanists to (a) search the ancient literature for references to healing properties of plants; (b) visit herbariums, which contain firsthand accounts of observations made by plant collectors; and (c) do fieldwork. (Schultes spent almost 12 years studying plants in the northwest Amazon and collected nearly 24,000 specimens.)

Animals may provide clues about which plants are useful. Jane Goodall observed that chimpanzees often seek out leaves of a shrub, Aspilia, as soon as they wake up in the morning. Rodriguez et al. (1985) searched for unusual chemicals in the plant and isolated a previously unknown substance, thiarubrine-A, that is an extremely powerful antibiotic.

In 1989 a group of scientists formed Shaman Pharmaceuticals, a California company that aims to commercialize the pharmaceutical uses of plants. They believe that demand for medicinal plants within the Amazon rain forest alone will eventually add up to a multibillion-dollar-a-year retail market ("Lost Tribes," 1991).

4. A related approach involves testing compounds made naturally by microorganisms such as fungi, viruses, and molds. Scientists grow the microorganisms in special broths, one type per broth.

5. Chemists systematically modify the structure of a known drug so they can develop **congeners** (related drugs) with better properties. These might include reduced side effects, a greater margin between therapeutic and toxic doses, better absorption when taken orally, shorter latency of onset, different duration of action, fewer interactions with other substances, and so forth. Shulgin (1983) noted that most of the approximately 200 known psychedelics can be classified structurally into one of two groups, the phenethylamines and the indoles. The neurotransmitter dopamine is a phenethylamine, serotonin an indole. For about

35 years, Shulgin has used phenethylamines and indoles as starting points for designing, preparing, and evaluating new psychotropic drugs.

Albert (1987) discussed methods for increasing the selectivity of drugs:

a. Many toxic substances can be taken safely because they distribute selectively. For example, radioactive iodine taken orally accumulates in the thyroid gland and is used to attack tumors there. Particle size can affect distribution: inhaled particles above 5 micrometers in diameter remain in the nasal passages; those above 2 micrometers lodge in the larger bronchial areas; and only those smaller than 1 micrometer reach the small bronchi and alveolar sacs as is necessary for effective medication by aerosol nasal sprays.

b. **Prodrugs** are inert substances converted within the body into the parent drugs. Prodrugs may taste better, be more soluble for making injectable solutions, or have selective affinity for specific tissues. The prodrug L-dopa enters the brain and is converted to dopamine, which helps to relieve the symptoms of Parkinson's disease. The prodrug gamma-glutamyl-dopamine accumulates in the kidney and is converted to dopamine, which is valuable for treating shock (Hiller, 1991).

c. Organs and tissues are made up of highly differentiated cells, each kind adapted to a particular task. Their different structures offer opportunity for selectivity. For example, nerve-blood vessel junctions have wide synaptic gaps that permit activity of only small quantities of norepinephrine upon nerve stimulation; so antiadrenergic drugs easily interrupt neurotransmission there. By contrast, the nictitating membrane and vas deferens have small synaptic gaps, so norepinephrine often reaches 100 times its threshold concentration; thus, antiadrenergics have little effect on such tissues.

6. Side effects of known drugs may have therapeutic potential. Promethazine, at one time used during surgery to control shock, produced unwanted sedation and drowsiness. The surgeon Laborit speculated that related compounds might cause similar but more specific and desirable effects. Many syntheses were attempted and led eventually to the development of chlorpromazine, the first major antipsychotic drug.

7. Alexander Fleming observed by chance that bacterial cultures contaminated by a common mold stop growing. Florey and Chain followed up and isolated the substance responsible: penicillin. Many other potentially important observations have not been exploited. For example, some users of certain drugs experience depression as a side effect. If their unique predisposing characteristics could be identified,

researchers might have a clue toward finding a treatment for depression in all people

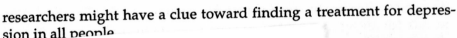

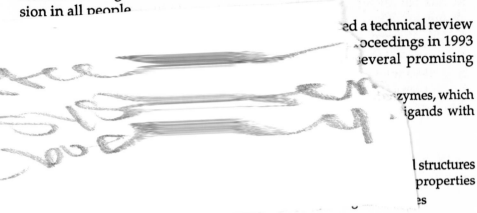

ed a technical review
...oceedings in 1993
several promising

zymes, which
igands with

l structures
properties
es

※ Screening Techniques

Once isolated, substances must be tested for therapeutic effectiveness and safety. Given the vast number developed each year, there is a premium on rapid, inexpensive tests. Tests may be conducted in **vitro** (in the test tube), on subhuman animals, or on humans.

IN VITRO TESTING

In vitro experiments involve testing compounds for their effects on enzymes or cell cultures. The tests, generally brief, simple, and inexpensive, may suggest ways of modifying a compound's chemical structure to improve its performance. Owicki and Parce (1990) described an instrument called a silicon microphysiometer that detects the ability of chemical agents to alter metabolic rates of cells. The device helps screen for new therapeutic drugs. Pillai and Watson (1990) reviewed several in vitro techniques for evaluating effects of drugs of abuse on the immune system.

ANIMAL TESTING

If in vitro testing shows that a compound is biologically active, its pharmacokinetics, potency, and toxicity are studied in living animals. Researchers compare the minimum dose needed to produce desired effects in the least sensitive recipients with the minimum toxic dose in the most sensitive. Scheuplein, Shoaf, and Brown (1990) discussed the value of collecting various other types of data. Computing a drug's half-life helps determine dosing regimens. Examining organs and tissues to learn where a drug concentrates discloses areas of potential toxicity. Also, drugs that concentrate in non-eliminating tissues may act over prolonged periods even though undetectable elsewhere within the body. Analyzing pharmacokinetic data from different animals indicates the degree of population variability in drug disposition and, often, the source of the variability. Measuring the percentage of drug excreted unchanged can indicate if metabolism or excretion is more variable.

Choice of Subjects

Government regulations require that animal studies be conducted on at least one rodent and one nonrodent species. The outcome of a screening test may depend heavily on the choices, and unsuitable choices may lead to tragedy. Routine testing of the hypnotic drug thalidomide with several species had revealed no harmful effects, so it was released for sale in Europe and widely marketed from 1958 to 1961. But thalidomide is not safe for humans, especially developing fetuses. Thousands of babies whose mothers took it early in pregnancy were born without arms or legs.

Mice are usually the first animals tested. Rats and mice are inexpensive to buy and maintain, easily handled, and well adapted to laboratory conditions. Their short generation spans enhance their value for teratological work. (A **teratogen** is a substance that increases the likelihood that offspring will be born malformed.) And scientists have accumulated much data on responses of certain strains of mice and rats to carcinogens (Scheuplein et al., 1990).

Other species are picked for specific purposes. Hamsters, highly sensitive to the teratological effects of nitriles, are routinely used for testing those chemicals. Cats and humans react similarly to many drugs. (The oral dose is approximately three times as great for cats as humans; but narcotic analgesics, antihistamines, and meprobamate-like drugs stimulate cats and depress humans.) Of the common laboratory animals, pigs are most similar to humans metabolically. Offsetting the obvious advantages of monkeys are the costs to buy and maintain them. Also, monkeys are relatively insensitive to drug-induced neurologic impairment (Irwin, 1966).

Testing a new drug on a sufficient number of rats costs a great deal of money, and dogs and monkeys are even more expensive. Shulgin (personal communication, 1988) said that companies are reluctant to spend huge sums on unpromising drugs, so animal screens are often preceded by tests on one or a few people. "The animal screen confirms human use for legal purposes."

Choice of Tests

The choice of **screening tests** should depend on research objectives and types of drugs. One useful procedure is simple observation. Animals can be observed for alertness or stupor; stereotyped behaviors; excessive grooming, which often indicates stimulation; vocalizations, which suggest pain; startle responses to loud noises; motor incoordination; changes in pupil size, which may reflect altered autonomic nervous system activity; urination or salivation, which indicates muscarinic activity; and changes in heart rate.

TOXICITY SCREENING TESTS

Noel (1973) recommended a minimum of four dose-level groups for screening studies.

1. High dose: a dose impractical to exceed in clinical practice, for demonstrating toxic signs that could be encountered on repeated dosage
2. Low dose: computed from pharmacological and metabolic data including comparisons with similar compounds, for studying the effects of a reasonable maximum human intake
3. Intermediate dose: for estimating safety margins and establishing the minor changes that precede more serious toxic ones (so users can discontinue the drug before the more serious toxicity occurs)
4. A control group of undrugged animals

Toxicity tests measure teratogenicity, carcinogenicity, and **dependence liability.** The LD50—the dose of drug lethal to 50% of test animals—is often calculated. Determining the LD50 requires sacrificing large numbers of animals, generally for nonessential information. Animal rights activists argue, in my view reasonably, against the use of LD50s.

Tests for Teratogenicity

Teratogens are a major cause of serious birth defects and spontaneous abortions. Screening drugs for teratogenicity might seem straightforward—administer the drug to a pregnant animal and observe its offspring for defects—but in actual practice, many problems arise. See Chapter 8.

Tests for Carcinogenicity

The National Cancer Institute published guidelines for carcinogenicity testing in 1976. Each drug should be tested in both males and females of two different rodent species. The routes of administration should approximate the human route, and at least two dose levels should be used: the highest dose level that does not shorten the animal's life span from effects other than cancer; and either one half or one quarter of that dose. The drug should be administered for the life of the animal.

Almost all substances that cause cancers in humans also cause them in animals, but tumor induction in test animals does not reliably predict human carcinogenicity (Maugh, 1978). Mason et al. (1990) discussed recent developments in short-term carcinogenicity testing in rodents.

Many people disregard newspaper reports on drug-induced cancers in laboratory animals, but Lijinsky (1977) offered the disconcerting view that animal tests are conservative; they are more likely to miss a carcinogen than to give a **false positive**. A carcinogen administered in a low enough dose won't produce tumors, but humans are exposed daily to low doses of many carcinogens whose effects may be additive or even **synergistic**. Also, the best way to induce tumors is to administer small doses at frequent intervals over a long period; but tumors often take several years to develop, and mice and rats live for only about 2 years, so the more common laboratory method is to administer one or a few large doses. But most substances owe their carcinogenic actions to metabolites, and large doses overload metabolic systems; so the substances are excreted mostly unchanged. Furthermore, if a drug is toxic to 1% of experimental animals, then about 295 animals must be tested to give a 95% probability of observing the effect in at least one animal (Barnes & Denz, 1954).

Weissman (1990) offered a different perspective. He noted that screening tests have been validated almost exclusively with drugs harmful to humans. There is little proof that they can show that safe drugs are safe. Some screening tests detect changes of no relevance to humans; they seem useful only because researchers have improperly cited rare adverse effects of the drugs in humans. For example, cimetidine reliably disrupts the behavior of rats on a particular test; Rastogi and McMillan (1984) concluded that the test is valuable and used as evidence a report that "neural dysfunction in the form of confusion, delirium and hallucination have been observed with higher doses of cimetidine in humans." Weissman pointed out that the report was on a single person, and the prevailing view is that cimetidine produces few adverse effects. Weissman (1990) wrote, "If one assumes that *any* behavioral effect is a *toxic* behavioral effect, it will be necessary to discount the fact that many useful, safe drugs produce behavioral effects at extraordinarily low doses."

Lijinsky (1977) was right in asserting that screening tests are sometimes not sensitive enough. Weissman was also right. Some tests are too sensitive and may cause potentially valuable drugs to be jettisoned needlessly. Many indispensable medicines, including penicillin, digitalis, ipecac, cinchona bark, ether, and chloroform, are available only because they were introduced prior to the development of elaborate screening procedures.

Tests for Dependence Liability

Tests for dependence liability usually involve some form of self-administration procedure. Animals are implanted with venous catheters attached to a remotely operated pump. When they press a bar or make some other predesignated response, drug solution is injected directly into their veins. An increase in responding is taken to mean that the drug is rewarding. Giving animals continuous access to a drug allows for assessment of toxicity, tolerance, physical dependence, and changes over time at self-regulated doses. Most drugs that increase responding and are used by humans are abused by humans. Johanson, Balster, and Bonese (1976) gave monkeys continuous access to cocaine, d-amphetamine, or d-methamphetamine. Few survived more than 5 days, none more than 15.

Once an animal self-administers at a stable rate for a standard drug such as cocaine or morphine, other drugs may be substituted. Patterns of responding are compared for the standard, the test drug, and saline. Except for various psychedelic drugs, the substitution procedure accurately identifies drugs likely to be abused by humans (Johanson & Balster, 1978). The number of times an animal presses a bar for a single infusion of a drug, the more reinforcing the drug is assumed to be. Some monkeys pressed more than 12,000 times for a single 0.5 mg/kg cocaine dose (Yanagita, 1973).

The Committee on Problems of Drug Dependence (1984) elaborated on many additional procedures for using animals to assess dependence liability. A particularly sensitive technique, **drug discrimination**, requires animals to respond differently to different drug states. To receive food, a hungry rat might be required to turn right in a maze if pretreated with morphine and left after saline injection. Animals can be trained to respond with nearly 100% accuracy to drugs that produce strong subjective effects in humans; and once trained, they readily identify pharmacologically similar drugs. The rat trained to turn left under the influence of morphine will turn left to heroin, right to saline, and randomly to amphetamine (Browne, 1986; Browne & Fondren, 1978). Overton (1973) assembled evidence showing a strong relationship between the discriminative properties of a drug, that is, the ease with which subjects distinguish between the drug and no-drug conditions, and the drug's abuse potential.

Discrimination tests can identify possible drug antagonists. For example, Browne (1986) trained rats to discriminate phencyclidine (PCP) from saline; then he administered PCP plus various test compounds. Most failed to antagonize the PCP discrimination, but a few analogs of adenosine did. Although adenosine is not an antidote for PCP intoxication in humans, Browne argued that the discrimination procedure is likely to uncover one.

Tests to Indicate Behavioral Effects

If a known therapeutic drug induces a change in an easily measured and reliable behavior, then drugs with similar therapeutic actions are likely to induce a similar change. So, identifying and measuring such behaviors is a good strategy for developing screening tests. The tests described below do not require complex apparatus. For detailed information on screening tests, see Domer (1971) or Weissman and Koe (1987).

Tests for CNS Depression

1. Thirsty animals are trained to run down a runway for water. When times to exit from the starting box have stabilized, the animals are injected with the test substance. CNS depressants retard exit latency.
2. Animals are injected with the test substance and placed on their backs; failure to right themselves within 30 seconds indicates CNS depression.
3. After drug administration, the cornea and conjuctiva of both eyes are touched with a fine hair; CNS depressants block the normal reflex.

Tests for Central Stimulation

1. The dose of pentobarbital that kills 99% of a group of mice is determined. A new group is injected with pentobarbital and the test drug under identical conditions. Many stimulants protect against pentobarbital-induced deaths.
2. Hungry rats are injected with the test substance, and then their food intakes are measured. Not all stimulants depress appetite, but almost all appetite depressants are stimulants.

Tests for Antianxiety Effects

1. Rats trained to bar-press for food are exposed to a clicking sound that lasts for 3 minutes and is immediately followed by electric shock. After several pairings of click and shock, the rats reduce their responding as soon as the click sounds. Antianxiety drugs attenuate the response decrement (Millenson & Leslie, 1974).
2. Rats show a startle response to loud sounds that becomes stronger in fear-provoking situations. After repeated exposure to a light followed by electric shock, they learn to fear the light alone. Then, their startle response to a loud sound is measured in the presence of the light alone. Most drugs that reduce anxiety in humans decrease the fear-potentiated startle response in rats; in nonfearful situations, that is, without light or shock, the drugs don't affect startle. Yohimbine and piperoxane, which provoke anxiety in humans, increase potentiated startle (Davis, 1990).

Tests for Antipsychotic Effects

1. High doses of antipsychotic drugs retard movement so profoundly that drugged animals can be molded into bizarre positions and will remain there. The duration of the immobility correlates with antipsychotic efficacy in humans. (Clozapine, a relatively new and effective antipsychotic, induces little or no immobility.)

See Donner 1971

Or

Weissman and Kve 1987

CIRCULATING BOOK STACK LOCATIONS

A-	**General Work**	**3rd**
AE	Encyclopedias	
AI	Indexes	
AY	Almanacs	
B-	**Philosophy/Psychology/Religion**	**3rd**
B-BD	Philosophy	
BF	Psychology	
BL-BX	Religion	
C-	**History: Related Fields**	**3rd**
CC	Archaeology	
CD	Archives	
CT	Biography	
D-	**History:** (except America)	**3rd**
E-	**History:** America & U.S. (General)	**3rd**
F-	**History:** U.S. (Local) & North American, Central America, and South American	**3rd**
G-	**Geography/Anthropology/Recreation**	**3rd**
G-GF	Geography	
GN	Anthropology	
GR	Folklore	
GV	Recreation	
H-	**Social Sciences**	**3rd**
HA	Statistics	
HB-HE	Economics	
HD	Labor (Professions)	
HF	Commerce, Accounting, Advertising	
HG	Finance	
HM	Sociology	
HQ	Family, Marriage, Women's Studies	
HV	Social Pathology, Welfare & Criminology	
HX	Socialism, Communism $ Anarchism	
J-	**Political Science**	**3rd**
JK	United States	
JX	International Law	
K-	**Law**	**3rd**
KF	Law of the U.S.	
KFN	Law of North Carolina	
L-	**Education**	**3rd**
LA	History of Education	
LB	Theory & Practice of Education	
LC	Special Aspects of Education	
M-	**Music**	**3rd**
M	Musical Score	
ML	Literature of Music	
MT	Musical Instruction and Study	

N-	**Fine Arts**	**2nd**
N	Visual Arts	
NA	Architecture	
NB	Sculpture	
NC	Drawing	
ND	Painting	
NE	Print Media	
NK	Decorative Arts	
NX	Arts in General	
P-	**Languages and Literature**	**3rd**
P	Philology, Linguistics, Communication	
PA	Classical Languages & Literatures	
PB-PH	Modern European Languages	
PE	English Language	
PN	Literary History and Collections	
PQ	Romance Literature	
PR	English Literature	
PS	American Literature	
PT	Germanic Literature	
Q-	**Science**	**2nd**
QA	Mathematics (including Computer Sciences)	
QC	Physics	
QE	Geology	
QH	Natural History (including General Biology)	
QK	Botany	
QL	Zoology	
QP	Physiology	
QR	Microbiology	
R-	**Medicine**	**2nd**
RA	Public Aspects of Medicine	
RC	Internal Medicine and Practice of Medicine	
RT	Nursing	
S-	**Agriculture**	**2nd**
SB	Plant Culture	
SD	Forestry	
SH	Aquaculture	
T-	**Technology**	**2nd**
TD	Environmental Technology	
TP	Chemical Technology	
U-	**Military Science**	**2nd**
V-	**Naval Science**	**2nd**
Z-	**Bibliography and Library Science**	**2nd**
Folio-	**Oversized Books**	**2nd**
REF-	**Reference**	**1st**

2. Rats hear a tone that precedes an electric shock and can avoid the shock by jumping a hurdle. Antipsychotic drugs inhibit the avoidance response. The rats escape as soon as the shock begins, showing that its painful properties remain. Barbiturates and related drugs do not block avoidance except at doses large enough to impair all motor activity.

Tests for Hallucinogenic Activity

1. Mice, rats, and cats stand in abnormal postures after receiving LSD-like drugs.
2. Normal cats flick their paws only to shake off foreign substances. LSD-treated cats frequently raise their paws and shake them rapidly. The number of limb flicks per unit time is a measure of a test drug's LSD-like activity.

Test for Analgesic Activity

A rat in a restraining device is exposed to a hot, painful beam of light. The measure used is the latency with which the animal moves its tail out of the light with and without the drug.

Test for Hypnotic Activity

The test drug is injected along with a subhypnotic dose of a short-acting barbiturate. Latency and duration of anesthesia are measured.

TESTING ON HUMANS

If warranted, results of animal tests plus **protocols** for the conduct of human clinical studies are described in an Investigational New Drug (IND) application to the FDA. (Some animal testing continues after human tests begin, to learn whether long-term use of the drug may cause cancer or birth defects. Also, more animal data may be needed if human tests turn up unexpected effects. And new therapeutic uses may be found by continued animal studies.) Human testing involves three phases:

1. Healthy volunteers, usually fewer than 100, are exposed for about one month to a limited number of doses. The goals are to evaluate toxicity and pharmacokinetics. To test for abuse liability, volunteers are asked to discriminate between drugs and allowed to self-administer. If animal studies have shown that a drug concentrates in a specific target

organ, that organ is monitored for altered function. About 70% of IND submissions successfully pass **Phase I.**

2. A few hundred sick people are given the drug for a few months while matched controls receive placebo. The goals are to ensure that the drug works without causing serious toxicity and to identify side effects. About 33% of IND submissions successfully pass **Phase II.**

3. Thousands of people are tested in settings almost identical to those in which the drug will be used if released for general marketing. The drug's actions on special groups such as the elderly or people with impaired kidney function may be investigated. About 25%-30% of IND submissions successfully pass **Phase III.**

Problems With Volunteers

The practice of using volunteers in Phase I studies raises both scientific and ethical problems. From a scientific standpoint, the problem is one of confidence in generalizations. Volunteers differ in many ways from nonvolunteers, especially for drug studies (Esecover, Malitz, & Wilkens, 1961; Lasagna & von Felsinger, 1954; Rosenthal & Rosnow, 1969).

The ethical problems are complex. On the one hand, many crucial medical advances originated from experiments that sacrificed human volunteers. Walter Reed's isolation of the *Aedes* mosquito as the carrier of yellow fever is a prominent example. Public health would suffer if dangerous experiments were banned. Tests for possible toxicity of drugs and chemical additives would be disallowed—they entail risks but no direct gain for participants. No treatment, having once gained acceptance, would ever be withheld to further test its value. Thus, useless, painful, time-consuming, and dangerous treatments would persist even longer than they do now.

On the other hand, terrible things have been done to people in the name of science. See Leavitt (1991) for many examples. Today, institutional review boards require that researchers obtain the informed consent of prospective subjects. Gray (1975), however, reported that people are often tricked into consenting. He interviewed 51 women who had signed a consent form to receive a new labor-inducing drug. Fewer than half had understood that they would be research subjects, were not required to participate, would be subjected to special monitoring procedures, and might be exposed to hazards. Upon hearing that the drug was new, they assumed it to be superior, not experimental.

Many volunteers are prison inmates with few options. They are bored, have limited opportunities to earn money, and may improve their chances of early release by participating in experiments. Meyer (1975) observed that the use of prisoners reduces the costs of research to sponsoring pharmaceutical firms, which means that the correctional system subsidizes the pharmaceutical industry. Researchers prefer to work with stable populations, so correctional and rehabilitative programs may be undermined and alternatives to prison ignored.

A researcher who offered ice cream to a child for permission to remove her thymus gland would be excoriated. He'd fare little better by choosing an institutionalized schizophrenic. The outrage would stem from awareness that such donors are incapable of rational choice. By extension, perhaps adults who volunteer for painful and hazardous experiments, even if apparently normal, should be disqualified as irrational.

An ethical dilemma. Several years ago, I served on a three-person committee to review a large grant proposal. The applicants were the head of the Department of Medicine and the head of the Department of Toxicology at a large hospital. Attached to the proposal was a document indicating that the hospital ethics committee had approved the proposal unanimously.

The rationale for the study was that, once a drug is approved for human use, physicians can prescribe whatever doses they choose. Although dosage recommendations are given in the literature, physicians' personal experiences often take precedence. The grant proposers wanted to establish proper starting doses for every drug used in the hospital, which physicians could then modify according to patients' characteristics. They designed the study in two parts.

Part I. They would review hospital records for the previous 20 years for a select group of drugs, correlating dosage with outcome. For each drug, they would find the dose associated with the best outcome. (The results would have been inconclusive because of nonrandom assignment of patients to doses. If, for example, the sickest patients had received the highest doses, their poor outcomes might not have been due to improper dosing.)

Part II. Physicians within the hospital would randomly assign their patients for the next several months to one of three dosage groups. Patients would not be told they were research subjects. (Otherwise, some might refuse to participate, compromising the randomness of the groups.)

I opposed the proposal on ethical grounds but was outvoted two to one. A year later, the researchers submitted a progress report; they had learned a great deal, including confirmation of previous beliefs about optimal dosage for one drug: More patients survived who received that dose than any other. I voted against extending the study for another year and was again outvoted. That ended my involvement.

I'd vote the same way today, but two points weaken my position. First, nobody was sure of the best dose or the study would have been unnecessary; and educated guesses about which of two treatments is superior are wrong about 50% of the time (Gilbert, Light, & Mosteller, 1975). Second, in the long run such studies save far more lives than they cost. Suppose that the best guesses about survival rates for 1, 5, and 10 mg doses of a particular drug are 40%, 70%, and 50%, respectively. Suppose the best guesses are correct. Then, of 300 patients given the 5 mg dose, an expected 210 would survive. If the patients were instead assigned randomly, 100 to each dosage group, the expected number of survivors would be 160 [$(100 \times 0.4) + (100 \times 0.7) + (100 \times 0.5)$]. Fifty would die who could have been saved.

Suppose, in this hypothetical but realistic case, that the drug is prescribed for a disease affecting 10,000 people worldwide each year; and that 10% of physicians normally prescribe each of the suboptimal doses. Then the annual survival rate would be $(1,000 \times 0.4) + (8,000 \times 0.7) + (1,000 \times 0.5) = 6,500$. But if research had clearly established the proper dose, the survival rate would be $10,000 \times 0.7 = 7,000$. Every year—forever, because without proper experimentation there would be no way to learn the proper dose—500 extra people would die.

After completing Phase III work, a drug company can submit a new drug application (NDA), requesting FDA approval to market the drug. FDA reviewers must decide if the drug is both effective and safe.

THREE IMPORTANT CONCERNS

Some Groups Are Underrepresented in Drug Testing

Gender, age, and race affect response to drugs, yet women, the elderly, and minorities are inadequately represented in drug trials. In 1986, the National Institute of Health began promoting the inclusion of greater numbers of women in clinical studies; however, the U.S. General Accounting Office reported in 1990 that underrepresentation of women continues. Some scientists worry that, because women's behavior and physiology change throughout the menstrual cycle, the inclusion of women subjects would introduce too much experimental variability. A recent study investigating the potential of aspirin to prevent coronary heart disease used 22,071 subjects, all men. Robert Temple of the FDA ("Is There Gender Bias," 1991) contended that, with the exception of the aspirin study, recent data indicate that women are tested in about equal numbers as men. Nevertheless, the Congressional Caucus on Women's Issues plans to introduce legislation barring the use of federal funds to support research that arbitrarily excludes women (Segawa, 1990).

Svensson (1989) examined 50 recently published studies of drug tests and concluded that African Americans are generally underrepresented. No official remedy is pending. The FDA issued guidelines asking manufacturers to determine if a drug is likely to have significant use among the elderly; if so, the manufacturers were advised to include adequate numbers of elderly subjects in clinical trials ("Testing Drugs in Older People," 1990).

Insufficient Research Is Conducted
Toward Developing Drugs to Treat Rare Diseases

About 5,000 rare diseases are known that affect fewer than 200,000 people each. Until recently, pharmaceutical companies had little incentive to develop drugs to treat these diseases. New legislation allows the government to give tax credits, marketing exclusivity rights, and other inducements for developing "orphan" drugs. As of June 1990, 49 orphan drugs had been approved (Haffner, 1991).

The Drug Testing Process May Take Too Long

The requirement that drugs be proved safe and effective prior to marketing protects the public; but it also delays release of valuable drugs and increases their prices. In other countries, different weights are assigned to benefits and costs of testing. Lasagna (1972) reported that the FDA received 72,200 pages of information on the drug ketamine; in Switzerland, Germany, and the United Kingdom, three places where life expectancies are comparable to those in the United States, the numbers of required pages were 159, 159, and 857 respectively. The FDA, responding to criticism that testing sometimes takes too long, reduced regulatory guidelines and offers help to sponsors planning clinical research. It recently approved an AIDS drug for marketing that had not been thoroughly tested in clinical trials; and it allows patients to import unapproved drugs into the country for personal use. FDA commissioner Dr. David Kessler said, "In the past the agency saw its mission as keeping unsafe drugs off the market. Of late the agency has recognized that it must get safe and effective drugs on the market" (MacNeil/Lehrer Report, 1991). Still, in December 1989 new drug applications averaged 31 months even though the FDA is required by law to process them within 6 (Hilts, 1989).

▓ Profits in the Drug Industry

Pharmaceutical companies are in business to make money, and they do very well. According to a report released by U.S. Senate Aging Committee Chairman David Pryor (*The Washington Post*, August 27, 1991), the top 10 drug companies had an average profit on sales in 1990 of 15.5% compared to 4.6% for the average *Fortune* 500 industry. The results of a congressional study released in early 1993 indicated that the industry earns at least $36 million more than development costs on each new drug (*Oakland Tribune*, February 26, 1993). Drug companies have used three questionable strategies to increase profits.

CUTTING LABORATORY COSTS

The *FDA Consumer* (1990) cited the estimate of economist Steven Wiggins that drug companies spend about $65 million on average to develop a new drug. The temptation to reduce costs by cutting corners is great and not always resisted. In the past two decades, several major and minor scandals have damaged public confidence in the pharmaceutical industry. Each monthly issue of *FDA Consumer* has a section listing recent agency actions against companies that have improperly tested, labeled, advertised, or marketed drugs. Since October 1985, FDA investigators have turned up serious deficiencies in 7% of their audits.

Levy (1992) reported that many and perhaps the majority of investigations of drug effectiveness are designed by pharmaceutical company staff. They control the data and decide whether and what to publish. Levy reviewed several analyses of the medical literature in which new drugs (protected by patent law and so commanding higher prices) and older ones were compared. The following conclusions were overwhelmingly supported:

- The new drug was reported to be more effective.
- The new drug was reported to have fewer adverse effects.
- Studies that favored a new drug were much more likely to have received pharmaceutical industry financial support. "In no case was a therapeutic agent manufactured by the sponsoring company found to be inferior to an alternative product manufactured by another company."
- Statistical errors and bias were common and almost always favored the new drug.

About 12,000 clinical investigators in the United States regularly conduct Phase II testing of drugs. Kohn (1986) reported that several investigators, paid by the drug manufacturers, were grossing more than one million dollars a year. Investigators who repeatedly turn in negative reports are unlikely to remain on the payroll, which establishes a clear conflict of interest. Several investigators were found guilty of submitting false claims.

Levy (1992) discussed a related problem. Scientists submit studies with positive results (the drug and control groups differed) more frequently than they do negative studies (no difference between groups) to scientific journals. And journal reviewers accept positive studies more readily than equally well-designed negative ones. Thus, a serious bias (not unique to the drug industry) is introduced. For example, published studies showed longer survival times for patients undergoing a particular form of cancer chemotherapy. Simes (1986) tracked down unpublished studies and did a combined analysis of the published and unpublished results; contrary to what the literature suggested, the new therapy offered no significant advantages.

CHARGING HIGH PRICES

Patent laws give the developer of a drug exclusive marketing rights for 17 years, so the developer can charge high prices with no fear of direct competition. Industry spokespersons justify the high prices by claiming that drug development entails great risks, as in drilling for oil or sponsoring a Broadway play. But about three-fourths of research money goes toward developing insignificant variants of existing drugs. At least 22 different penicillins are marketed in the United States; and new classes of drugs such as beta blockers and cephalosporins, which were introduced by a single drug about 15 years ago, are now large families (Health and Public Policy Committee, 1988). As the expiration date on a patent draws close, manufacturers often promote related drugs heavily—even if they offer no advantages over the original (cf. Greenblatt & Shader, 1974). Physician Sidney Wolfe in an article in *Time* magazine said that 70% to 90% of newly approved drugs are not important therapeutic advances. But companies charge more, often much more, for the newer drugs ("Cheaper Can Be Better," 1991). The article cited two examples involving drugs only marginally better than established ones, but widely sold at more than 10 times the price.

PROMOTING DRUGS

Most new drugs offer little to distinguish them from their competitors. A recent congressional study revealed that 58% of the drugs introduced between 1975 and 1989 were "me-too" products that offered no therapeutic gains (*Oakland Tribune*, February 26, 1993); and few physicians have the time or resources to study subtle distinctions. The formal pharmacological education of physicians occurs almost exclusively in the second year of medical school, at which time they learn about drugs for treating diseases they have never seen in clinical situations. Five years usually elapse between the pharmacology course and completion of a 3-year residency, during which time about 100 new drugs become available. So physicians frequently prescribe drugs about which they have received no formal education. In 1987, physicians who had graduated from medical school in 1960 were writing 85% of their prescriptions for drugs they did not study in medical school. And most hospitalized patients receive the most recent and novel drugs, although such usage is often inappropriate (Health and Public Policy Committee, 1988).

After medical school, physicians receive no systematic, informed exposure to unbiased assessments of drug therapy. Under the circumstances, drug company promotions greatly influence sales; and the drug industry spends almost as much on promotion as is spent by all U.S. medical schools. For example, free promotional meals plus $100 for "time and participation" were provided for an estimated 175,000 physicians a year in the late 1980s ("AMA, Pharmaceutical Association," 1991, pp. 2304-2305).

Most physicians must take continuing medical education (CME) credits each year, and much of the financial support for CME courses is provided by the drug industry. In 1988, 16 companies sponsored 34,688 symposiums at a cost of almost $86 million (Kessler, 1991). The symposiums feature well-known speakers and attract large audiences.

Companies pick speakers whose opinions match their marketing needs, and they pay well. The authors of a *Consumer Reports* article ("Pushing Drugs to Doctors," 1992) claimed that experts can identify the type of drug being promoted at symposiums merely by hearing the speakers' names. The director of a small teaching hospital was quoted:

> We had a speaker for grand rounds last month, talking about patients who come into the emergency room with severe headache. Roche sponsored his presentation. The speaker mentioned only three drugs by name during his lecture, all of which were made by Roche. I was absolutely in awe that he was able to work all of them in.

The authors also cited a study by Bowman, who analyzed the content of two CME courses on the same topic but sponsored by different companies. In each case, the sponsoring company's drug was presented more favorably. In follow-up work, Bowman found that physicians began prescribing more of the drug made by the company that sponsored the course they took.

Orlowski and Wateska (1992) interviewed physicians invited on all-expense-paid trips to attend symposia to promote two drugs. Most claimed that their prescribing habits would be unaffected. But pharmacy inventory usage reports showed that attending physicians prescribed both drugs significantly more following the symposia, and significantly differently from national patterns.

Below are examples of other drug company promotions (from "Cheaper Can Be Better," 1991):

- Wyeth-Ayerst Laboratories gave physicians 1,000 frequent-flyer points each time they placed a patient on Wyeth's new hypertensive drug.
- Roche paid physicians $1,200 for prescribing a new Roche antibiotic to 20 patients.
- Connaught Labs awarded points redeemable for merchandise to physicians who bought Connaught vaccines.
- Ciba-Geigy offered Caribbean vacations to physicians who attended a few lectures on Ciba-Geigy's estrogen patch.

On December 3, 1990, the ethics committee of the American Medical Association issued guidelines severely limiting the freedom of physicians to accept gifts. Three days later, the Pharmaceutical Manufacturers Association incorporated the guidelines into its ethics code of marketing practices. Still, gift-giving continues. One company recently arranged to send the 55 dermatologists who purchased the largest volume of injectable collagen during a specified time period on an all-expenses-paid South Pacific cruise ("AMA, Pharmaceutical Association," 1991, p. 2305).

Promotions Directed at Health Professionals

Physicians learn about new drugs by reading the scientific literature, attending seminars, and consulting with friends. They also learn through free films created by drug companies to sell their products. And through pharmaceutical sales representatives—1 for every 12 prescribing physicians in the United States (Drake & Uhlman, 1993). Sales reps visit physicians with free samples and (often) slanted product information. Direct advertisements, sometimes in the guise of supplements to reputable, objective journals, also play a big role. For example, a supplement to the *Journal of Clinical Psychiatry* (September 1991) on selection of an appropriate sleeping pill was heavily slanted toward one drug—the one manufactured by the supplement's sponsor.

Stimson (1977) analyzed 591 separate ads and concluded that they are severely deficient as information sources. Only 43% listed active ingredients by quantity; 14% listed the recommended dose; 4% mentioned side effects and special precautions; and 6.3% gave the cost. All the information is important, yet 49% of the ads had none of it and only 0.5% had all. Mehta, Sorofman, and Rowland (1989) analyzed 665 advertisements for oral hypoglycemics over the period 1963 to 1986. They found a steady decline in space devoted to scientific support for the products, such as reference to clinical tests or experiments or other statistical information.

Wilkes, Doblin, and Shapiro (1992) asked reviewers to evaluate 109 full-page pharmaceutical ads appearing in 10 medical journals. Each ad was sent to two experienced physicians in the relevant clinical area and one clinical pharmacist. At least two of the three reviewers

in 30% of cases, disputed the advertiser's claim that the drug was the "drug of choice."

in 40% of cases, believed that information on efficacy was not balanced by information on side effects and contraindications.

in 44% of cases, believed that physicians guided only by information presented in the ad would prescribe improperly.

in 57% of cases, believed that the ads had little or no educational value.

Table 6.1

	Minimally Important in Influencing My Prescribing Habits	Very Important in Influencing My Prescribing Habits
Drug ads	68%	4%
Detail men	54%	20%
Patient preferences	74%	2%
Academic sources	4%	62%
Advice from colleagues	12%	48%
Practitioner's own training and clinical experiences	1%	88%

References, when presented, are misleading. Wade, Mansfield, and McDonald (1989) wrote to 10 international pharmaceutical companies and asked them to supply their best evidence in support of marketing claims for 17 products. They received 15 replies citing a total of 67 references. Only 31 supplied relevant original data, and 17 of those were proceedings of symposia, either unpublished or published in nonreviewed supplements. Only 13 of the 31 studies were controlled and all had one or more serious methodological flaws.

But the ads work. One expert claimed that promotional dinners result in a marked increase in the sales curve about 80% of the time ("AMA, Pharmaceutical Association," 1991, pp. 2304-2305). Avorn, Chen, and Hartley (1982) asked a random sample of physicians in the greater Boston area how much advertising affects their prescribing habits; the results are presented in Table 6.1. He also studied their attitudes toward two drugs shown by controlled studies to be at best minimally better than nonprescription alternatives. Although scientific support was lacking, the manufacturers had heavily promoted the drugs as being effective. And despite what physicians claimed about the minimal influence of advertisements, 49% of them believed that the heavily promoted propoxyphene (Darvon) is more effective than aspirin against pain; 71% believed that reduced cerebral blood flow (for which heavily promoted drugs were available) is a cause of senile dementia.

Drug ads have several insidious effects. They are a major source of revenue to medical journals, leading to the charge that drug manufacturers influence medical policy. Challem (1979) wrote that journals are reluctant to publish articles on vitamin therapy for mental illness, because unpatentable vitamins are not big profit-makers. Articles on effectiveness of vitamins would be antagonistic to the interests of the industry.

The ads lead to poor prescribing. Biron (1973) reported that 55% of physicians who prescribed a particular drug combination and 44% who prescribed a second, could not name the active ingredients. During 1973, Bendectin was promoted as a drug for curing nausea and vomiting during pregnancy, even though none of its components had been proven effective. An older, effective drug was available at one fourth the cost, yet three fourths of prescriptions were for Bendectin (Subcommittee on Health, 1974).

The ads lead to overprescribing. In the United States, about two thirds of physician visits lead to prescription of a drug; and U.S. patients receive about four times more medication than patients with the same complaint in Scotland. Almost two thirds of antibiotic prescriptions in hospitals are unnecessary or for the wrong dose (Health and Public Policy Committee, 1988). Advertisers encourage physicians to extend drug use into inappropriate areas, a practice that FDA commissioner David Kessler wants stopped (Kessler, 1991).

Drug companies aim about 75% of their promotion efforts at physicians, but they don't neglect other health professionals. They try to influence pharmacists, nurses, and hospital administrators who pick the drugs used within the hospital.

Promotions Directed at Laypeople

Drug companies promote alcohol, tobacco, and over-the-counter drugs. The tobacco industry is the eighth largest source of magazine advertising revenue in the United States (*Advertising Age* magazine, cited in the *Oakland Tribune*, January 30, 1992). Warner, Goldenhar, and McLaughlin (1992) found that magazines, especially women's magazines, that make the most money from cigarette advertising are least likely to report on the dangers of smoking. Television commercials encourage people to self-prescribe over-the-counter drugs but rarely mention side effects, contraindications, or the possibility that the symptoms treated may indicate a serious condition requiring competent medical help. In recent years, companies have begun advertising prescription drugs like the hair restorer minoxidil (Rogaine). The August 11, 1991 *Parade Magazine* had an advertisement for the antihypertensive drug atenolol; people taking atenolol could send in a coupon to receive free books, a free sample of coffee, and discounts on health-related products, frozen dessert, compact discs, and film. One result of such promotions is that nearly one third of prescriptions for new products are written at the request of patients ("Miracle Drugs or Media Drugs?" 1992). A professor of medicine was quoted in *Time* ("Just What the Patient Ordered," 1990): "There is no question that certain physicians are being influenced to issue prescriptions that they would not otherwise write."

The authors of a two-part *Consumer Reports* article ("Miracle Drugs or Media Drugs?" 1992; "Pushing Drugs to Doctors," 1992) described several unethical promotional tactics of drug companies:

- The companies offer to pay freelance writers to develop stories on their products and place them in national magazines—without telling the magazine's editors about the arrangement.
- The companies threaten to withhold advertising if a magazine publishes articles unfavorable to its products.
- The companies pay substantial fees to attractive, articulate physicians to act as spokespeople for new products. The physicians are taught to handle hostile questions and charm the media. Then they are booked as medical experts on talk shows, with no disclosure of their financial ties with the company.
- Celebrities are enlisted who pretend to campaign for a disease rather than a specific product. For example, former star football running back Earl Campbell toured the country telling medical groups, consumer organizations, newspapers, and radio and television audiences that panic disorder is treatable. The Upjohn Company paid him and claimed that the campaign was solely educational. But Upjohn marketed the only drug approved for treating panic disorder.

▧ A Quixotic Alternative

Fresle (1992) reported that, several years ago, a WHO (World Health Organization) committee of experts developed a list of drugs needed to ensure a reasonable degree of health care for as many people as possible. The list, periodically updated and expanded to incorporate new discoveries, now includes about 270 entries of proven safety, efficacy, and well-understood therapeutic qualities. Most are no longer protected by patent so could be produced inexpensively. Although advocating such a system for the United States is quixotic, the advantages to public health of a limited drug list far outweigh the disadvantages. A limited list would be more economical, cause fewer mistakes, and make for easier ordering, storing, and distributing. Physicians, pharmacists, and patients would all be more likely to remember both therapeutic and adverse effects.

Summary

Several strategies are available for developing new drugs:

1. Compounds are tailored to act on the biochemical pathways that are affected by a disease.
2. Active metabolites of drugs become starting points for molecular modifications leading to better ones.
3. Plants used by people in other cultures are studied.
4. Compounds made by microorganisms are studied.
5. The structure of a known drug is systematically modified.
6. Prodrugs are created from active drugs.
7. Side effects of known drugs may have therapeutic potential.
8. Interesting effects are observed by chance.

Screening tests include both in vitro and live animal testing. In vitro tests are usually inexpensive and easy. Animal tests provide pharmacokinetic and other crucial data. Although animal screening tests are crucial, they are considerably less than 100% accurate in predicting how drugs act in humans. It is likely that tests underpredict carcinogenic potential of drugs.

Before a drug is released for general medical use, it must pass the animal screen, then be tested for toxicity on human volunteers, and then demonstrate safety and efficacy in controlled human studies. The latter two phases create serious problems, both scientifically and ethically.

Concerns have been raised about the underrepresentation of certain groups in drug testing, the insufficient research on diseases that strike only small numbers of people, and the length of the drug testing process.

Pharmaceutical companies are in business to make money. Many have attempted to increase profits inappropriately, by one of three broad strategies:

1. They have not collected or have falsified data, thus cutting laboratory costs.
2. They charge excessively high prices.

3. They take advantage of the impossible task that physicians face in trying to keep up with the medical literature. The drug companies advertise, offer financial inducements, and present misleading information about their products.

Mini-Quiz: New Drugs

Related drugs are called _____.

congeners

Inert substances that are converted within the body into parent drugs are called _____.

prodrugs

In vitro tests are conducted in _____.

test tubes

Which animal species is usually the first used in testing a new drug?

mice

T/F: Thalidomide was released for sale without first being screened on animals.

false (but rats and mice aren't affected by it and humans are)

Substances that increase the likelihood that offspring will be born malformed are called _____.

teratogens

Animals are given the opportunity to self-administer drugs in order to test the drug's _____ in humans.

abuse potential

In the technique known as _____, animals must respond differently to different drug states.

drug discrimination

T/F: Animal tests are more likely to miss a human carcinogen than to give a false positive.

true

Who are the subjects in each phase of new drug testing with humans?

Phase 1: a small number of healthy volunteers

Phase 2: a few hundred sick people receive drug while matched controls receive placebo

Phase 3: thousands of people in settings like those that will be used if the drug is approved

Why does the use of volunteers in drug testing raise concerns about the validity of the findings?

volunteers often differ from nonvolunteers in important ways

Drugs used to treat rare diseases are called _____ drugs.

orphan

Name the three ways listed in the text by which drug companies have tried to increase profits.

cut lab costs; charge high prices; expand the market

Drug company employees who visit physicians with free samples are called _____.

detail men

Critics of current practices have charged that medical journals are reluctant to publish articles on vitamin therapy because _____.

vitamins can't be patented so have limited potential as profit-makers

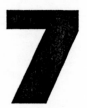
By the time you finish reading this chapter, you should be able to answer the following questions:

Why is the question, "Is drug X dangerous?" not a very good one?

What is a therapeutic window?

Why is it important to distinguish between experimental and correlational studies?

Why must results from case studies be interpreted cautiously?

What special dangers affect people who inject (smoke) drugs?

Why does Leavitt believe that the dangers of both physical and psychological dependence are overrated?

Which of the following drugs cause physical dependence: alcohol, cocaine, heroin, LSD, marijuana, nicotine?

What is one beneficial effect of alcohol (cocaine, heroin, LSD, marijuana, nicotine)?

On the average, who lives longest: abstainers from alcohol, moderate drinkers, heavy drinkers?

Chronic, high dose use of which drug leads to a state almost indistinguishable from paranoid schizophrenia?

Who would be more likely to benefit from caffeine—an asthmatic or a person with a heart problem?

Which drug did polydrug abusers rate as the one they could least do without?

Pharmacological Dangers and Benefits of Psychoactive Drugs

Contents

When we absorb a new drug, entirely different in composition, it is always with a delicious expectancy of the unknown. Our heart beats as at a first assignation. To what unknown forms of sleep, of dreams, is the newcomer going to lead us? He is inside us now, he has the control of our thoughts. In what fashion are we going to fall asleep? And, once we are asleep, by what strange paths, up to what peaks, into what unfathomed gulfs is he going to lead us? With what new grouping of sensations are we to become acquainted on this journey? Will it bring us in the end to illness? To blissful happiness? To death?

Marcel Proust—*Remembrance of Things Past*

In light of the terrible harms caused by many psychoactive drugs, discussion of their beneficial effects may seem frivolous. But by 1991, an estimated 75.4 million Americans age 12 and older had used illicit drugs (NIDA, National Household Survey, 1991), and millions more use legal substances like caffeine, tobacco, and alcohol. Let's hope that not all are irrational or suicidal. The benefits from illicit drugs often parallel those from licit ones. Both morphine and antianxiety drugs make harsh environments more bearable, and both cocaine and antidepressants at least temporarily relieve depression. Refusal to acknowledge anticipated benefits sabotages strategies designed to prevent and treat harms, partly by making assessment of the harms less clear. Except by examining reasons for use, how could judgment be made on dangers of the following?

1. Strychnine, a deadly poison that improves memory when taken in very small doses.
2. The essential nutrients Vitamins A and B-1, which in large doses cause toxic and even fatal reactions.
3. Methotrexate, used to treat acute leukemias but with many toxic effects. The margin between therapeutic and toxic doses is smaller for methotrexate than strychnine.
4. Aspirin, which upsets the stomach and causes ringing in the ears of many users.

The strychnine and vitamin examples point to the importance of dose. All substances are dangerous at sufficiently high doses, and doses exist below which virtually all substances are safe. The fact that some people are harmed by excessive use of a drug is not by itself reason to call the drug dangerous.

Evaluating benefits is simple for drugs like methotrexate, much less so when the user's intent is to enhance creativity, memory, or sexual or other pleasures; promote religious experiences; relieve pain, stress, or anger; satisfy curiosity. Many people, believing that drug-induced enhancements of normal functioning are unacceptable, refuse to count any of the foregoing as benefits. Yet, on medical grounds alone, stress relief is valuable. A substantial scientific literature shows that psychological stress increases the risk of a variety of illnesses (cf. Cohen, Tyrrell,

& Smith, 1991; Stone et al., 1987; Young, Richter, Bradley, & Anderson, 1987). Inadequate relief of physical pain increases the morbidity of hospitalized patients (Camp, 1991); and psychological pain, which can be relieved temporarily by a variety of drugs, probably also increases morbidity.

Determining the likelihood that a drug will produce harm is even more problematic. Estimates of frequency and patterns of use are probably not very accurate, especially for illicit drugs; and many users who experience adverse effects probably don't report them. But figures on major adverse outcomes can probably be trusted. Table 7.1 gives information from the Drug Abuse Warning Network (DAWN) on drug mentions in emergency rooms in 21 U.S. metropolitan areas and a national panel of emergency rooms over a recent 3-year period. Table 7.2 lists the most frequently mentioned drugs over a 6-month period. Tables 7.3 and 7.4 present selected medical examiner (coroner) data from 27 metropolitan areas. Figure 7.1 gives nationwide estimates of deaths and includes those attributed to tobacco.

Adverse effects originate in a variety of ways:

- Sometimes, beneficial and adverse effects occur at similar doses, that is, a drug produces **side effects.** Amphetamine given to control appetite increases blood pressure and causes insomnia.
- All drugs have a **therapeutic window**—a range between the therapeutic and toxic doses. Because people vary, doses within one person's therapeutic window may be toxic to another.
- Extremely potent drugs may be dangerous despite having a wide therapeutic window. For example, the recreational dose of LSD is about 50 to 100 micrograms. The small spice tins sold in supermarkets hold one ounce (about 28 million micrograms); so a spice tin can hold enough LSD for 280,000 100-microgram trips. Sensitive equipment and great care are required to discriminate 100 from 1,000 micrograms; and an LSD overdose is more serious than an overdose of oregano.
- Many drugs, safe when taken by themselves, interact adversely with other drugs or foods.
- Certain drugs, such as penicillin, produce serious **hypersensitivity reactions** in some users.
- Some drugs, such as tobacco, produce few or no **acute** adverse effects in experienced users but great harm when taken chronically.
- Many drugs taken during pregnancy affect the developing fetus. These will be discussed in Chapter 8.

(text continued on page 127)

Table 7.1 Total DAWN System—Emergency Room Data Trends in Number of Drug Mentions in Emergency Room Episodes by Selected Drug Category: January 1987-December 1989

Drug Groups: Therapeutic Class by Drug Category (Examples of commonly encountered brands are provided if applicable)	January-June 1987	July-December 1987	January-June 1988	July-December 1988	January-June 1989	July-December 1989
TRANQUILIZERS						
Diazepam (Valium)	2,659	2,446	2,271	2,120	1,848	1,571
Alprazolam (Xanax)	1,294	1,221	1,302	1,305	1,250	1,195
Chlordiazepoxide (Librium)	451	391	381	357	314	289
Clorazepate (Tranxene)	205	180	160	145	150	121
Lorazepam (Ativan)	507	490	436	486	485	583
Meprobamate (Equanil, Miltown)	93	90	71	70	53	48
NARCOTIC ANALGESICS						
Heroin/Morphine	7,062	8,021	7,968	8,744	8,543	8,440
d-Propoxyphene (Darvon, Darvocet N)	543	521	531	506	475	464
Methadone	838	767	709	700	676	628
Oxycodone (Percodan, Percocet 5)	394	351	407	388	386	293
Codeine	405	409	330	313	270	234
Meperidine HCl (Demerol)	151	113	86	100	98	101
Hydromorphone (Dilaudid)	172	190	136	132	116	105
NON-NARCOTIC ANALGESICS						
Aspirin	1,954	1,748	1,877	1,889	1,901	1,604
Acetaminophen (Tylenol)	2,213	2,062	2,097	2,206	2,383	2,157
Pentazocine (Talwin)	175	121	74	74	44	72
Butalbital combinations (Fiorinal)	287	277	275	248	259	219

NONBARBITURATE SEDATIVES						
Methaqualone (Quaalude)	84	72	50	76	50	67
Flurazepam (Dalmane)	419	325	316	282	264	227
O.T.C. sleep aids (Sominex, Nytol, Sleep-eze)	607	569	612	652	641	582
Ethchlorvynol (Placidyl)	116	100	83	71	63	50
Glutethimide (Doriden)	220	225	180	142	89	46
Chloral hydrate (Noctec)	52	37	48	47	36	27
ANTIDEPRESSANTS						
Amitriptyline (Elavil)	824	705	674	679	662	546
Amitrip. combination (Triavil, Limbitrol, Etrafon)	183	172	158	135	121	84
Doxepin (Sinequan, Adapin)	381	337	321	285	292	255
Fluoxetine (Prozac)	N/A	N/A	37	150	246	339
Imipramine (Tofranil)	320	273	312	272	290	239
Desipramine (Norpramin)	175	169	162	167	197	169
Nortriptyline (Pamelor, Aventyl HCl)	119	125	161	172	193	174
ANTIPSYCHOTICS						
Chlorpromazine (Thorazine)	255	265	243	224	220	236
Thioridazine (Mellaril)	306	263	240	244	240	237
Haloperidol (Haldol)	425	356	420	369	379	407
Trifluoperazine (Stelazine)	140	108	96	133	106	108
BARBITURATE SEDATIVES						
Phenobarbital	473	481	449	445	391	364
Secobarbital/Amobarbital (Tuinal)	59	55	41	46	26	19
Secobarbital (Seconal)	86	61	47	57	54	24
Amobarbital (Amytal)	14	2	10	7	3	3
Pentobarbital (Nembutal)	37	28	29	22	22	6
AMPHETAMINES						
Amphetamine	442	433	532	476	388	354

(continued)

Table 7.1 Continued

Drug Groups: Therapeutic Class by Drug Category (Examples of commonly encountered brands are provided if applicable)	January-June 1987	July-December 1987	January-June 1988	July-December 1988	January-June 1989	July-December 1989
Methamphetamine/Speed (Desoxyn, Methedrine HCl)	1,059	1,031	1,146	1,311	1,175	990
HALLUCINOGENS						
PCP/PCP combinations	3,552	4,317	3,530	3,105	2,294	1,483
LSD	457	505	450	423	440	478
OTHER DRUG CLASSES						
Alcohol-in-combination	13,763	15,198	16,309	17,860	17,933	16,761
Cocaine	14,604	19,284	21,599	24,098	24,286	21,398
Marijuana/Hashish	3,120	3,536	3,792	3,584	3,584	3,154
Diphenylhydantoin sodium (Dilantin)	523	534	627	525	484	424
Diphenhydramine (Benadryl)	570	522	563	569	574	582
O.T.C. diet aids (Dexatrim)	170	146	154	129	141	130
ALL OTHER DRUGS	10,806	9,927	10,734	10,369	10,536	9,757
DRUG UNKNOWN	5,719	6,598	7,386	7,321	6,937	6,199
Total drug mentions	79,483	86,157	90,622	94,230	92,608	84,043
Number of episodes	50,790	55,376	58,288	60,763	60,086	54,012

SOURCE: NIDA, Drug Abuse Warning Network (March 1990 imputed data file).

Table 7.2 Weighted Emergency Room Estimates. Drugs mentioned most frequently by emergency rooms in 1990 (Drugs with fewer than 200 weighted mentions are excluded)

Rank	Drug Name	Number of Mentions	Percentage of Total Episodes	Rank	Drug Name	Number of Mentions	Percentage of Total Episodes
1.	Alcohol-in combination	115,162	31.02	26.	Phenobarbital	3,668	0.99
2.	Cocaine	80,355	21.65	27.	Doxepin	3,457	0.93
3.	Heroin/Morphine	33,884	9.13	28.	Cyclobenzaprine	3,453	0.93
4.	Acetaminophen	25,422	6.85	29.	Haloperidol	3,415	0.92
5.	Aspirin	19,188	5.17	30.	Amphetamine	3,362	0.91
6.	Ibuprofen	16,299	4.39	31.	Naproxen	3,210	0.86
7.	Alprazolam	15,846	4.27	32.	Unspecified Benzodiazepine	3,165	0.85
8.	Marijuana/Hashish	15,706	4.23	33.	Flurazepam	3,064	0.82
9.	Diazepam	14,836	4.00	34.	Carbamazepine	3,061	0.82
10.	Amitriptyline	8,642	2.33	35.	Trazodone	3,003	0.81
11.	Acetaminophen W Codeine	8,222	2.21	36.	Imipramine	2,871	0.77
12.	O.T.C. Sleep Aids	7,984	2.15	37.	Erythromycin	2,836	0.76
13.	Lorazepam	7,625	2.05	38.	Theophylline	2,660	0.72
14.	D-Propoxyphene	7,417	2.00	39.	Carisoprodol	2,643	0.71
15.	Fluoxetine	6,917	1.86	40.	Methadone	2,617	0.70
16.	Diphenhydramine	6,483	1.75	41.	Temazepam	2,595	0.70
17.	Methamphetamine/Speed	5,236	1.41	42.	Butalbital Combinations	2,573	0.69
18.	Oxycodone	4,526	1.22	43.	Chlordiazepoxide	2,398	0.65
19.	PCP/PCP Combinations	4,408	1.19	44.	Caffeine	2,370	0.64
20.	Lithium Carbonate	4,402	1.19	45.	Chlorpromazine	2,311	0.62
21.	Clonazepam	4,335	1.17	46.	Nortriptyline	2,272	0.61
22.	Hydantoin	4,026	1.08	47.	Thioridazine	2,251	0.61
23.	Hydrocodone	3,921	1.06	48.	Hydroxyzine	2,182	0.59
24.	LSD	3,869	1.04	49.	Pseudoephedrine	2,133	0.57
25.	Triazolam	3,801	1.02				

Table 7.2 Continued

Rank	Drug Name	Number of Mentions	Percentage of Total Episodes	Rank	Drug Name	Number of Mentions	Percentage of Total Episodes
50.	Codeine	2,037	0.55	96.	Phenylpro/Bromph/Phenyle	480	0.13
51.	Benztropine	1,962	0.53	97.	Phenylpropanolamine	478	0.13
52.	Clorazepate	1,876	0.50	98.	Promethazine	473	0.13
53.	Propanolol HCl	1,779	0.48	99.	Meclizine	470	0.13
54.	Desipramine	1,648	0.44	100.	Sulindac	466	0.13
55.	Amoxicillin	1,582	0.43	101.	Penicillin V Potassium	463	0.13
56.	Cimetidine	1,515	0.41	102.	Secobarbital	448	0.12
57.	Amitriptyline Combinations	1,498	0.40	103.	Prochlorperazine	446	0.12
58.	Metoprolol	1,418	0.38	104.	Pseudoephed/Dexbromphen	435	0.12
59.	Thiothixene	1,352	0.36	105.	Chlorpheniramine	434	0.12
60.	Meperidine HCl	1,335	0.36	106.	Hydrochlorothiazide	425	0.11
60.	O.T.C Diet Aids	1,335	0.36	107.	Prednisone	417	0.11
62.	Trifluoperazine	1,311	0.35	108.	Amantadine HCl	416	0.11
63.	Brompheniramine Maleate	1,247	0.34	109.	Disulfiram	386	0.10
64.	Tetracycline HCl	1,217	0.33	110.	Dimenhydrinate	381	0.10
65.	Perphenazine	1,214	0.33	111.	Ferrous Sulfate	376	0.10
66.	Pseudoephed/Triprolidine	1,195	0.32	112.	Household/Commercial Subs	364	0.10
67.	Chlorzoxazone/Acetamin	1,091	0.29	113.	Ethchlorvynol	363	0.10
68.	Insulin	1,090	0.29	113.	Phenazopyridine	363	0.10
69.	Fluphenazine HCl	1,068	0.29	115.	Clomipramine	346	0.09
70.	Penicillin G Potassium	1,058	0.28	115.	Clonidine HCl	346	0.09
71.	Butabarbital Combination	993	0.27	117.	Trihexyphenidyl HCl	329	0.09
72.	Ampicillin	954	0.26	118.	Clidinium Brom/Chlordiaz	328	0.09
73.	Methocarbamol	935	0.25	119.	Meperidine Combination	320	0.09
74.	Trimethoprim/Sulfamethox	921	0.25				
75.	Ephedrine	907	0.24				
76.	Cephalexin	838	0.23				

	Drug	Estimate	Percent
77.	Hydromorphone	718	0.19
78.	Digoxin	683	0.18
79.	Indomethacin	673	0.18
80.	Meprobamate	667	0.18
81.	Methaqualone	639	0.17
82.	Pentazocine	628	0.17
83.	Phenylpro/Chlorphen Mal	623	0.17
84.	Triamterene	614	0.16
85.	Metronidazole	598	0.16
86.	Levothyroxine Sod	592	0.16
87.	Loxapine	585	0.16
88.	Furosemide	576	0.15
89.	Doxycycline	562	0.15
90.	Guaifenesin	545	0.15
91.	Atrop/Scopo/Hyoscy/Pheno	531	0.14
92.	Oxazepam	515	0.14
93.	Mushrooms	495	0.13
94.	Tolmetin Sodium	492	0.13
95.	Prazepam	481	0.13
120.	Glutethimide	315	0.08
121.	Nitroglycerin	282	0.08
121.	Phenelzine	282	0.08
123.	Metoclopramide	281	0.08
124.	Chloral Hydrate	274	0.07
125.	Methylphenidate	271	0.07
126.	Butalbital	263	0.07
127.	Nitrofurantoin	262	0.07
128.	Diphenoxylate/Atropine	250	0.07
129.	Amoxapine	247	0.07
130.	Carisoprod/Phenacet/Caff	245	0.07
131.	Phenylpro/Chlorphen/Aspi	242	0.06
132.	Phenylpro/Phenyltol/Acet	237	0.06
133.	Dicyclomine	236	0.06
134.	Phenylpro/Chlorph/Isopro	207	0.06
135.	Terbutaline	205	0.05
136.	Maprotiline	204	0.05
137.	Quinine	203	0.05
138.	Chlorzoxazone	202	0.05

SOURCE: NIDA, Drug Abuse Warning Network (May 1991 data file).
NOTE: These estimates are based on a representative sample of non-federal short-stay hospitals with 24-hour emergency rooms in the coterminous United States.

Table 7.3 Drugs Mentioned Most Frequently by Medical Examiners in 1990 (Drugs with less than 10 mentions are excluded)

Drug Name	Number of Mentions	Percentage of Total Episodes	Drug Name	Number of Mentions	Percentage of Total Episodes
1. Cocaine	2,483	42.59	36. Temazepam	42	0.72
2. Alcohol-in-combination	2,304	39.52	37. Chlorpheniramine	41	0.70
3. Heroin/Morphine[a]	1,976	33.89	38. Chlorpromazine	39	0.67
4. Codeine	682	11.70	39. Meperidine HCL	35	0.60
5. Diazepam	502	8.61	40. Theophylline	34	0.58
6. Methadone	421	7.22	41. Carbamazepine	31	0.53
7. Amitriptyline	393	6.74	41. Glutethimide	31	0.53
8. Nortriptyline	327	5.61	43. Mesoridazine	27	0.46
9. D-Propoxyphene	258	4.43	44. Carisoprodol	26	0.45
10. Diphenhydramine	224	3.84	45. Ethchlorvynol	25	0.43
11. Acetaminophen	209	3.58	45. Oxycodone	25	0.43
12. Marijuana/Hashish	209	3.58	45. Trazodone	25	0.43
13. Methamphetamine/Speed	197	3.38	48. Lithium Carbonate	24	0.41
14. Lidocaine	156	2.68	48. Oxazepam	24	0.41
15. Desipramine	143	2.45	50. Triazolam	23	0.39
15. Doxepin	143	2.45	51. Amobarbital	22	0.38
17. Unspecified Benzodiazepine	138	2.37	51. Dextromethorphan	22	0.38
18. PCP/PCP Combinations	128	2.20	53. Benztropine	21	0.36
19. Phenobarbital	127	2.18	53. Pentobarbital	21	0.36
20. Amphetamine	111	1.90	55. Amoxapine	20	0.34
20. Aspirin	111	1.90	55. Haloperidol	20	0.34
22. Chlordiazepoxide	105	1.80	57. Hydroxyzine	19	0.33
			57. Phenylpropanolamine	19	0.33

23.	Fluoxetine	103	1.77		
24.	Imipramine	90	1.54		
25.	Alprazolam	74	1.27		
26.	Hydantoin	65	1.11		
27.	Quinine	64	1.10		
28.	Thioridazine	63	1.08		
29.	Secobarbital	62	1.06		
30.	Flurazepam	60	1.03		
31.	Butalbital	57	0.98		
32.	Caffeine	54	0.93		
33.	Meprobamate	52	0.89		
34.	Hydrocodone	45	0.77		
35.	Doxylamine Succinate	44	0.75		

59.	Cyclobenzaprine	18	0.31
59.	Ephedrine	18	0.31
61.	Promethazine	16	0.27
61.	Pseudoephedrine	16	0.27
63.	Lorazepam	15	0.26
64.	Hydromorphone	14	0.24
64.	Propanolol HCL	14	0.24
66.	Ibuprofen	13	0.22
67.	Digoxin	12	0.21
67.	Oxymorphones	12	0.21
69.	Pyrimethamine	11	0.19
70.	Alcohol substitutes	10	0.17

SOURCE: NIDA, Drug Abuse Warning Network (May 1991 data file).

NOTES: a. Includes opiates not specified as to type.

In using this table the reader should be aware that individual drugs are frequently mentioned in combination with other drugs and that the population at risk of an adverse consequence relating to the abuse of any particular drug is unknown, i.e, the number of people abusing a particular substance, either alone or in any combination, is unknown. Thus the relative frequency of mentions of any drug pertains only to the DAWN system and not to the larger population at risk.

Table 7.4 Medical Examiner Data. Two-way drug combinations mentioned most frequently in drug abuse deaths: 1991 (Based on episodes involving two or more drugs)

Frequency	Drug Combination	Heroin/ Morphine	Cocaine	Codeine	Amitriptyline
		Drug Involvement Key			
1,005	Alcohol-in-combination - Cocaine		x		
884	Alcohol-in-combination - Heroin/morphine	x			
726	Cocaine - Heroin/morphine	x	x		
506	Codeine - Heroin/morphine	x		x	
249	Alcohol-in-combination - Codeine			x	
246	Amitriptyline - Nortriptyline				x
200	Cocaine - Codeine		x	x	
172	Cocaine - Methadone		x		
157	Alcohol-in-combination - Diazepam				
128	Diazepam - Heroin/morphine	x			
120	Alcohol-in-combination - Methadone				
116	Alcohol-in-combination - Amitriptyline				x
111	Heroin/morphine - Methadone	x			
103	Cocaine - Diazepam		x		
100	Alcohol-in-combination - Marijuana/hashish				
97	Alcohol-in-combination - Nortriptyline				
89	Diazepam - Methadone				
88	Amphetamine - Methamphetamine/speed				
81	Cocaine - Lidocaine		x		
75	Alcohol-in-combination - d-Propoxyphene				
73	Codeine - Diazepam			x	
71	Alcohol-in-combination - Diphenhydramine				
69	Amitriptyline - Cocaine		x		x
64	Diazepam - Unspecified Benzodiazepine				

Count	Drug A		Drug B				
58	Desipramine	-	Imipramine				
58	Amitriptyline	-	Methadone	x			
58	Cocaine	-	Nortriptyline			x	
58	Acetaminophen	-	Alcohol-in-combination				
58	Alcohol-in-combination	-	Doxepin		x		
57	Amitriptyline	-	Heroin/morphine				x
56	Alcohol-in-combination	-	PCP/PCP combinations				
55	Heroin/morphine	-	Lidocaine				x
55	Diphenhydramine	-	Heroin/morphine				x
53	Amitriptyline	-	Diazepam				x
53	Heroin/morphine	-	Nortriptyline	x			
52	Acetaminophen	-	d-Propoxyphene				
52	Methadone	-	Nortriptyline				
52	Alcohol-in-combination	-	Methamphetamine/speed				x
51	Acetaminophen	-	Heroin/morphine				x
51	Acetaminophen	-	Codeine				x
50	Heroin/morphine	-	Quinine				x
48	d-Propoxyphene	-	Diazepam				
47	Cocaine	-	Marijuana/hashish			x	
47	Alcohol-in-combination	-	Chlordiazepoxide			x	
45	Cocaine	-	Diphenhydramine			x	
43	Heroin/morphine	-	Methamphetamine/speed				x
43	Alcohol-in-combination	-	Unspecified Benzodiazepine				
41	Amitriptyline	-	Codeine	x	x		
40	Diazepam	-	Nortriptyline				
38	Alcohol-in-combination	-	Desipramine				
37	Cocaine	-	PCP/PCP combinations			x	
37	Alcohol-in-combination	-	Lidocaine				
36	Heroin/morphine	-	PCP/PCP combinations				x
36	d-Propoxyphene	-	Heroin/morphine				x

(Continued)

125

Table 7.4 Continued

Frequency	Drug Combination	Heroin/ Morphine	Cocaine	Codeine	Amitriptyline
		Drug Involvement Key			
36	Alcohol-in-combination - Phenobarbital				
35	Chlordiazepoxide - Diazepam				
35	Acetaminophen - Diazepam				
34	Cocaine - d-Propoxyphene		x		
33	Cocaine - Methamphetamine/speed		x		
32	Acetaminophen - Cocaine		x		
32	Codeine - d-Propoxyphene			x	
30	Amitriptyline - d-Propoxyphene				x
30	Codeine - Methadone			x	
30	Heroin/morphine - Unspecified Benzodiazepine	x			
30	Alcohol-in-combination - Imipramine				
29	Codeine - Glutethimide			x	
29	Alcohol-in-combination - Quinine				
27	Diazepam - Diphenhydramine				
27	Alcohol-in-combination - Aspirin				
27	Alcohol-in-combination - Alprazolam				
25	Mesoridazine - Thioridazine				

SOURCE: NIDA, Drug Abuse Warning Network (May 1991 data file).
NOTES: These estimates are based on a representative sample of nonfederal short-stay hospitals with 24-hour emergency rooms in the coterminous United States.
Drug abuse episodes involving more than two mentions contribute multiple pairs to the data in this table. Three-drug episodes generate three paired entries; four-drug episodes, six entries. For example, an episode in which cocaine, heroin, and alcohol are mentioned results in three entries: alcohol-cocaine, alcohol-heroin, and cocaine-heroin. Within pairs, drugs are listed alphabetically.
It should be noted that the benzodiazepine category includes benzodiazepines other than alprazolam, bromazepam, chlordiazepoxide, clonazepam, clorazepate, diazepam, flurazepam, lorazepam, nitrazepam, oxazepam, prazepam, triazolam, and temazepam.
Mentions of heroin/morphine include opiates not specified as to type.
Excludes cases in which AIDS was reported.

126

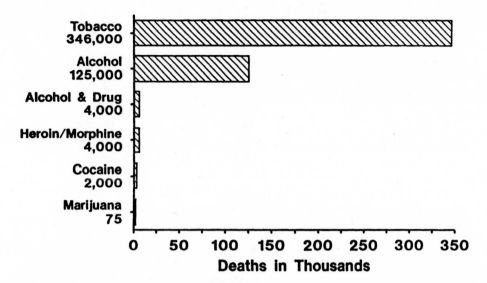

Figure 7.1. Estimated Annual U.S. Deaths From Various Drugs
SOURCE: Crowley (1988).

░ Evaluating Evidence on the Dangers of Drugs

EXPERIMENTAL VERSUS CORRELATIONAL STUDIES

Consider a hypothetical research project in which 50 volunteers are given caffeine pills and 50 are given placebos. While waiting for the caffeine to take effect, the researcher asks the subjects about their smoking patterns. Half of the people in each group are nonsmokers and half smoke exactly one pack per day. (Hypothetical data are great to work with.) The people are asked to lift weights, with the results shown in Table 7.5.

Comparing groups 1 and 2 with 3 and 4 gives the difference between caffeine and placebo, independent of subjects' smoking habits. Comparing 1 and 3 with 2 and 4 gives the difference between smokers and nonsmokers, independent of caffeine.

Question 1. Assuming that the study was well done (another virtue of hypothetical research) and the data are statistically significant, what conclusions can be drawn? My answers to this and the two questions below are on pp. 148-150.

Table 7.5 Results of a Hypothetical Research Project

Group	Maximum Weight Lifted (lbs)
1. caffeine/smoker	100
2. caffeine/nonsmoker	80
3. placebo/smoker	80
4. placebo/nonsmoker	60

The November 4, 1985 edition of the *Oakland Tribune* carried a story under the headline, "Study Shows Major Role of Alcohol in Crimes."

More than half of jail inmates convicted of violent crimes had been drinking before committing the offenses, the government said yesterday in a grim study of alcohol's role in fueling crimes of passion. . . . While there has been much publicity in recent years about the problem of drunk driving, the study released yesterday provided a new insight into the impact alcohol has on a wide range of other crimes. Nearly 7 out of 10 people convicted of manslaughter—68%—had been drinking before the offense, while 62% of those convicted of assault had been drinking. The survey found that 49% of those convicted of murder or attempted murder had been drinking. The findings were based on personal interviews.

Question 2. Is it reasonable to assume that the data are accurate?

Question 3. If they are accurate, what do they mean?

The questions illustrate a major difficulty in assessing dangers of drugs. Only results from carefully controlled experiments justify statements such as "Drug X causes symptom Y." Nonexperimental comparisons between users and nonusers are misleading, because the two groups differed before they ever tried a drug. It is a logical necessity. Unless some factor(s) had been differentially operative, either everybody or nobody would use. Those factors, rather than the drug, might account for other differences between users and nonusers. Consider two real examples.

1. Eysenck (1977) reported that **extroverts** are more likely than **introverts** to both develop cancer and smoke tobacco. He argued that extroversion, rather than smoking, may be an important factor in the development of cancer. (Eysenck's criticism, although valid, should not dissuade smokers

from quitting. Converging evidence from many sources clearly demonstrates the detrimental health consequences of smoking—see p. 147.)

2. Concerned about evidence linking coffee drinking to coronary heart disease, Puccio, McPhillips, Barrett-Connor, and Geniats (1990) asked people about their caffeine consumption and other habits. Drinkers of caffeinated coffee were more likely than nondrinkers to smoke tobacco, and they drank more alcohol, had more saturated fats and cholesterol in their diets, and exercised less. Any of those factors, rather than the caffeine, might have accounted for health differences between coffee and non-coffee drinkers.

Correlational research is often an important first step in establishing causal connections. The correlation between smoking and lung cancer suggests one of three possibilities: (a) smoking causes cancer; (b) cancer causes people to smoke; or (c) some other factor(s) causes both smoking and cancer. The correlation cannot conclusively prove the first hypothesis but makes it more plausible. The ideal follow-up would be a well-controlled **experiment** on long-term drug effects of smoking on humans. Some people selected at random would be required to smoke a specified number of cigarettes per day, others to refrain from smoking. Volunteers would be hard to find.

Experiments can be conducted on nonhuman animals. Among the advantages are that animals such as rats and mice are inexpensive to buy and maintain, have known histories, can be placed in fully controlled environments, and raise fewer ethical concerns. Many of the findings discussed in this book are on nonhumans. But all species have unique patterns of response to drugs, so results from experiments with nonhumans do not conclusively establish effects on humans.

CASE STUDIES

Kolansky and Moore (1971) published a highly influential paper in which they cited 38 cases showing that, "moderate to heavy use of marijuana in adolescents and young people without predisposition to psychotic illness may lead to ego decompensation ranging from mild ego disturbance to psychosis." Two years later, Altman and Evenson (1973) published a superficially similar paper. The latter pair questioned inmates arriving at mental institutions until 38 were identified who had used marijuana prior to showing psychiatric symptoms.

Table 7.6 Number of Patients Whose Psychiatric Symptoms Were
Subsequent to Use of Marijuana and Other Variables
(Total Number of Patients = 158)

Variable	Number of Patients
Marijuana	38
Growing long hair	54
Masturbation	54
Driving a car	64
Sex education	66
Sexual intercourse	76
Beer drinking	85
Dancing	94
Tobacco	107
Kissing	112
Late TV movies	123

SOURCE: From "Marijuana Use and Subsequent Psychiatric Symptoms: A Replication" by H. Altman & R. Evenson, 1973, *Comprehensive Psychiatry*, 14, pp. 415-420. Copyright 1973 by *Comprehensive Psychiatry*. Used by permission.

Altman and Evenson gave several capsule case histories of the patients, such as the following:

> CASE 3. A 15-year old white male who began using marijuana at age 12; no previous problems; always seemed very bright. Presenting complaint by patient was flashbacks, feeling nervous, afraid of losing self-control, and performing hostile acts. No family history of mental illness.

The second study seemed to confirm the first, and most of the psychiatric residents taught by Altman and Evenson initially thought so. But Altman and Evenson had questioned 158 patients before finding 38 whose marijuana use had preceded psychiatric symptoms, and all 158 were also asked whether each of 18 other events had preceded psychiatric symptoms. Table 7.6 lists 10 that elicited more positive responses than did marijuana. The psychiatric residents did not conclude that kissing causes psychosis.

Medical researchers have made many important discoveries by investigating people with unusual symptoms; but unless they follow up the case studies with experiments, statements about causes are premature—and so are weaker statements, about correlations. The reason is that case studies use only a small part of the necessary information. In the marijuana study, people could have been placed in one of four groups:

1. Users who developed symptoms.
2. Users who did not develop symptoms.
3. Nonusers who developed symptoms.
4. Nonusers who did not develop symptoms.

As long as Group 1 contains some subjects, an *apparent* case can be made for relating drug use to development of symptoms. But no matter how large the number, conclusions are unwarranted without data on the other groups. With 38 people in the first group, suppose the numbers in Groups 2, 3, and 4 were one million, one million, and zero, respectively?

BIAS IN SCIENCE

The idea that scientists dispassionately test their theories and quickly discard them if results are unfavorable—is a myth. I give two personal anecdotes to introduce the topic of bias in science.

1. Several years ago I co-taught a class entitled "Altered States of Consciousness." My colleague was an enthusiast, I a skeptic, as we evaluated various popular movements. Discussion was lively and the class, mostly true believers, listened with amused tolerance to my attempts to expose methodological flaws in works they had regarded as definitive. But they became increasingly aware of the need to analyze data properly. Then my colleague brought in a tape made by a man who claimed that plants, measured by their responses to an electroencephalograph hook-up, show emotions. The plants responded not only when he pulled off their leaves but even when he merely thought of injuring them. They were compassionate, responding strongly when he boiled shrimp in their presence or stirred up yogurt (thereby killing millions of innocent bacteria). When the tape ended, the class looked at me expectantly. I said, "As far as I can tell, the controls and statistical analysis were more sophisticated than in most published work, and the automated procedures for stimulating and recording eliminated the possibility of experimenter bias. But I don't believe any of it."

2. I invited a well-known crusader against drugs to speak to my psychopharmacology class. He had written several influential books on the subject and held a powerful position in the drug hierarchy within his state. He

gave an impassioned speech condemning marijuana, one charge being that it causes users to become apathetic toward work. That consequence alone, he argued, was sufficiently serious to justify criminal penalties against users. He had written as much in his books. At dinner that night, I questioned his data on the amotivational syndrome and said that I'd attended several parties with hard-working, occasionally renowned scientists, who had spent much of their time passing around marijuana cigarettes. His response startled me: "Fred, I realize that educated people can use it without any problems. It's the students I worry about."

Because the drug field is so emotionally charged, biases are substantial. One type of evidence comes from scientists' collected works. Unbiased observers would be expected to find adverse effects of drugs under certain circumstances and positive effects under others. But some of the most productive scientists have, regardless of topic, reported exclusively positive or exclusively negative effects.

Wesley Hall (*San Francisco Chronicle*, March 2, 1971), a former president of the American Medical Association, drew newspaper headlines by announcing that marijuana promotes birth defects and "makes a man of 35 sexually like a man of 70." He later retracted (*San Francisco Chronicle*, April 3, 1971), admitting that his statement was issued to reduce marijuana use and not based on evidence.

Bias intrudes in other ways. Research requires financing, and funding sources like the National Institute on Drug Abuse grant more money for studying adverse rather than beneficial effects of drugs. Also, reports of adverse effects are more likely to be published. Koren, Graham, Shear, and Einarson (1989) studied all abstracts submitted to one scientific journal between 1980 and 1989 on maternal cocaine use and fetal health. Of 49 reporting negative consequences, 27 (57%) were accepted; of nine reporting no adverse effects, one (11%) was accepted, even though as a group the nine were better controlled than the 49. Researchers who report adverse effects are more likely to receive repeated government funding.

▓ General Dangers of Drugs

DRIVING

In the United States, injury from accidents is the fourth leading cause of death in all age groups and the leading cause for people between the ages of 1 and 44; about half of those are due to automobile accidents ("Counseling," 1991). Many drugs impair psychomotor skills, so there is reason for concern about their effects on driving. But conclusive evidence is hard to come by. Questionnaire studies comparing violation and accident rates in users and matched controls, and measures of drug concentrations in accident victims are correlational. Laboratory experiments on drug-induced changes in visual acuity and reaction time, factors assumed to contribute to skillful driving, may have little relevance to routine driving performance. Teenaged drivers as a group have the best reaction times and visual acuity but are not the safest drivers.

Experiments with driving simulators are not equivalent to driving in real traffic. Many drugs impair ability to maintain full attention on the road during long, dull stretches of driving. But users remain capable of performing under scrutiny in the laboratory. Subjects in such experiments have generally been experienced users who probably wanted favorable drug outcomes; if they knew whether they had received drug or placebo, they would have had a chance to exert their biases. Given the above caveats, the following statements can be made.

1. In most jurisdictions, the legal limit for alcohol intoxication is a **blood alcohol concentration** (BAC) of 0.10 or greater. Fell (1987) estimated that the risk of a fatal crash, per mile driven, is about eight times higher for legally drunk drivers than sober ones; and 38% of drivers killed in traffic accidents had BACs of 0.10 or greater (National Highway Traffic Safety Administration [NHTSA], 1988). Yet survey data indicate that 6.1% of U.S. adults drive at least once a month when they've had too much to drink (Bradstock et al., 1987); and Wolfe (1986) reported that 3% of U.S. drivers randomly stopped and given a roadside breath analysis had BACs higher than .10. Since 1977, the annual number of arrests for driving under the influence of alcohol has always exceeded 1,000,000 (*Bureau of Justice Statistics Sourcebook*, 1992).

2. Marijuana impairs driving performance (Klonoff, 1974; Rafaelson, 1973).

3. Of 643 drivers who died within 2 days of a car accident, 18.2% had used cocaine; of the 379 who died within 2 hours, 8% tested positive for cocaine alone, 11% for alcohol and cocaine, and 50% for alcohol alone (Skolnick, 1990).

4. About one third of patients brought to a trauma center as the result of motor vehicle or nonvehicular accidents tested positive for marijuana, another one third for alcohol (Soderstrom, Trifillis, Shankar, & Clark, 1988).

5. Among drivers stopped and charged for driving under the influence of drugs, 47% tested positive for phencyclidine, 47% for marijuana, 22% for benzodiazepines, 15% for barbiturates, 11% for opiates, and 9% for cocaine (Poklis, Maginn, & Barr, 1987).

6. Among drivers stopped and charged for driving under the influence of drugs over a 5-year period, 65% tested positive for a benzodiazepine, 38% for an opiate. Drivers involved in an accident were more likely to have used antidepressants than other drugs (Christensen, Nielsen, & Nielsen, 1990).

PROBLEMS CAUSED BY INJECTIONS

Following oral administration, potentially dangerous impurities in drugs are rendered ineffective by stomach enzymes or other mechanisms. But many drug abusers inject impure drugs with unsterile needles. Illicitly manufactured drugs often contain filler substances that don't dissolve properly; they may lodge in the lungs and cause small lesions. Subcutaneous and intramuscular injections may cause multiple ulcerating lesions (see Figures 7.2 and 7.3) that often lead to tetanus. Injecters are susceptible to hepatitis, endocarditis, embolic pneumonia, and septicemia. Intravenous drug use or sexual contact with an IV user accounts for more than 80% of AIDS cases in women; and nearly 60% of pediatric AIDS patients were affected from either a mother who injected intravenously or whose sex partner did (Third Triennial Report to Congress, 1991).

PROBLEMS CAUSED BY SMOKING

Smokable drugs enter the bloodstream and brain rapidly, producing intense effects. So inhalation is a preferred route of administration: tobacco, cocaine, opium, free-base heroin, marijuana, methamphetamine, and phencyclidine are all smoked. In a monograph edited by Chiang and Hawks (1990), several authors noted that drugs undergo chemical reactions when exposed to high temperatures in the presence of air, and the resulting compounds often have different toxicities than the parents.

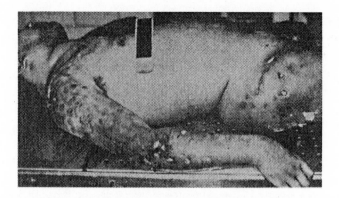

Figure 7.2. Subcutaneous or intramuscular self-administration of narcotics is called skin popping. It may be accomplished in any accessible location. Note the multiple ulcerating lesions and keloids of arms and right hip.

SOURCE: Hirsch (1972). Reproduced with permission of *Human Pathology.*

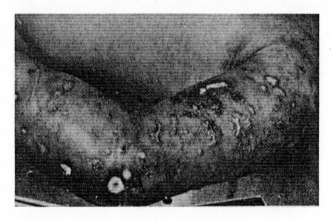

Figure 7.3. Close-up of six sites of skin popping on arm.

SOURCE: Hirsch (1972). Reproduced with permission of *Human Pathology.*

Habitual smoking of any of a number of substances leads to pulmonary problems.

ESCAPE FROM REALITY

It is often stated that drugs enable alienated, depressed people to escape from reality.[1] If the phrase means nothing more than a drug-induced respite of several hours from the demands of everyday living, then it applies to all forms of relaxation. Television, books, and attendance at sporting events fulfill the same needs. If it refers specifically to perceptual distortions, hallucinations, or disjointed thought, then not all psychoactive drugs produce escape. Marijuana enhances ability to attend to sensory stimuli; LSD, psilocybin, and amphetamine all improve certain aspects of sensory acuity; MDMA sessions frequently elicit confrontations with previously suppressed personal problems; and heroin's effects on thinking and perceptual processes (except the perception of pain) are small.

Some people, however, use drugs to avoid confronting problems. Adolescence is a time of special vulnerability. In most societies, adolescents must make often irreversible decisions concerning lifetime goals. The process is stressful, and inability or unwillingness to cope with it has been suggested as one factor in the rapid spread of drug usage among young Americans. Unfortunately, using drugs as a way of postponing decisions may reduce alternatives.

Drugs may give the illusion of coping. Hendin et al. (1987) administered a battery of tests and extensively interviewed 15 people who smoked marijuana daily. The most striking finding was the discrepancy between perceptions of users and observers. Marijuana smokers claimed that the drug improved their relationships, but Hendin et al. reported that it produced detachment rather than closeness. Unfortunately, Hendin et al. had no control groups, that is, they didn't study relationships of nonsmokers or of people who used drugs other than marijuana.

A friend told an interesting story. Before MDMA was given Schedule I status, a friend of his took some to help with a personal problem. Afterwards, he reported that he'd had a profoundly enlightening insight. About 2 months later, a second problem arose and he took some more. Again, he proclaimed the trip a great success. A month later, he had a new problem. Then another. On his 10th or 11th trip within a 2-year period, he had a final insight—he enjoyed MDMA so much that he had created problems to have an excuse to take the drug.

DRUG DEPENDENCY

Some drug users, because they crave repeated experiences, are called *psychologically dependent*. The World Health Organization (WHO) defines *drug dependence* as "a state of psychic or physical dependence, or both, on a drug, arising in a person following administration of that drug on a periodic or continuous basis." The definition owes its existence to arguments about drug legalization. Opponents asserted that drugs like heroin should remain illegal because they produce physical addiction. But some drugs were found not to be physically addicting; to justify sanctions against them, the concept of psychological dependence was introduced. In the U.S. Department of Justice (1989a) publication *Drugs of Abuse,* the following comments are made:

- Although no evidence of physical dependence is detectable when the drugs [hallucinogens] are withdrawn, recurrent use tends to produce psychic dependence, varying according to the drug, the dose, and the individual user.
- Because of the intensity of its pleasurable effects, cocaine has the potential for extraordinary psychic dependency.

A fundamental psychological principle states that living organisms try to repeat pleasurable experiences. Many drugs are harmful, and for a variety of reasons, but the fact that they give pleasure should not be one of them. If drugs are bad because they stimulate desire for more, then so are tasty foods, concerts, and friends.

The concept of physical dependence, evoking visions of desperate users impelled to commit vicious crimes or writhing in the agonies of withdrawal, also rests on a slippery foundation. Many drugs of abuse— cocaine, LSD, amphetamine, and marijuana among them—produce no or mild physical dependence. Others, such as the narcotic antagonists, produce physical dependence but are not abused. Patients made temporarily dependent on morphine in hospitals are not considered threats to society; but detoxified and hence no longer dependent heroin addicts are still regarded as addicts. Physical dependence occurs to heroin, alcohol, benzodiazepines, and insulin, with different consequences in each case. All of us are physically dependent on food and air.

Drug dependence, whether psychological or physical, is of concern any time it interferes with normal functioning. But people impaired by repeated voluntary self-administration of drugs must have had problems that preceded drug use. Dependence with impairment is a symptom rather than a cause.

DANGERS OF SPECIFIC DRUGS

Alcohol

Tolerance and Withdrawal. After chronic use, tolerance and withdrawal symptoms invariably occur. The well-known hangover is a withdrawal symptom; severe cases are marked by trembling, seizures, hallucinations, delirium, and even death.

Adverse Effects. Laboratory animals fed diets containing large amounts of alcohol suffer liver damage. In humans, alcohol contributes to fatty liver, alcoholic hepatitis, and cirrhosis. In 1986, cirrhosis mortality was the ninth leading cause of death in the United States (Seventh Special Report to U.S. Congress on Alcohol and Health [Seventh Special Report], 1990).

Regular alcohol use is associated with increased risk of esophageal and other cancers, cardiovascular disorders, hypertension, neurological problems, and accidents such as burns (Howland & Hingson, 1987) and falls (Hingson & Howland, 1987).

In a prospective study of middle-aged women, Hernandez-Avila et al. (1991) found a dose-response relation between alcohol consumption and incidence of both hip and forearm fractures.

Beneficial Effects. When emotional factors inhibit or cause excessive eating, alcohol can normalize appetite (Goetzl, 1953; Lolli, 1962). Alcohol reduces the pain and frequency of occurrence of attacks of angina pectoris (Helwig, 1940). Viruses such as those that cause polio, herpes simplex, and different types of gastrointestinal disorders are inactivated by incubation with red and, to a lesser extent, white wine (Maugh, 1977). Alcohol facilitates social interactions, especially in elderly people. Osler called it "the milk of old age," and Brooks said, "Either as a food, as a medicine, or for its comfort-giving qualities, alcohol properly administered is one of the greatest blessings of old age" (both cited in Leake & Silverman, 1966).

Pearl (1926) reported that both men and women who abstain from alcohol have longer average lifespans than heavy drinkers—but moderate drinkers live longest of all. The finding is difficult to interpret, as abstainers are often former heavy drinkers (Knupfer, 1987) with family histories of alcohol problems (Hughes, Stewart, & Barraclough, 1985) and less education and lower incomes than moderate drinkers (Goodwin et al., 1969). There is little experimental data. Schmidt, Popham, and Israel (1987) mixed alcohol in varying concentrations into the water of male mice; mice receiving moderate amounts lived the longest.

From January 1978 through December 1985, people who registered for health exams at the Kaiser Medical Center in Northern California were asked to fill out questionnaires that included questions about drinking.

By December 1988, 4,501 of the 128,934 respondents had died. Klatsky, Armstrong, and Friedman (1992) found that self-reported heavy drinkers (more than three drinks per day), whether they preferred liquor, beer, or wine, had the highest mortality rate. The study is correlational, so cannot conclusively show that heavy drinking caused premature deaths. In fact, heavy drinkers tended to engage in other life-impairing behaviors such as smoking. Still, statistical analyses that adjusted for risky behaviors indicated that the heaviest drinkers were 50% more likely to die that lighter drinkers. The effect was greater in women than men. People who had more than one drink per month but less than one per day had the lowest mortality rate.

Drinking more than three drinks per day increased mortality in all age groups but especially in people under 40. They were twice as likely to die as light drinkers of the same age.

Colsher and Wallace (1989) analyzed the key issues in the debate over whether small amounts of alcohol promote health. Several, but not all, studies show that moderate drinkers (in both total consumption and amount drunk per drinking episode) have fewer health problems than either heavy drinkers or abstainers. With the probable exception of coronary heart disease (conflicting reports exist), no specific conditions are improved by moderate drinking.

Amphetamine

Tolerance and Withdrawal. Most stimulants do not produce tolerance, but amphetamine and structurally related drugs are exceptions. After occasional use, mild sleep disturbances are the only annoying withdrawal symptoms; but high-dose bingeing leads to a dramatically different pattern. A period of depression, anxiety, and agitation gives way to craving for sleep and then to a period of decreased mental and physical energy that may last for weeks (Ellinwood, 1973).

Adverse Effects. The main problems following oral, moderate use are insomnia and irritability. Sustained, high-dose, intravenous use leads to a psychotic state almost indistinguishable from paranoid schizophrenia (Rang & Dale, 1987). Continual tooth grinding ends in ulcers of the lip and tongue (Ashcroft, Eccleston, & Waddell, 1965). Amphetamine damages neurons containing dopamine (Ricaurte & McCann, 1992).

Beneficial Effects. The appetite-depressing effect of amphetamine made it popular among dieters. It increases alertness, elevates mood, improves ability to concentrate, and diminishes fatigue.

Caffeine

Tolerance and Withdrawal. Tolerance develops to some of the effects of caffeine but not to the central stimulation. Goldstein, Kaizer, and Whitby (1969) randomly assigned 18 non-coffee drinkers and 38 heavy drinkers to receive coffee containing 0, 150, or 300 mg of caffeine; each subject was tested three times with each identically tasting preparation under double-blind conditions. When the heavy drinkers drank the caffeine-free preparation, they reported nervousness, irritability, and lack of alertness; so did the nondrinkers when they received caffeine.

No preference for caffeinated over decaffeinated coffee was exhibited by people who had drunk lots of decaffeinated coffee during the previous week; but those who had drunk lots of caffeinated coffee preferred caffeinated. This suggests that people drink caffeinated beverages at least in part to relieve withdrawal symptoms (Griffiths, Bigelow, & Liebson, 1986).

Adverse Effects. Several unpleasant side effects occur following ingestion of as little as one gram of caffeine (7 to 10 cups of coffee). These include insomnia, restlessness, ringing in the ears, muscle tenseness and tremor, cardiac irregularities, exacerbation of the symptoms of peptic ulcer, and diarrhea. Reimann (1967) concluded that many instances of unexplained illness are caused by excessive ingestion of caffeine.

Veleber and Templer (1984) randomly assigned volunteers to receive low, medium, or high doses of caffeine. One hour later, the subjects filled out questionnaires about their moods. A strong positive correlation was found between caffeine intake and self-reported increases in anxiety, depression, and hostility.

Although doses of 200-300 mg caffeine increase blood pressure in both caffeine users and nonusers, other studies show a slight inverse correlation between blood pressure and self-reported coffee consumption (Myers, 1988). Rosmarin and colleagues (Rosmarin, Applegate, & Somes, 1990a, 1990b) randomly assigned healthy men to drink three or more cups of coffee per day for 3 months and then to abstain for 2 months, or to abstain first and then drink. During the drinking phase, the men averaged 3.6 cups of coffee per day. Monthly measurements revealed no differences between the coffee-drinking and abstention phases in systolic or diastolic blood pressure, total cholesterol, or high- or low-density lipoprotein cholesterol. The study was not done blind, and no precautions were taken to ensure that the subjects drank coffee when they were supposed to and did not drink caffeine or substitutes during the abstention phase. Nevertheless, the most plausible interpretation is that moderate amounts of caffeine have weak or no adverse effects on coronary heart disease. But the issue is not settled: A correlational study of 1,130 men showed a strong relationship between coffee consumption and the risk of coronary heart disease even after adjustment for possible confounding factors like cigarette smoking (LaCroix et al., 1986).

Grossarth-Maticek and Eysenck (1991a, 1991b) tested the hypothesis that stimulant drugs protect against cancer but promote coronary heart disease (CHD), and CNS depressants have the opposite effect. They did two correlational studies. First, they found that, among coffee drinkers who averaged 10 cups per day, 4% died of cancer and 12% of CHD; among diazepam users, 28% died of cancer and 1% of CHD. Then they compared people who had drunk between two and three liters of Coca-Cola daily for at least 10 years with a control group matched on age, gender, cigarette and alcohol consumption, and personality type. Coca-Cola drinkers had about one fourth the mortality from cancer and about four times the mortality from CHD (and higher overall mortality).

In a correlational study described above, Klatsky, Armstrong, and Friedman (1993) evaluated questionnaires from 128,934 people. Heavy coffee drinkers (more than four cups per day) had a slightly increased risk of death from heart attack, but mortality rates from all causes combined were independent of levels of coffee and tea drinking. One surprising finding was that the risk of suicide decreased with increasing daily coffee intake. Klatsky et al. suggested that chronic caffeine consumption might have an antidepressant effect. (Chronic users become tolerant to the acute depressing effects.)

In a prospective study of middle-aged women, Hernandez-Avila et al. (1991) found a positive relation between caffeine intake and incidence of hip fractures.

Beneficial Effects. Caffeine is a bronchodilator, so it helps asthmatics. Lieberman et al. (1987) instructed coffee drinkers and nondrinkers to swallow a pill, which contained caffeine in one of various dosages, on each of several consecutive mornings. Then, shortly afterwards, the volunteers took a series of tests of mental performance, including reaction time and vigilance. The more caffeine they had taken, the better they did.

Cocaine

Tolerance and Withdrawal. Withdrawal from cocaine is similar to that from amphetamine.

Adverse Effects. Cocaine in low doses increases blood pressure and heart rate, so is contraindicated in people with hypertension or cardiac problems. Combined with alcohol, cocaine increases heart rate three to five times as much as when either drug is given alone (Foltin & Fischman, 1989b). Stress also potentiates cocaine's cardiovascular effects (Foltin et al., 1988). About 90% of cocaine-induced heart attack victims have no known history of heart disease (Bunn & Giannini, 1992). Frequent snorting inflames the mucous membranes of the nose. In men, cocaine use for 5 years or more was associated with a low sperm count and large number of abnormally shaped sperm (Bracken et al., 1990).

If cocaine powder from which adulterants have not been removed is mixed with water and baking soda and boiled until the water has evaporated, the residue is a waxy substance that can be smoked to produce almost immediate, intensified, effects. Called crack, it has become the most popular form of cocaine for many users. Smart (1991a) cited case studies, subject to the limitations of all case studies (see above), reporting crack-induced seizures, intracerebral hemorrhage, sudden death, psychosis, stroke, and cardiac abnormalities. These have also been reported in users of other forms of cocaine. Two types of adverse reactions specific to crack are pulmonary disease and neurological symptoms due to passive inhalation of crack smoke.

Beneficial Effects. Cocaine is a powerful antifatigue agent. It increases alertness, improves performance on a variety of tasks, and may relieve depression unresponsive to other drugs (Smith & Wesson, 1978).

Marijuana

Tolerance and Withdrawal. Moderate use of marijuana produces little tolerance or withdrawal symptoms. Tolerance and mild withdrawal symptoms, including nausea, irritability, and decreased appetite, occur after sustained, high-dose use (Hollister, 1986; Jones, 1983).

Adverse Effects. Perhaps in no scientific arena are biases more clearly displayed than that on adverse effects of marijuana. The fabrications of the former AMA president were mentioned above. Tennant and Groesbeck (1972) characterized heavy users as suffering from apathy, dullness, lethargy, and impairment of judgment, with the implication that marijuana was the cause. But heavy use was defined as smoking 17 to 200 marijuana cigarettes per day (200 per day over 16 waking hours is about one every 5 minutes). The amount is so excessive that the pre-marijuana judgment of the people should certainly have been questioned.

Adverse effects do occur. Marijuana increases heart rate, temporarily weakens heart muscle contractions, and reduces delivery of oxygen to the heart (Prakash & Aronow, 1976; Gottschalk, Aronow, & Prakash, 1977), so people with coronary disease should refrain from using. Chronic smoking damages the pulmonary system (Gong, Fligiel, Tashkin, & Barbers, 1987). Effects on sperm formation, menstrual cycles, and other reproductive functions have been reported, but their significance is not clear (Dewey, 1986). Block, Farinpour, and Schlechte (1991) and several other recent researchers (references in Block et al., 1991) found no significant hormonal changes in chronic marijuana users. Although chronic use may suppress functioning of the immune system, users do not appear more susceptible to infections, AIDS, or other diseases (Hollister, 1988).

Marijuana temporarily impairs memory (see Chapter 15) but probably has no long-term adverse consequences on cognition. Schaeffer, Andrysiak, and Ungerleider (1981) gave IQ tests to 10 people who had been very heavy users for the previous 7 years. Their scores were virtually identical with their IQ test scores from 15 to 20 years earlier.

Beneficial Effects. The primary beneficial effect is an increased sense of well-being. Anecdotal evidence suggests that the following conditions respond favorably to marijuana: pain, anxiety, insomnia, cough, excessive menstrual bleeding, withdrawal from narcotics and alcohol, poor appetite, and epilepsy (Snyder, 1971). Marijuana reduces intraocular pressure, so helps in treating glaucoma (Green, Kim, & Bowman, 1976). Kleiman and Doblin (1991) surveyed more than 1,000 oncologists about its usefulness in controlling nausea and vomiting caused by cancer chemotherapy. Forty-four percent said they had recommended it to at least one patient, 63% said it was effective, 48% said they would prescribe it if it were legal, and 77% said it is more effective than legally prescribed synthetic marijuana tablets.

Opioids

Tolerance and Withdrawal. Some people use morphine, opium, or heroin intermittently over a period of many years and eventually quit without difficulty (Chein & Wilner, 1964). But except for opium, continuous use leads to rapid development of tolerance to the euphoriant effects. So most addicts keep increasing dosages. Withdrawal is painful and prolonged, with peak effects occurring about 3 days after the last dose and some persisting for 7 to 10 days. Cross tolerance develops between the different opioids.

Adverse Effects. Brecher (1972) argued that both heroin and morphine are much less harmful than generally believed. He devoted an entire chapter to "eminent narcotics addicts"—highly successful people with long-standing addictions. He quoted a 1956 unpublished study in which the authors claimed that they had been unable to locate even one scientific study on the proved harmful effects of addiction; nor were eminent research workers or officials of the United Nations Commission on Narcotic Drugs able to cite a single study or offer any data on harmful effects.

The above reassurances notwithstanding, heroin addicts under 30 have an annual death rate estimated at 17.0 per thousand (the nonuser rate is between 1.0 and 2.3 per thousand). For users over 30, the estimate is 30.7 annual deaths per thousand (Duvall, Locke, & Brill, 1963). How can a benign drug do so much damage?

Recent findings have shown that opioids depress immune system functioning, probably resulting in increased susceptibility to many different infections and diseases including AIDS (Arora, 1990; Bryant, Bernton, & Holaday, 1990; Donahoe, 1990; Kreek, 1990). Because opioids reduce sensitivity to pain, users may not be alerted to symptoms of various diseases. Street heroin is never pure, and diluents such as quinine cause tissue injury and severe skin lesions. Some diluents are poorly soluble, and intravenous injection of incompletely dissolved substances may cause a fatal reaction (Eiseman, Lam, & Rush, 1964). Addicts who share needles are at great risk for AIDS and almost invariably develop hepatitis (Cherubin, 1967).

Beneficial Effects. The famous physician William Osler called morphine "God's own medicine." It and other opioids are highly effective in relieving both physical and mental pain.

Over-the-Counter (OTC) Drugs

Tolerance develops and withdrawal effects occur after prolonged use of many nonprescription drugs. The original symptoms may worsen following extensive use of nasal decongestants and headache remedies. Tolerance develops to the stimulating property of caffeine pills, and increasing the dose causes insomnia and anxiety.

Phenylpropanolamine (PPA), closely related to amphetamine, is the active ingredient in most diet pills and many cold remedies and cough syrups. It is the fifth most used drug in the United States. Since 1965, 142 adverse drug reactions to PPA have been reported and many more may go unrecognized. PPA elevates blood pressure leading to severe headache and, in 8 cases, death (Lake, Rosenberg, & Quirk, 1990). Anxiety and irritability often occur with PPA and also with various OTC asthma drugs.

Phencyclidine (PCP)

Tolerance and Withdrawal. Weak tolerance develops to the depressant effects of PCP, less to the stimulant effects (Balster & Woolverton, 1981). Withdrawal signs in humans are minimal or nonexistent (Burns & Lerner, 1981).

Adverse Effects. Street doses of PCP reduce appetite and cause weight loss; chronic users treated for overdose had averaged less than one meal per day for an extended period (Lerner & Burns, 1978). Other problems included insomnia, constipation, long-lasting memory and speech difficulties, anxiety, depression, and auditory hallucinations. For reasons not yet understood, a small proportion of users become psychotic. Some people intoxicated with PCP have committed serious acts of violence, leading to the charge that it induces violence (Wright, 1980). But analyses of clinical reports of PCP intoxication (Brecher, Wang, Wong, & Morgan, 1988) and of men arrested for criminal activity (Wish, 1986) do not support this view. Experiments with animals suggest that PCP generally reduces aggression (cf. Balster, 1987). Users reported that positive effects occurred in 60% of intoxications, adverse effects in 100% (Siegel, 1978a).

Beneficial Effects. Chronic users describe the PCP experience as very intense, exhilarating, and euphoric. They say that it provides a perfect dream world (Lerner & Burns, 1978).

Psychedelics

Tolerance and Withdrawal. Tolerance develops rapidly to LSD, mescaline, and psilocybin, and they are all cross tolerant. Withdrawal symptoms are minimal.

Adverse Effects. Not all drug experiences turn out as anticipated, and unpleasant outcomes occur often enough to make the phrase *bad trip* part of the drug culture lexicon. Any potentially enjoyable event may disappoint, as when rainy weather spoils a picnic. The special quality of drug-induced bad trips is that they cannot easily be terminated. Concerns have been raised that LSD damages chromosomes (Cohen, Marinello, & Back, 1967), causes brain damage (Acord & Baker, 1973), and leads to prolonged psychosis (Abraham, 1983). The weight of the evidence indicates that the concerns are unfounded (Dishotsky et al., 1971; McWilliams & Tuttle, 1973; Strassman, 1984).

Beneficial Effects. LSD users wax lyrical about its ability to promote insights into everyday problems, enhance creativity, and provide mystical and religious experiences. These claims are evaluated in appropriate chapters.

Steroids

Anabolic steroids—synthetic derivatives of male hormones—help counter serious medical conditions such as breast cancer in women and bone marrow associated anemias. They are also used to enhance athletic performance and muscular appearance. But their many side effects include liver cancer, cardiovascular problems, sterility, testicular atrophy, and, in female users, development of masculine characteristics such as facial hair, enlarged clitoris, and deepened voice. Behavioral effects include depression, irritability, and unpredictable, uncontrollable rage reactions.

Tobacco

Tolerance and Withdrawal. Both tolerance and withdrawal symptoms occur with tobacco, with nicotine the causative agent. The most prominent symptoms are drowsiness, nervousness, anxiety, headaches, and energy loss. Tobacco accelerates the metabolism of caffeine, so blood caffeine levels increase sharply during withdrawal from tobacco and may contribute to the symptoms (Benowitz, Hall, & Modin, 1989). In a survey of polydrug abusers, nicotine was rated above heroin, methadone, amphetamine, barbiturates, LSD, marijuana, alcohol, and caffeine as the drug they could least do without (Russell, 1971c).

Adverse Effects. Tobacco use is a major cause of cancer, heart disease, and chronic obstructive lung disease (U.S. Department of Health and Human Services, 1982a, 1982b). Smokers are more likely than nonsmokers to develop and die from peptic and duodenal ulcers (Surgeon General's Report, 1979; Kurata, Elashoff, Nogawa, & Haile, 1986). Tobacco is responsible for about one sixth of deaths from all causes in the United States, more than the combined total from AIDS, cocaine, heroin, alcohol, fire, automobile accidents, homicide, and suicide (Davis, 1987; U.S. Department of Health and Human Services, 1989; Warner, 1987). Benowitz (1992), from rates of emergency department mentions and medical examiner cases, estimated that the yearly death rate per 1,000 users is about 10 times higher for tobacco than for cocaine or phencyclidine.

Smokers are more likely than nonsmokers to have accidents, die in fires, and experience early disability (Kristein, 1983). Tobacco depletes vitamin C levels in the blood, resulting in deficiencies in more than 25% of U.S. smokers (Schectman, Byrd, & Hoffman, 1991). Tobacco interacts with many drugs, reducing the effectiveness of various analgesics, antianxiety agents, antidepressants, and antipsychotics among others; it increases the risk of serious complications associated with the use of oral contraceptives (American Pharmaceutical Association, 1986).

In the next chapter I argue that victimless crimes should not be crimes. Ironically tobacco, legal, heavily promoted, and widely available, is one drug that routinely victimizes nonusers. The health consequences of passive smoking are substantial, including cognitive impairment (Osborne, 1983) and increased risk of respiratory infections (Harlap & Davies, 1974), lung cancer ("Smoking Attributable Mortality," 1991), and heart disease (Steenland, 1992). Steenland observed that the excess risk of heart disease deaths due to passive smoking is much greater than that used in determining environmental limits for other toxins.

Beneficial Effects. Even nicotine isn't all bad. Jarvik (1991), reviewing the positive effects, cited all of the following: Nicotine reduces appetite while increasing metabolic activity, thus promoting weight loss. It facilitates performance, learning, and memory. It may protect against Parkinson's disease and benefit victims of Tourette's syndrome, ulcerative colitis, Alzheimer's disease, and obstructive sleep apnea. Jarvik wrote, "Thus, the principal virtue of nicotine is its ability to make people feel good. And, unlike alcohol, cocaine, or heroin, it does so without impairing thinking or performance. If this property could be dissociated from the harmful effects of tobacco it could be an ideal drug."

RELATIVE DANGERS OF VARIOUS PSYCHOACTIVE DRUGS

Gable (1993) found 350 articles that estimated lethality of 20 abused drugs. He selected 4 or 5 articles per drug to estimate the LD50 and ED50 for each. ED50 was defined as the median amount of drug capable of serving as a reinforcer for self-administration or of eliciting a verbal self-report of a desired subjective state such as euphoria.

As Gable acknowledged, his estimates are uncertain. In addition, the significance of a therapeutic index (ratio of LD50/ED50) depends partly on the route of administration. For a given therapeutic index, smoked drugs are generally safer than either ingested or injected ones, because smoking involves gradual increments in dosage whereas drugs taken by the other routes are typically administered all at one time. (Oral caffeine, however, is usually taken in gradual increments.) Also, the therapeutic index does not indicate long-range harmful effects. Nevertheless, Table 7.7, adapted from Gable, offers an interesting perspective on relative safety of various abused drugs.

ANSWERS

Question 1. Subjects randomly assigned to experimental or control groups are assumed equivalent prior to treatment. Subsequent differences can, within the limits of statistical error, be attributed to the treatments. So, the researcher could appropriately conclude that caf-

Table 7.7 Therapeutic Indexes of Various Psychoactive Drugs

Drug	Therapeutic Index (LD50/ED50)
Heroin (intravenous)	7.5
Morphine (intramuscular)	9
Opium (smoked)	8
Secobarbital (oral)	25
Diazepam (oral)	1,000
Alcohol (oral)	10
Methaqualone (oral)	133.3
Amphetamine (oral)	20
Caffeine (oral)	100
Cocaine (intranasal)	25
Cocaine (smoked crack)	25
Nicotine (smoked)	60
Ketamine (intramuscular)	26
Nitrous oxide (inhaled)	24
Phencyclidine (smoked)	40
LSD-25 (oral)	280
MDMA (oral)	15
Mescaline (oral)	17.1
Psilocybin (oral)	3,500
Marijuana (smoked)	2,667

feine improves weight lifting ability. But subjects were not randomly assigned to the smoking/nonsmoking groups, so pretreatment equivalence should not be assumed. They, themselves, had decided long before participating in the research project whether or not they would smoke. They were influenced by factors such as genetics, stress, or desire to project a certain image, and those same or other unknown factors might account for differences in weight lifting abilities. It would be safe to conclude that smokers lift more weight than do nonsmokers, but not safe to conclude that smoking is the cause.

Question 2. Interview data are often unreliable, partly because people forget, partly because they misinterpret or don't understand the meanings of questions, partly because they tend to answer in ways that relieve themselves of responsibility for undesirable acts (Leavitt, 1991).

Question 3. Because the data are correlational rather than experimental, they do not prove the government's contention that alcohol has an impact on crimes. Many alternatives are possible. For example:

- The genes that predispose some people to drink excessively also predispose to criminality.
- Stressful environments promote both drinking and criminality.
- People who intend to commit crimes drink to fortify themselves or give themselves an excuse.
- Young men are the biggest drinkers, and they are also the most aggressive.
- People drink a lot in sports bars, and sporting events often incite violence.
- Hostile, tense people drink to *reduce* their aggressive tendencies. It works, but not always.

Summary

Dangers of drugs should be evaluated in relation to benefits, as part of cost-benefit analyses.

Adverse effects of drugs arise in a variety of ways: as side effects; dosing errors, especially likely with extremely potent drugs; as a result of interactions; hypersensitivity reactions, as a result of small chronic insults; and in pregnant women, harm to the developing fetus.

Correlational data, including data from case studies, may strongly suggest that a drug causes harm; but the only research method that can conclusively demonstrate causal relationships is experimentation.

Bias is a serious problem in science and may be especially powerful in the drug field.

Many drugs impair psychomotor skills and probably contribute to motor vehicle crashes.

Injected drugs may contain materials that do not dissolve properly and lodge in the lungs. Injections may cause ulcerating lesions. Unsterile needles are a vehicle for transmitting a variety of serious diseases including AIDS.

Smoking anything is likely to cause lung problems and may be carcinogenic.

Some people use drugs to avoid confronting difficult decisions. This may reduce their options while giving them a false sense of security.

Drug dependency—whether psychological or physical—is not a useful concept.

Withdrawal symptoms are severe after chronic use of alcohol. Chronic alcoholism is associated with liver damage and several other serious problems. Moderate use may be beneficial.

High-dose bingeing of amphetamine inevitably leads to depression and anxiety during withdrawal.

Intake of more than seven cups of caffeine per day may cause several unpleasant physical and mental effects. Chronic high dose caffeine use is associated with coronary problems.

Cocaine increases heart rate and blood pressure, especially in people under stress. Many cases of sudden death have been attributed to cocaine use.

Marijuana is dangerous to people with heart problems. Chronic smoking damages the pulmonary system.

Withdrawal from opiates is painful. Opiates depress immune system functioning. Impurities in street heroin cause tissue injury, and sharing of needles leads to the spread of many infectious diseases.

Over-the-counter drugs occasionally produce unpleasant and even dangerous reactions.

Phencyclidine abusers often suffer from malnutrition. A small proportion become violent.

The major documented danger of psychedelics is occurrence of bad trips.

Anabolic steroids cause many physical effects including liver damage and testicular atrophy; and behavioral effects such as depression and violence.

Tobacco is a major cause of cancer, heart disease, and lung disease. Mere exposure to cigarette smoke causes health problems.

▓ Note

1. Lily Tomlin offered her own perspective: Reality is a crutch for people who can't cope with drugs.

Mini-Quiz: Dangers and Benefits

Both _____ and antidepressants relieve depression at least temporarily.

cocaine

T/F: Drugs such as marijuana may in some cases improve physical health by reducing stress.

true

Insomnia produced by amphetamine is an example of a _____.

side effect

The range between the therapeutic and toxic doses of a drug is called its _____.

therapeutic window

The only research design that justifies conclusions of the type "Drug X causes symptom Y" is the _____.

experiment

Give two reasons why it is dangerous to infer causes from case studies.

1. The data are correlational, not experimental.
2. Case studies use only part of the necessary information.

T/F: There is strong experimental evidence that alcohol impairs driving.

false—but there is a great deal of correlational evidence

List dangers faced by drug abusers who inject but not by drug abusers who administer orally.

1. Dangerous impurities are not destroyed by stomach enzymes.
2. Insoluble filler substances may lodge in the lungs.
3. Injections may cause lesions.
4. Sharing needles may transmit a variety of serious diseases including AIDS.

T/F: Marijuana smokers claimed that marijuana improved their relationships.

true

T/F: The authors of the study in which marijuana smokers claimed that marijuana improved their relationships agreed with the smokers' assessments.

false

Which of the following drugs cause strong physical dependence: cocaine, LSD, amphetamine, marijuana, narcotic antagonists, heroin, alcohol?

narcotic antagonists, heroin, alcohol

According to the text, psychological dependence is (choose one):
a. a symptom of an underlying problem.
b. a cause of drug abuse.

a

Alcohol harms the _____ and, in moderation, may benefit the _____.

liver; heart

Withdrawal following high-dose amphetamine use is marked by _____.

depression, agitation, and reduced energy

The stimulant _____ is a bronchodilator, so it helps people suffering from _____.

caffeine; asthma

A theory cited in the text is that stimulant drugs protect against _____, and CNS depressants protect against _____.

cancer; coronary heart disease

Withdrawal symptoms are similar from amphetamine and _____.

cocaine

Cocaine and _____ combine to increase heart rate much more than when either drug is given alone.

alcohol

T/F: Opioids damage the immune system.

true

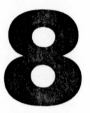

By the time you finish reading this chapter, you should be able to answer the following questions:

What are teratogens?

Why is it not a simple matter to screen drugs for teratogenicity?

What are the different methods by which investigators seek to identify teratogens?

In humans, when is the period during which teratogens are most likely to produce gross anatomical malformations?

What are the different mechanisms by which drugs can affect fetuses?

What is the most frequent and clearly documented adverse outcome associated with fetal exposure to alcohol, nicotine, and illicit drugs?

T/F: Most substances in the maternal blood cross the placenta.

T/F: Drugs taken by males prior to mating may affect fetal development.

T/F: Many drugs produce effects similar to those of fetal alcohol syndrome.

Effects of Drugs on the Embryo, Fetus, and Developing Young

Contents

The main point of this chapter can be summarized in a single sentence: *As much as possible, drugs should be avoided during pregnancy.* What follows is mere detail.

▨ A Few Statistics

More than half of human conceptions are lost in the first 30 weeks of gestation and almost 80% before term (Hertig, 1967). Of the survivors, about 1% to 3% are born with gross structural defects and a similar percentage with more subtle abnormalities (Cook, Petersen, & Moore,

155

1990). The causes of spontaneous abortions, miscarriages, stillbirths, and live born with abnormal conditions are often unknown, but the use of drugs during pregnancy is the major preventable cause. Drug-exposed infants are also much more likely than unexposed to have withdrawal symptoms and be infected by syphilis and human immunodeficiency virus (HIV).

Rudd and Brazy (1988) reported that women use an average of 10 drugs throughout pregnancy. Chasnoff, Schnoll, Burns, and Burns (1984) found that 3% of women enrolling for routine prenatal care had sedative-hypnotics in their urine at the time of admission. Sixty percent of women of childbearing age drink alcohol, 30% smoke during the period of conception, and 25% smoke throughout pregnancy (cited in Cook et al., 1990). In San Francisco, 70% of addicted women were mothers (Rosenbaum & Murphy, 1984). Unmarried pregnant adolescents, compared with high school seniors, reported similar or higher lifetime use rates for alcohol, marijuana, cocaine, inhalants, stimulants, sedatives, barbiturates, tranquilizers, and cigarettes. Upon learning they were pregnant, they reduced but did not discontinue drug use (Gilchrist, Gilmore, & Lohr, 1990). The National Institute on Drug Abuse estimated that 5 million women of childbearing age used illicit drugs in 1988 (General Accounting Office [GAO], 1990). Making matters even worse, pregnant women require higher doses of certain drugs to achieve plasma concentrations equivalent to those in nonpregnant women.

Cocaine was detected in urine specimens of 10% of newborns (cited in Cook et al., 1990). Of women receiving prenatal care at Boston City Hospital, 18% had used cocaine at least once (Zuckerman, Amaro, & Cabral, 1989; Zuckerman, Frank, Bauchner et al., 1989; Zuckerman, Frank, Hingson et al., 1989). Chasnoff (1989) observed that hospitals with rigorous detection procedures identified 16% of infants as drug-exposed, whereas hospitals with less rigorous procedures identified only 3%.

⊠ Methodological Issues

ANIMAL STUDIES

Substances that increase the likelihood that offspring will be born malformed are called *teratogens*. Although new drugs are routinely tested for teratogenicity on pregnant laboratory animals, Rudd and Brazy (1988) claimed that most known human teratogens were identified only after many children had been injured by prenatal exposure. The following are some reasons why lab tests are rarely definitive:

- In most cases, teratogens do maximal damage when administered during the earliest stages of embryonic development. Some, however, act only in later stages. The potential of a drug to produce serious consequences may go undetected if the drug is administered to a laboratory animal outside the critical period.
- Some malformations are not present at birth (cited in Clegg, 1971).
- Dosage is crucial. For most drugs, if a given dose kills or malforms half the embryos, a dose one to three orders of magnitude below that will have no discernible effect (Brent & Beckman, 1990). Total dosage is sometimes less important, sometimes more, than peak concentrations (Nau, 1986; Pierce & West, 1986a, 1986b).
- Many laboratory animals eliminate defective fetuses in utero, so researchers who ignore litter size may fail to detect potential teratogens.
- People use several different routes of administration, whereas laboratory animals typically receive drugs through implanted catheters or mixed in food.
- Rare defects may not show up in small samples or may be attributed to other causes.
- The developing organism is so sensitive to unusual stimuli that anything in large doses may be dangerous. A better question than, "Is drug X teratogenic?" is, "What is the relationship between the therapeutic dose in the mother and toxic doses for the embryo and fetus?"
- Species differences are important. Thalidomide is not teratogenic to mice or rats.
- Pregnant rats given chlorpromazine behave abnormally toward their babies; pups exposed in utero and reared by their mothers were more strongly affected than littermates reared by foster mothers (Ordy et al., 1966). In this case, the animal research has clear human parallels. The likelihood of mental impairment among children exposed prenatally to methadone or heroin increases greatly if they are raised in a drug-abuse environment (Hans, 1989; Wilson, 1989). Such environments often involve violence toward the mother during her pregnancy (Amaro, Fried, Cabral, & Zuckerman, 1990), physical abuse of the children, and exposure of the children to violence directed at others (van der Kilk, 1988). Women recovering from phencyclidine abuse interact immaturely with their children (Howard, Beckwith, & Rodning, 1990).

SURVEYS

Surveyors have asked pregnant women questions about their drug use and, following delivery, examined their babies. They've also questioned mothers of babies with birth defects about drug use during pregnancy. But survey research is limited by respondents' imperfect memories and attempts to give socially desirable answers. For example, Hingson et al. (1986) asked two groups of pregnant women about their marijuana use. Those told that their urine would be tested for marijuana reported more use than women not so told, yet less than what the urine assays showed. Zuckerman, Amaro, and Cabral (1989) recruited 1,226 women from a prenatal clinic and questioned them about cocaine and marijuana use. Sixteen percent of marijuana and 24% of cocaine users denied use but were identified by urine analyses.

A second limitation of survey research is that it may fail to detect rare birth defects. A third is that the work is correlational: Pregnant drug abusers and nonabusers differ in many ways including age, nutritional status, general health, and receipt of prenatal care.

SURVEILLANCE SYSTEMS

Surveillance systems for monitoring birth defects and relating them to maternal drug abuse are a potentially valuable source of information. At present, however, standards are inconsistent. Martin and Edmonds (1991) reported striking differences in rates of major birth defects according to data source. The number of defects per 10,000 births varied from 88.9 (from birth certificates) to 415.0 (National Birth Defects Monitoring Program) to 830.0 (physical examination of infant).

▓ Mechanisms of Action

Susceptibility to teratogens varies throughout gestation. In the first stage (in humans, until about the 17th day after conception), the embryo has few cells. Most drugs kill either so many cells that the embryo dies or so few that they can be completely replaced. Pregnant laboratory animals given teratogens during the first stage bear fewer but normal young. The period of greatest susceptibility to gross anatomic malformations is, in humans, days 18 through 60. After day 60, teratogenic agents are most likely to cause growth retardation and mental and behavioral deficits. Many drugs, especially CNS depressants, induce subtle behavioral deficits that can be detected in precisely controlled laboratory studies but are unlikely to be noticed in humans (cf. Armitage, 1952; Hoffeld, McNew, & Webster, 1968; Werboff & Havlena, 1962).

Some drugs are directly toxic to the fetus, and others interfere with fetal metabolism. Some exert effects on the fetus similar to those on the mother. (The so-called placental barrier is considerably less formidable than the defensive line of the Chicago Bears. Most substances in the maternal blood cross the placenta and, because fetal metabolism is inefficient, some reach higher concentrations in fetal than maternal circulation. Alcohol, opioids, and cocaine transfer very rapidly across the placenta, marijuana much more slowly [Abrams et al., 1985; Brien, Clarke, Richardson, & Patrick, 1985; Golub, Eisele, & Anderson, 1986; Woods, 1989]).

Drugs may impair development through direct effects on neurotransmitters. Indirect effects like contraction of smooth muscle may cause umbilical cord spasms that impair fetal nutrition and oxygen supply. Nutrition may be affected by reduction of amniotic fluid volume and blood flow from uterus to placenta; and oxygen supply may be reduced by smoked drugs that increase carbon monoxide levels. Some drugs harm fetuses indirectly by altering the mother's endocrine balance or nutritional status. Whenever pregnant addicts experience withdrawal symptoms, so do their fetuses.

Some drugs have delayed effects. Diethylstilbesterol (DES), a synthetic estrogen, caused vaginal cancer in a high proportion of daughters of women who took it during pregnancy to prevent miscarriage; almost all the cancers occurred after the girls reached age 14 (Herbst, Scully, & Robboy, 1975).

Lifschitz and Wilson (1991) asserted that low birth weight is the most frequent and clearly documented adverse outcome associated with fetal exposure to opioids, nicotine, alcohol, marijuana, and cocaine. The primary reason is impaired fetal growth, but increased occurrence of premature births plays a role. Growth often remains retarded after birth. Contributing factors include maternal undernutrition and poor weight gain, absence of prenatal care, preeclampsia (a toxic disease of pregnancy), chronic maternal illness, and intrauterine infections.

Women do not bear the sole burden for the health of their babies. Drugs taken by men prior to mating may affect fetal development by damaging sperm, changing the volume or composition of seminal fluid, remaining within the seminal fluid, or reducing the man's body weight or testosterone level (Joffe, 1979). Adverse effects to fetuses occur following paternal exposure to thalidomide (Lutwak-Mann, 1964), lead, morphine, methadone, alcohol, caffeine, or cocaine (Abel et al., 1989; Joffe, 1979; Joffe, Peruzovic, & Milkovic, 1990). Butler (1977) reported increased mortality in children of men who smoked more than 10 cigarettes per day; and clinical studies show that lead, anesthetic gases, and caffeine affect the fetus through its father (Joffe, 1979). Yazigi, Odem, and Polakoski (1991) demonstrated that cocaine binds to human spermatozoa, raising the possibility that the sperm may then transport cocaine into an ovum.

▓ Drug Effects

Below are summarized findings on the effects of prenatal exposure to various drugs. For research prior to 1985, consult Lee and Chiang (1985). They constructed a comprehensive table of drug effects on the fetus and developing young.

ALCOHOL

Maternal alcoholism is associated with high rates of spontaneous abortion, miscarriage, and stillbirth. Infants of even moderate drinkers have sleep disturbances (Scher et al., 1988). Women who average seven ounces or more of absolute alcohol a week during pregnancy greatly increase their chances of giving birth to low birth weight infants of shorter than normal length and with smaller head and chest circumference measurements (Cook et al., 1990). In 1973, Jones and Smith described a cluster of symptoms in infants of alcoholic mothers. Called **fetal alcohol syndrome** (FAS), it is the leading known cause of mental retardation. The diagnosis of FAS, which occurs in about 2.5% of live births of alcoholic women (Abel, 1984), requires at least one feature from each of three categories:

1. Prenatal and postnatal growth retardation: abnormally small weight, length, and/or head circumference
2. Central nervous system disorders: abnormal brain functioning, delays in behavioral development, and/or intellectual impairment

3. Two or more of the following: small head, small eyes or short eye openings, poorly developed groove above the upper lip, thin upper lip, short nose, flattened midfacial area

When only some of the criteria are met, the infant may be diagnosed as having **fetal alcohol effects** (FAE). Abel (1984) estimated that FAE occurs about four times as often as FAS in the alcohol-abusing population. Infants whose mothers drink moderately throughout pregnancy often experience more subtle neurobehavioral and growth deficits (Coles, Smith, Lancaster, & Falek, 1987); and some alcohol-induced deficits persist at least until age 7 (Streissguth et al., 1986).

Zuckerman (1991) argued that the focus on alcohol as the specific cause of FAS has obscured other possible causes. They include antianxiety drugs, barbiturates, marijuana, opioids, and other central nervous system depressants.

ANALGESICS AND ANESTHETICS

Drugs given to mothers to relieve pain during labor and delivery depress fetal respiration, heart rate, and other physiological functions. Aleksandrowicz (1974) noted that peak drug effects occur $3\frac{1}{2}$ to 4 hours after administration, so they may not be observed by doctors who examine babies only at delivery. All commonly used **obstetric drugs** reduce alertness, habituation, and responsiveness to visual and auditory stimulation, some effects persisting for at least one month (Aleksandrowicz, 1973). Rudd and Brazy (1988) advised doctors to administer intravenous drugs during contractions; then the drug enters and is distributed to the maternal circulation before entering the fetus, thus minimizing fetal exposure.

Regular use of aspirin prolongs pregnancy and delivery. Aspirin taken close to term may cause bleeding in the newborn, but low-dose aspirin improves **perinatal** outcome for several conditions (Barton & Sibai, 1991). Streissguth et al. (1987) reported that, among 1,529 pregnant women, aspirin and acetaminophen were the two drugs taken most during the first half of pregnancy. Examination of the offspring at 4 years of age revealed no effects of either drug on physical size, and acetaminophen use was uncorrelated with their intellectual performance. But maternal aspirin use was significantly related to IQ and attention decrements in the children at age 4. The effect was greater for girls than boys.

CAFFEINE

Caffeine consumption during pregnancy has been associated, in a dose-dependent manner, with decreased birth weight (Caan & Goldhaber, 1989; Martin & Bracken, 1987). Caffeine withdrawal symptoms have been reported in infants of mothers who consumed large amounts of caffeine during pregnancy (McGowan, Altman, & Kanto, 1988).

COCAINE

Cocaine abuse increases the likelihood of complications during pregnancy and delivery. Cocaine constricts blood vessels, and one major consequence is that the fetus suffers oxygen deprivation. Cocaine-exposed infants are often growth-retarded and excessively irritable with rigid limbs and hand and arm tremors (Chasnoff, 1988). Hume et al. (1989) reported abnormal breathing patterns. Despite media reports that cocaine-exposed babies are born addicted, no withdrawal syndrome has been documented (Zuckerman, 1991).

MARIJUANA

Infants of marijuana users have a lower average birth weight than infants of nonusers and are more likely to have features similar to those of FAS (Hingson et al., 1982). They suffer sleep disturbances (Scher et al., 1988) and jitteriness (Parker et al., 1990). Marijuana taken during pregnancy increases the ratio of male to female offspring (Fried, 1982; Tennes et al., 1985). Hutchings, Brake, and Morgan (1989), after comparing the number of implantation sites in female rats that had been exposed to marijuana with the number and sex of their stillborn and live pups, concluded that high doses are selectively lethal to female fetuses. Fried (1985) reported several perceptual and motor decrements in infants born to heavy marijuana smokers, but no differences were detected at age 2.

OPIOIDS

Heroin babies often have small heads (Vargas, Pildes, & Vidyasagar, 1975) and intellectual impairment (Lifschitz & Wilson, 1991). School-age children who were exposed to opioids are prone to hyperactivity, poor attention span, and motor dyscoordination (Hans, 1991).

Methadone-maintained women tend to have infants with lower birth weight than those of nonaddicted controls. Nevertheless, methadone infants have much less severe problems than do infants of heroin addicts. In addition, participation in a methadone program makes a woman available for prenatal care, nutritional counseling, and parenting skills classes. Thus, Zweben and Sorensen (1988) supported the administration of methadone to pregnant addicts.

NICOTINE

In 1988, 2,552 infant deaths were attributed to the mothers' smoking (U.S. Department of Health and Human Services, 1989). Recent studies have shown that paternal smoking is also harmful. Women married to smokers, whether or not they themselves smoke, are at much greater risk of delivering a low birth weight baby (Cook et al., 1990).

PRESCRIPTION AND OVER-THE-COUNTER DRUGS

Antibiotics

Streptomycin taken at even late stages of pregnancy may cause hearing damage in the child. Tetracycline causes permanent staining of the baby teeth (Zamula, 1989).

Antianxiety Drugs

Reports that benzodiazepines cause fetal defects, especially cleft palate and malformations of the heart, were not confirmed by later studies (American Psychiatric Association, 1990). Newborns whose mothers have been taking benzodiazepines do, however, show withdrawal symptoms. On the other hand, benzodiazepines relieve stress; and stress during pregnancy increases the risk of fetal damage (Platt, Anand, & Aynsley-Green, 1989; Rothberg & Lits, 1991).

Anticonvulsants

Several antiseizure drugs have been associated with a variety of birth defects, but women who need such drugs should continue taking them. Otherwise, they are prone to seizures that threaten the health of the fetus even more.

Antihypertensive Drugs

Drugs for maternal hypertension elevate neonatal blood pressure and heartbeat (Rudd & Brazy, 1988). Prenatal exposure to the antihypertensive drug clonidine has been associated with sleep disturbances (Kellog & Guillet, 1988).

Corticosteroids

Dexamethasone and other corticosteroids are frequently administered to pregnant women to prevent neonatal respiratory distress syndrome. Uno et al. (1990) gave pregnant rhesus macaque monkeys doses of dexamethasone comparable to those given to humans. The fetuses showed severe abnormalities in the hippocampal region of the brain.

Isoretinoin

The antiacne drug isoretinoin (Accutane) was introduced in 1982. As of November 1988 the FDA had received 85 reports of fetuses and infants with malformations attributable to isoretinoin exposure during pregnancy (Chairperson, Public Affairs Committee, 1991).

Lithium

Lithium is teratogenic at therapeutic doses. It induces malformations in about 10% of exposed fetuses (Brent & Beckman, 1990).

PHENCYCLIDINE

Howard, Kropenske, and Tyler (1986) reported that all of 12 infants exposed prenatally to PCP developed deviant neurobehavioral symptoms within the first 24 hours after birth. Eight of the infants had one or more medical problems during the perinatal period, and they continued to have problems a year later. Complicating interpretation of the results is that 10 of the women were polydrug users, most had medical problems of their own, and none of the infants was discharged from the hospital to the care of its mother.

SEXUAL HORMONES

Many behavioral differences between men and women are influenced by cultural stereotypes and learning, but many are due to genetically programmed differential secretion of sex hormones. Most of the evidence comes from animal research: Even after identical rearing, male and female rats, hamsters, guinea pigs, and monkeys behave differently in many situations. The key factor is presence or absence of **androgens** (male hormones, the most important of which is **testosterone**); sufficient testosterone during a critical period early in life results in an animal with male characteristics, and low levels result in feminization. The early presence or absence of testosterone affects morphology, sexual preferences, sexual behavior, aggressiveness, activity level, exploratory tendencies, body weight and length, stance during urination, oxygen consumption, maze learning, and food preferences (see Adkins-Regan [1988], Ehrhardt [1984], and Quadagno, Briscoe, & Quadagno [1977] for reviews).

For several years beginning in the 1940s, physicians prescribed **estrogen** or **progesterone** (ovarian hormones with some testosterone-like effects) to pregnant women with a history of miscarriage. Some girls born to such women had masculinized external genitalia and were declared at birth to be boys. Even when raised as girls, they were more likely than controls to be identified as tomboys: They had more male friends, enjoyed more intense outdoor play, and had lower interest in doll play, baby care, and the role of wife and mother. Their behaviors were, however, within the range of normal variation (Ehrhardt & Meyer-Bahlburg, 1979). Dorner (1988) argued for the highly controversial view that women prenatally exposed to excess androgens, and men exposed to abnormally low androgen levels, are likely to become homosexual.

POLYDRUG ABUSE

Over a period of several years, Van Baar and colleagues (Van Baar, 1990; Van Baar, Fleury, Soepatmi et al., 1989; Van Baar, Fleury, & Ultee, 1989) compared development in offspring of polydrug-using and non-drug-using mothers. The drugs included combinations of methadone, heroin, cocaine, amphetamine, and tranquilizers. The newborns of drug-using mothers did worse on a neurological examination, had a greater incidence of abnormal electroencephalograms, and experienced withdrawal symptoms (80% had to be treated). By the age of 9 months, most differences had disappeared. But at 24 to 30 months, difficulties in early language development appeared in the offspring of drug-using mothers. Van Baar noted that the drug abusers lived in more difficult social circumstances than did the comparison group.

▩ Dose-Response Relationships

There are few all-or-none drug effects. Testosterone at levels too low to masculinize their genitalia nevertheless affected developing female mice. Vom Saal and Bronson (1980) reported that females that had developed in utero between two males had higher concentrations of testosterone in their blood and amniotic fluid compared with females that had developed between two females. They had larger anogenital spaces at birth and were more aggressive as adults. Adult male mice preferred females that had developed between two females.

Many drugs that are teratogenic at high doses have smaller effects at lower ones. For example, children of alcoholics may show fetal alcohol syndrome or the less severe fetal alcohol effects. Even more subtle decrements may occur—in one study, children of moderate drinking mothers averaged 5 IQ points less than children of nondrinkers (Bower, 1989)—forcing the conclusion that pregnant women should abstain as much as possible. In some cases, as when taken to relieve severe stress, drugs may increase the likelihood that a baby will be born healthy.

Summary

The use of drugs during pregnancy is the major preventable cause of spontaneous abortions, miscarriages, stillbirths, and liveborn with abnormal conditions. Yet a significant proportion of women of child-bearing age use drugs.

Substances that increase the likelihood that offspring will be born malformed are called teratogens. The methods for identifying potential teratogens—animal experiments, surveys, and surveillance systems—all have limitations. As a result, most teratogens become known only after they have harmed many developing fetuses.

The effects of teratogens vary with dose and period of gestation. Some are directly toxic to the fetus, others exert indirect effects. Most substances in the maternal blood cross the placental barrier.

Low birth weight is the most frequent and clearly documented adverse outcome associated with fetal exposure to a great many drugs. Drugs taken by males may also adversely affect fetuses.

Mini-Quiz: Pregnancy

T/F: When women were asked about their drug use during pregnancy, their answers corresponded closely with the results of urine analyses.

false; urine assays indicated heavier drug use

List three limitations of survey research for determining whether or not a drug is dangerous to the fetus if taken during pregnancy.

a. Responses to surveys may not be accurate. See previous question.
b. Survey research may not detect rare birth defects.
c. Survey research is correlational.

T/F: Susceptibility to teratogens is pretty constant throughout pregnancy.

false

T/F: The placental barrier prevents the passage of most drugs from the maternal to the fetal circulation.

false

Daughters of women who took _____ during pregnancy were highly susceptible to vaginal cancer.

diethylstilbestrol

The most frequent adverse outcome associated with fetal exposure to a wide variety of drugs of abuse is _____.

impaired fetal growth

T/F: Fetal development may be affected by paternal drug use.

true

The leading known cause of mental retardation is _____.

fetal alcohol syndrome

T/F: Many central nervous system depressants cause defects similar to those of fetal alcohol syndrome.

probably, though the research is correlational

T/F: Rats given high doses of marijuana have mostly male offspring.

true

Fetuses exposed to sufficient _____ during the critical period develop male characteristics.

testosterone

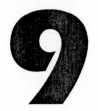

By the time you finish reading this chapter, you should be able to answer the following questions:

In Leavitt's view, who benefits from the laws against drugs: users, potential users, the general populace?

Are there any beneficiaries of the drug laws?

T/F: The number of people convicted of drug crimes has decreased steadily during the past 10 years.

T/F: The length of sentences imposed on convicted drug offenders has decreased during the past 10 years.

T/F: The drug laws help prevent the spread of AIDS.

The Question
of Legalization

Contents

John Stuart Mill asserted that no behavioral practice should be proscribed unless it interferes with the lives of others. Activities that don't victimize others, including bungee jumping, mountain climbing, running with the bulls at Pamplona, being grossly overweight, and living in Los Angeles, should not be crimes. Crimes committed while under the influence of drugs should be prosecuted, not drug use alone. Adherents of Mill's philosophy, even if they acknowledge that many drugs are dangerous, believe that government intrusion into the private lives of citizens is a greater evil. They may try to persuade tobacco smokers to stop, but they oppose bans on tobacco advertising.

I accept Mill's philosophy but am uneasy when it is applied to legalization of drugs. Drunken drivers do not hurt others, accidents hurt; drunken drivers are punished because they make accidents more likely. I support punishment for drunken drivers, and that conflicts with Mill's position. It also weakens my argument that other drugs should be legalized even if they have the potential to harm innocents. Furthermore, many drugs harm subtly, and drug-related impairments have consequences for others besides the immediate victims. They impact on the health, welfare, and educational systems and the burden of taxpayers.

The following questions, to which I have no satisfactory answers, increase my discomfort even more.

1. Should children be permitted to buy and use drugs?

> The obvious reason for answering "No" is that children cannot properly evaluate the dangers. But incompetent adults also exist, both inside and outside of mental institutions and Congress. Perhaps the very act of voluntarily administering a dangerous drug certifies a person as incompetent. Attempted suicide, whether by gun or chemical, is a sign of serious emotional disturbance. So too is a claim, against responsible medical opinion, that a drug is harmless.

2. Should people have the right to freely purchase (a) drugs; (b) handguns?

> Informal surveys have convinced me that most people respond oppositely to the two questions. They usually explain "Yes" answers on the grounds of individual freedom, "Noes" out of concern that the purchaser will cause harm. The inconsistency troubles me. (My own inconsistent answers are "yes," "no.")

3. Do people have the right to keep dangerous animals in their homes?

> Although the owner of a full-grown lion may have sufficient insurance to cover all accidental maimings and deaths, the neighbors may not be reassured. Some drugs, such as cocaine in large doses, may be chemical equivalents of dangerous animals.

Despite the foregoing, I support legalization of all drugs and would do so even if I did not subscribe to Mill's philosophy. The illegality of drugs causes more harm than their pharmacology, and the harm extends to people other than users. Thousands of people have exploited the laws to create criminal fortunes. Legalization would not eliminate the terrible consequences of drug abuse, and it would be irresponsible

Page 47: Classification

85: NEW DRUGS DEVELOP & Testing

171: The question of legalization

311: memory

327: Sexual Behavior
373 Aggression and Violence

Save 50%
on all Regular Priced items

*an unadvertised event for
our valued customers ...*

March Madness Sale!

March 5th - March 7th
Save 50%
on all Regular Priced Items!

Plus save over 70% on Doorbuster Specials

Everything in the store is on sale ...

While quantities last!

Premium Steaks	Chicken
Roasts	Seafood
Burgers	Pork
Appetizers	Desserts

In stock items only – sorry, no rain checks. Not available for mail order.
Cannot be combined with other offers. Expires March 7, 2010.

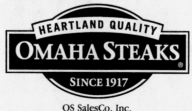

OS SalesCo, Inc.

©2010 OCG   11834

SRC 0029

to assert otherwise. But legalization is the best strategy for minimizing harms. (Legalization would present a new set of practical problems, such as determining age limits for users, penalties for driving while intoxicated, and what to do about the diminished capacity defense. Some promising solutions have been offered, e.g., in Trebach & Zeese [1990]).

▩ Consequences of Drug Laws for Users

The drug laws were not crafted to benefit users—obviously, or they would be less harsh. In 1975, a 19-year old Virginia boy was sentenced to 25 years in prison and a $10,000 fine for possession of marijuana with intent to distribute it; in 1991, a Florida man was sentenced to life imprisonment for selling marijuana (*San Francisco Examiner*, 1991); and at least 150 heroin junkies and small-time pushers were sentenced to life imprisonment within a one-year period in New York City (Fort & Cory, 1975). On the June 15, 1989, *Larry King Live* television show, a caller suggested to then-drug czar William Bennett that drug dealers should be beheaded. He replied, "I mean, what the caller suggests is morally plausible. Legally, it's difficult. . . . But . . . somebody selling drugs to a kid? Morally, I don't have any problem with that at all."

Most drug-using adults do not engage in other illegal activities (Chaiken & Johnson, 1988). But the prices of some illicit drugs, much higher than they would be in a free market, relegate virtually all habitual users to lives of crime. The average heroin addict commits about 1,000 crimes per year (Johnson et al., 1985).

Table 9.1 shows the number of people sentenced to prison for the years from 1980 to 1987 (Flanagan & Maguire, 1990). The number sentenced for drug offenses grew steadily both in absolute terms and as a percentage of the total of all offenders sentenced to prison. In 1990, the latest year for which data are available, the number of new court commitments for drug offenses reached a record high, about 103,800. More people were admitted for drug offenses than for property, violent, or public-order offenses. An estimated 32.1% of all new court commitments in 1990 were for drug offenses (Bureau of Justice Statistics Bulletin, 1992b).

Table 9.2 shows the average sentences imposed in 1980 and 1987. In both years, lengths of sentences were greater for drug than nondrug offenses. In fact, drug offenders received more severe sentences than

Table 9.1 Defendants Sentenced to Prison in U.S. District Court for Drug and Nondrug Offenses 1980-1987

	Total, All Offenders Sentenced to Prison		Offenders Sentenced to Prison for Nondrug Offenses		Offenders Sentenced to Prison for Drug Offense	
	Number	*Annual Percentage Change*	*Number*	*Annual Percentage Change*	*Number*	*Annual Percentage Change*
1980	13,766	—	10,091	—	3,675	—
1981	15,360	11.6	11,007	9.1	4,353	16.4
1982	17,481	13.8	12,343	12.1	5,138	18.0
1983	18,505	5.9	12,940	4.8	5,565	8.3
1984	19,125	3.4	12,638	−2.3	6,487	16.6
1985	20,605	7.7	12,831	1.5	7,774	19.8
1986	23,058	11.9	13,786	7.4	9,272	19.3
1987	23,579	2.3	13,383	−2.9	10,196	10.0

SOURCE: U.S. Department of Justice, Bureau of Justice Statistics, *Federal Criminal Cases, 1980-87*, Special Report NCJ-118311 (Washington, DC: U.S. Department of Justice, July 1989), p. 5, Table 9.

all other offenders except those convicted of murder, nonnegligent manslaughter, robbery, rape, kidnapping, transportation of stolen property, and racketeering. As the percentage of people held in prisons for drug offenses increased, reaching about 50% of all Federal offenders sentenced to prison in 1990, the prisons became severely overcrowded. By the end of 1992, the Federal system was operating at 37% over capacity and state prisons at 118% of their highest capacities (Bureau of Justice Statistics Bulletin, 1992a). At the end of 1990, probation and parole agencies were supervising more than 3.2 million adults in the United States—an estimated 1 of every 43 adults (Bureau of Justice Statistics Bulletin, 1992a). Neal Sonnett, chair of the American Bar Association's criminal justice section, said, "We have a criminal justice system in this country that is on a fast track to collapse because of the heavy emphasis on drug enforcement" (*Oakland Tribune*, February 8, 1993).

The mere threat of imprisonment increases the likelihood that users will develop paranoid feelings, have bad trips, and, because of reluctance to see physicians, allow minor problems to become serious. Because use violates the law, many landlords and employers regard it as sufficient reason for terminating contracts; a consequence is that many addicts are reluctant to seek cures. The unavailability of the

Table 9.2 Defendants Sentenced to Prison in U.S. District Courts for Drug and Nondrug Offenses and Average Sentence Imposed 1980 and 1987

Most Serious Offence	1980		1987		Percentage Change 1980-1987 in:	
	Number Sentenced to Prison	Average Sentence Imposed	Number Sentenced to Prison	Average Sentence Imposed	Number Sentenced to Prison	Average Sentence Imposed
Total	13,766	3.7 years	23,579	4.6 years	71.3%	24.6%
Nondrug offenses	10,091	3.6	13,383	3.8	32.6%	5.4%
Drug offenses	3,675	3.9	10,196	5.6	177.4%	43.9%

SOURCE: U.S. Department of Justice, Bureau of Justice Statistics, *Federal Criminal Cases, 1980-87*, Special Report NCJ-118311 (Washington, DC: U.S. Department of Justice, July 1989), p. 6, Table 11.

legal process increases the likelihood that disputes about drugs will end in violence.

Sellers of illicit drugs, undeterred by truth-in-packaging laws, frequently adulterate their products or substitute entirely different ones for what they claim to be selling. Many of the substitutes and diluents are directly harmful. In other cases, adverse effects occur when a user administers a drug different from what was expected or in a different dose. Treatment is difficult when the offending substance is unknown. Starting in 1979, drugs manufactured in underground laboratories and sold as heroin killed or crippled hundreds of people in California. Thousands of addicts throughout the country may still be regular, unsuspecting users (Straus, 1987). As inferred from the arrest records—see Table 9.3—the number of illegal laboratories is growing steadily.

A high proportion of current abusers (in contrast to users) have a history of mental disorder. Many live in overcrowded, impoverished neighborhoods and have limited employment prospects. If drugs were legally available and inexpensive, they would probably stay high much of the time. That would be tragic, but stiff criminal penalties do not improve their lot. The last thing they need is a "War on Drugs." Far more appropriate would be a "War on the Conditions That Breed Drug Abuse."

Illicit drugs are expensive and some drugs, such as alcohol and cocaine, may promote violence. So, imprisonment of abusers may benefit their families by preventing depletion of resources and protecting family members from physical harm. On the other hand, physically ill people often create a financial burden for their families, and the ethical solution is to help rather than abandon them. Legally available drugs would be much less expensive. Physical abuse is against the law with or without drugs.

▩ Consequences of Drug Laws for Potential Users

Many caring people, uninterested in abstract philosophical arguments, believe that laws protect the vulnerable from exposure to drugs. They may be right. The laws deter some potential experimenters and limit addicts' use. It is scary to contemplate what might happen if drugs were available in neighborhood pharmacies. Goldstein and Kalant (1990) summarized evidence showing that availability of drugs affects consumption.

Table 9.3 Seizures of Illegal Drug Laboratories (by type of drug manufactured, United States, fiscal years 1975-1991)

	Total Illegal Drug Laboratories Seized	PCP	Meth- amphetamine	Amphet- amine	Meth- aqualone	Hashish Oil	LSD	Cocaine	Other Hallu- cinogens	Other Controlled Substances[a]
Total	5,963	518	4,200	604	104	30	20	147	110	230
1975	32	15	11	2	1	0	0	3	0	x
1976	97	30	36	11	5	4	4	7	0	x
1977	148	66	46	10	10	6	1	2	7	x
1978	180	79	69	12	7	5	0	4	4	x
1979	235	53	137	10	9	4	2	5	15	x
1980	234	49	126	20	17	1	4	2	15	x
1981	182	35	87	14	13	2	4	5	10	12
1982	224	47	132	18	7	0	0	6	7	7
1983	226	39	119	25	10	4	0	11	11	7
1984	197	13	121	19	3	3	0	16	3	19
1985	419	23	257	67	5	0	1	29	2	35
1986	509	8	372	66	4	0	2	23	6	28
1987	682	13	561	68	1	1	1	17	2	18
1988	810	20	667	82	4	0	0	9	7	21
1989	852	13	683	101	5	0	0	1	0	49
1990	549	10	449	54	3	0	0	4	10	19
1991	387	5	327	25	0	0	1	3	11	15

SOURCE: Comptroller General of the United States. *Report to the Congress: Stronger Crackdown Needed on Clandestine Laboratories Manufacturing Dangerous Drugs* (Washington, DC: U.S. General Accounting Office, 1981), p. 37; and data provided to SOURCEBOOK (1992) staff by the U.S. Department of Justice, Drug Enforcement Administration.
NOTE: a. This category includes other controlled substances such as phenal 2 propanone, a precursor used in making methamphetamine and amphetamine, and methadone, an opiate-type heroin substitute.

1. During prohibition of alcohol in the United States, both alcoholism and deaths from liver cirrhosis declined considerably. More recently, several states lowered the legal drinking age, and alcohol-related driving accidents immediately increased. Several studies show that alcohol consumption varies inversely with price.
2. Physicians, dentists, and nurses have easy access to psychoactive drugs and a much higher per capita addiction rate than other professionals.
3. The imposition in New York State of an accurate record system for tracking benzodiazepine prescriptions produced a dramatic drop in consumption.
4. Tobacco smoking varies inversely with the price of cigarettes.
5. The cocaine epidemic in the United States has been attributed in part to the introduction of crack cocaine, which is much cheaper than cocaine salt preparations.

But the issue is complex. Other evidence suggests that current laws do not have a large deterrent effect.

1. Only 7.1% of nonusing high school students said they were deterred by the laws (cited in Stachnik, 1972). Drug dealers who had and had not been arrested were equally likely to quit or control their sales (Fish & Bruhnsen, 1979). Surveyors reported that about 23.7 million Americans have tried cocaine, 67.7 million, marijuana, and 2.9 million, heroin, although all are prohibited by law (NIDA, 1991). Clearly, factors other than legal status govern people's choices. The surveyors also found that, despite cocaine's reputation as an extremely addicting drug, fewer than 10% of people who ever used had used in the previous month.

2. Although legalization would encourage many current abstainers to experiment, the number of drug *abusers* would probably not change much—just as the number of suicide attempts would be little affected by repeal of laws against attempted suicide.

3. Sensation-seeking is one motive for using drugs (see Chapter 10), and illegality adds to the sensation. Illegality also forces casual users to come in contact with hardened criminals; they become more likely to try a variety of drugs and other criminal behaviors.

4. Drug sellers, like sellers of other products, continually strive to expand their markets. They try to get vulnerable people, especially children, hooked. Virtually all habitual heroin users recruit customers (Johnson et al., 1985). People who dispensed drugs legally in government stores would have much less incentive to increase sales.

5. Eleven states in the United States decriminalized marijuana in the late 1970s and experienced no subsequent increase in use (Nadelmann, 1988).

6. In the Netherlands, drug abusers are treated as sick people rather than criminals. Dutch policy makes therapy available whenever abusers want it and offers free needle exchange for intravenous users. Since the early 1970s, marijuana has been technically illegal but dispensed freely in Dutch coffee shops. People buy it even when police are around. The Dutch use as much or more alcohol and tobacco, but less of all the drugs that are illicit in the United States (Trebach & Zeese, 1990).

7. Legalizing need not send a message that drugs are safe. Tobacco is legal, and the tobacco industry advertises relentlessly; but efforts by the National Cancer Institute and Surgeon General's office to publicize its dangers have worked. Almost half of all living U.S. adults who ever smoked tobacco have quit (Trebach & Zeese, 1990). The antitobacco campaign accomplishes its objectives better than do the drug laws.

▓ Consequences of Drug Laws for the General Populace

People who cheer when police confiscate huge quantities of illegal drugs might be less enthusiastic if they understood the consequences. Successful drug raids drive up prices but rarely persuade habitual users to take up less expensive hobbies. Instead, they commit more crimes. Brown and Silverman (1974) developed a statistical model suggesting that a 10% increase in the price of heroin leads to a 3.6% increase in robberies, a 1.8% increase in burglaries, a 2% increase in petty larceny, a 2.5% increase in auto theft, and a 1.7% increase in taxicab robberies. Even when prices are stable, the potential profits from illegal drugs make violence inevitable. In both Washington, D.C., and New York City, the police attributed record numbers of assaults and homicides to drug dealers (Cooper, 1990). Taxpayers pay a heavy burden for criminalizing drug users. Ostrowski (1990) reported that drug-related law enforcement—courts, police, and prisons on all levels of government—costs about 10 billion dollars per year.

The view that marijuana is a stepping stone to more harmful drugs has been largely discredited (cf. Trebach, 1987). But unreasonable or unfairly administered laws, because they breed disrespect for other laws, are stepping stones of a different sort. More than 75 million U.S.

citizens have tried marijuana or other illicit drugs, but only a small fraction have been arrested. Whether caught or not, they have committed criminal acts. About half of the adult citizenry of our nation are criminals on the loose.

Enforcement of victimless crime laws is invariably discriminatory. Well-to-do violators act with relative impunity in their secluded homes and clubs, whereas the actions of poorer people are under much greater scrutiny. Beers (1991) noted that 80% of U.S. drug users are Caucasian but the majority arrested are African American. Drug prosecutions of white juveniles dropped 15% between 1985 and 1988 while jumping 88% for minority youth. Discrimination comes in other forms as well: Not only do law-abiding residents of inner cities live in terror from drug-related violence, they find it extremely difficult to get insurance or loans. Investors stay away. Inner-city children have few positive role models. The most successful people, if accumulation of material goods is the criterion, are the drug kingpins. The result is a subversion of education and morality. A 1991 Los Angeles Times story told of a 3-year-old girl who stood in front of her house and took orders for cocaine.

The Bill of Rights is a victim of the drug laws. New York Port Authority police identify people, generally lower-income African Americans and Latinos, who fit a "drug courier profile." The suspects are usually questioned and searched. Boston police have stopped hundreds of minority youth on the streets and searched them for drugs (Ellis, 1991). Tenants in public housing projects in Chicago were required to submit to repeated inspections of their apartments, including all personal belongings. Similar actions have been taken in Washington, D.C., New York City, Orlando, New Haven, Charleston, and Alexandria (Zeese, 1989).

The laws promote hypocrisy. As part of their punishment, many celebrities convicted of drug law violations have been required to publicly condemn use. The rationale is that celebrities are role models, thus highly persuasive. But discerning listeners might conclude that sufficiently well-connected people can minimize punishments by disavowing their true beliefs.

Related to hypocrisy are the suppression of information and spread of misinformation. Trebach (1991) reported being told that his book The Great Drug War had been banned from inclusion on a government archive computer disk because it disagreed with government policy. But a policy of disinformation sabotages the effectiveness of reports of real dangers. When stories about anabolic steroids first reached the sports pages, most authorities claimed that steroids do not improve athletic performance. Athletes, however, saw improvements and concluded that the experts were either lying or misinformed. So subsequent reports documenting very serious dangers were largely ignored, and steroid use escalated.

Many prominent U.S. citizens, among them President Bill Clinton, Vice President Albert Gore, Representative Newt Gingrich, Supreme Court Justice nominee Douglas Ginsburg, Supreme Court Justice Clarence Thomas, and Massachusetts Attorney General James Shannon (who now favors mandatory prison time for casual users), have admitted to youthful experimentation with illicit drugs; and ex-President George Bush and drug czar William Bennett both said that past marijuana-smoking should not disqualify someone from future high office (Kinsley, 1990). Three points need to be made. First, many crimes do disqualify people from future high office, so drug use must be viewed as somehow different. Second, President Clinton and his co-confessors presumably believe that the drugs produced no long-lasting harms. Third, people continue to be arrested for those same youthful indiscretions and face lengthy prison sentences.

Intravenous (IV) drug users are a very high-risk group for AIDS, and they spread the disease to sex partners and children, born and yet unborn. The virus that causes AIDS is transmitted when unsterile needles are shared, and sharing occurs largely because drug laws ensure that needles are hard to obtain. The Centers for Disease Control estimated that 27,000 AIDS cases in the United States as of mid-1989 were related to IV drug use (cited in Trebach & Zeese, 1990). By contrast, in Austria, England, and the Netherlands, three countries that allow addicts to exchange dirty for sterile needles, the numbers were, respectively, 104, 80, and 75.

The drug laws lead to corruption of government and banking officials, judges, and police. Cooper (1990) and Carter (1990) cited many cases and Carter, on the basis of several references, estimated that at least 30% of the nation's police officers have been involved with illicit drugs since being employed in law enforcement. According to *Time* magazine (October 11, 1993), "The deluge of cash that has flowed from the drug trade has created opportunities for quick dirty money on a scale never seen before."

▩ Beneficiaries of the Drug Laws

Ostrowski (1990) estimated annual sales of illegal drugs at 80 billion dollars. That means substantial profits for some. Entrepreneurs have started new businesses—Byrd Laboratories of Austin, TX, advertises in various newspapers, "Pamphlet: 'Conquering the Urine Tests,' $5. Our famous Drug Free Powdered Urine, $19.95. Guaranteed." Jones (1992) estimated that 20 million people in the United States had urine tests in 1991 at a cost of about $350 million.

Young children make about $15 a day turning in empty crack vials for recycling, older children earn far more than the minimum wage as lookouts protecting drug transactions, and some 12-year-olds make $1,000 per week selling crack (Cooper, 1990). Marijuana is so much more profitable than other crops that, between 1981 and 1987, production in the United States nearly tripled; the net profits make it the country's biggest cash crop (Cooper, 1990). Reuter (1990) estimated that crew members on ships coming up from Colombia earned about $15,000 each for smuggling 100-kilograms of cocaine; and pilots who flew 250-kilogram shipments of cocaine over the Mexican border received $250,000.

Employers of the pilots make vastly larger sums. A 1989 *Frontline* television show ("Who Profits From Drugs?") devoted exclusively to the laundering of drug money cited criminal cases within the United States extending from coast to coast and Florida to New England. People indicted or convicted of drug money laundering include U.S. congressmen, lobbyists, bankers and chairmen of boards of banks, lawyers, accountants, college professors, and trade unionists. According to officials within the Drug Enforcement Administration, only a small fraction of the participants are caught while the rest continue to benefit. Members of the business community, by accepting large cash payments, are an essential part of drug money laundering operations. Mentioned on the *Frontline* show were stores in Boston's Faneuil Hall Market Place, restaurants, brokerages, the Apache boat racing team, banks, nightclubs, commercial and residential real estate ventures, and a radio station.

The drug industry benefits from the drug laws. The nonprofit organization Partnership for a Drug-Free America creates and pays for antidrug messages, such as the television commercial with a fried egg and the words, "This is your brain on drugs." Cotts (1992) noted that the ads have frequently distorted, exaggerated, and relied on scare tactics rather than reliable evidence. The Partnership focuses on illegal drugs while overlooking the dangers of tobacco, alcohol, and prescription and over-the-counter drugs.

More than 50% of Partnership financial support—more than 5.4 million dollars—has come from manufacturers of legal drugs. Cotts inferred that, "The war on drugs is a war on illegal drugs, and the Partnership's benefactors have a huge stake in keeping it that way. They know that when schoolchildren learn that marijuana and crack are evil, they're also learning that alcohol, tobacco and pills are as American as apple pie."

Many government employees benefit from the drug laws, and the world press has noticed. The following is condensed from an article in the Wellington, New Zealand *Dominion Sunday Times* (September 27, 1992).

The 1985 drug forfeiture laws allow government agencies to confiscate assets of convicted traffickers. After a police officer from the seven-person force in Little Compton, RI, helped capture a major drug baron, the Little Compton force was awarded 3 million dollars. The police chief bought the heroic officer a Formula Firebird Pontiac, then added to the police fleet two new cruisers with video cameras on the dashboard. Soon, cars outnumbered officers. The chief—in a town of 3,400 where there has been no murder for 27 years—bought a computer system that gave immediate access to every crime record since 1960. He bought bulletproof vests, guns with laser sights, and a new tower to boost his radio system. After renovating his offices and commissioning architects to design a rifle range, he proposed building a $750,000 police and fire station complex. The town barber filed a lawsuit, however, and a judge froze the remaining money until the next year's town meeting.

Other government agencies have also spent freely, purchasing items such as giant-screen television sets, fitness centers, Christmas parties, amusement park tickets, and Las Vegas junkets. Opponents of the law are concerned that police confiscate assets from people who have committed minor offenses or are merely under suspicion. A New Hampshire family with three small children had their home seized for growing four marijuana plants in the back garden.

The article ended with a quote from Bo Edward, an attorney from Nashville, TN: "the whole forfeiture deal is nothing but legalized theft by the government."

▨ A Note on Laws Related to Tobacco and Alcohol Use

In sharp contrast to the laws that illegalize many drugs is legislation related to the two major drugs of abuse. The motivation has often been protection of special interest groups rather than concern for public health. Demoss (1992) wrote, "Ironically, the U.S. government spends billions of dollars on antidrug campaigns . . . while at the same time, it provides tobacco growers with $3 billion per year in subsidies and tax exemptions for cigarette advertising." The United States is the major world supplier of tobacco.

Summary

Although drug abuse is a serious problem, laws against drugs harm both users and abstainers.

Drug laws harm abusers—the laws inflict severe penalties that work against rehabilitation.

The laws are probably ineffective in deterring potential users.

The laws discriminate against minorities and subvert education, morality, and the Bill of Rights. They are a factor in the spread of AIDS. They create huge potential financial gains for police officers, business people, and politicians, which tempt such people to break laws.

Mini-Quiz: Legalization

List two reasons given in the text for retaining laws against use of various drugs. List four reasons for repealing the laws and making all drug use legal.

Reasons for keeping drugs illegal:
1. Legalization would increase availability, and increased availability would probably mean increased consumption.
2. The argument that drug abuse is a victimless crime is fallacious:
   a. People impaired because of drug abuse impose a burden on taxpayers.
   b. People intoxicated on some drugs may deliberately or accidently cause physical harm to innocent others.

Reasons for repealing the drug laws:
1. "The less government we have, the better" (Ralph Waldo Emerson).
2. Drug users suffer more than they would if drugs were legal.
3. The deterrent effect of drug laws is probably small.
4. The general populace suffers because of the drug laws.
   a. The laws increase crimes against nonusers.
   b. The laws are enforced in a discriminatory way, which breeds disrespect for other laws.
   c. Because of the laws, people who interact with drug abusers, and people who interact with them, are at increased risk for contracting various diseases.
   d. Many people become wealthy because of the laws, and they become role models for youths.
   e. The laws lead to corruption of public officials.

By the time you finish reading this chapter, you should be able to answer the following questions:

Why is it unsatisfactory to use only two categories for classifying people's drug habits?

What is a reasonable definition of drug abuse?

How is information gathered for estimating use of drugs?

What are the weaknesses of survey data?

How do men and women differ in drug use?

What types of evidence have been used to show that drug abuse has a genetic component?

What combination of traits in first graders is highly predictive of adult drug abuse?

How can animals be induced to voluntarily consume large quantities of alcohol and other drugs?

Why do people use drugs?

What is the self-medication hypothesis?

T/F: People who use any one drug excessively are likely to be heavy users of other drugs.

T/F: Many animals use drugs.

T/F: Drug use declines with age.

Users and
Abusers of Drugs

Contents

Some writers recognize only two categories of drug use: abusers and abstainers. They do not distinguish between one-time experimenters, occasional users, and heavy abusers. Blumenfield et al. (1972) defined abuse as any use of an illicit substance, Blum (1984) defined it as "the use of a drug that is not legally or socially sanctioned," and the Office of Substance Abuse Prevention [OSAP] (1989) wrote, "all use of illegal drugs and all use of legal drugs (specifically alcohol) by persons under the legal age is defined as abuse."

The dichotomy, although easy to apply, is misleading and unsatisfactory. It defines abuse by legal rather than medical standards and disregards that some drugs, even illicit ones, sometimes enhance overall functioning. For example, infrequent low-dose amphetamine use improves certain types of performance, and moderate alcohol drinking may increase longevity (although heavy use of either endangers both physical and emotional health). As discussed below, Jurich and Polson (1984) showed large differences between users and abusers in both personality and motivations for use.

An alternative approach is to define abuse by consequences such as physical complaints and impaired work habits and family relationships. Shifting the focus to consequences means that many of the 68 million Americans who have tried marijuana would no longer be classified as drug abusers—but virtually all of the 55 million current U.S. cigarette smokers would be.

░ Methods of Data Collection

Cole and Chiarello (1990) reviewed national programs for determining incidence and prevalence of use of prescription, over-the-counter, and illicit drugs. Individual researchers have used similar methods to study specific drugs. For legal drugs such as alcohol, the amount consumed is estimated from tax receipts and industry records.

SURVEY DATA

The National Prescription Audit monitors sales of prescriptions, and the National Disease and Therapeutic Index surveys prescription practices of a sample of physicians. According to Cole and Chiarello (1990), data from both are difficult to obtain and use.

The High School and Young Adult Survey is conducted annually. The National Household Survey on Drug Abuse, conducted every few years and most recently in 1991, provides data based on extensive interviews with a large cross section of the population. Most of the statistics on **incidence** and **prevalence** for this chapter come from the 1991 survey.

It is dangerous to place too much faith in survey data. Small differences in the wording of questions and statistical analyses often have large effects on estimates of drug use (cf. Room, 1990). In addition, survey data are subject to two important types of distortion. First, respondents and nonrespondents often differ in important ways including use of drugs. For the 1991 survey, about 16% of those approached refused to participate. Some segments of society with high rates of drug abuse are typically never even approached: the homeless, school absentees and dropouts, prisoners, and inmates of mental institutions. So, estimates of total use are likely to be low (Dryfoos, 1990; McKirnan & Johnson, 1986; Robertson, Koegel, & Ferguson, 1989; Smart & Adlaf, 1991). Contrast the 1990 National Household Survey estimates of heavy cocaine (662,000) and heroin users (200,000) with estimates from a study commissioned by the Senate Judiciary Committee (2.4 million and 1 million, respectively; Kelly, 1990). Kaufman and McNaul (1992) suggested that efforts during the past decade to prevent drug use may appear to have succeeded only because many abusers have been expelled from schools.

A second type of distortion occurs because respondents sometimes forget, lie, or answer inconsistently. Warner (1977) noted that public awareness of dangers of smoking had more impact on self-reports of smoking than on actual smoking behavior. Zuckerman et al. (1989) recruited 1,226 women from a prenatal clinic and questioned them about cocaine and marijuana use; 16% who gave positive urine analyses for marijuana and 24% who were positive for cocaine denied use.

Although self-report data from the National Household Survey on Drug Abuse indicate a 36% decline in marijuana use between 1985 and 1988, estimated U.S. domestic production and nondomestic production available for use in the United States during the same time period increased 119% and 58%, respectively (Sidney, 1990). The *Oakland Tribune* (1984) reported on a series of raids in northern Mexico leading to the seizure of more than 10,000 tons of marijuana destined for the United States: more than eight times the total that authorities had believed was produced yearly in all of Mexico and about as much as they believed was used in an entire year in the United States.

PATIENT DATA COLLECTION SYSTEMS

The Drug Abuse Warning Network (DAWN) covers 756 emergency rooms and 75 medical examiner's offices in 27 U.S. metropolitan areas.

DAWN collects data on people who have problems associated with non-medical drug use. The latest available data are from 1987.

The Client Oriented Data Acquisition Process provides data on drug treatment facilities that receive federal funds. Data are collected only on people who seek treatment in one of the facilities.

▓ Amounts of Use

In 1982, world drug use to treat medical problems, excluding herbal preparations, was estimated at 214 million kilograms (cited in Albert, 1987). The United States consumed 34% of the total, Western Europe 32%, Japan 4%, and the rest of the world 30%. (Their respective populations were 228, 336, 117, and 4,120 million.) In industrialized countries, about half the total resulted from physician prescriptions and half as over-the-counter remedies for minor ailments.

Table 10.1 provides an overview of past month, past year, and lifetime users of illicit drugs, alcohol, and caffeine. Based on surveys, about 12.6 million of the approximately 203 million (6.2%) in the U.S. household population aged 12 and older would admit to illicit drug use at least once during the previous month; 26 million (12.8%) to past year use; and 75.4 million (37%) to using an illicit drug at least once in their lifetimes. The difference between lifetime prevalence and past month use supports the view that use and abuse should be distinguished.

In 1989, U.S. pharmacies dispensed an estimated 880.8 million new prescriptions and 1.64 billion prescriptions overall (Burke, Baum, Jolson, & Kennedy, 1991). Svarstad (1983) reported that 90% of women and 83% of men said they had used at least one over-the-counter drug in the past month. The average daily caffeine consumption is 3 mg/kg for U.S. adults (Barone & Roberts, 1984).[1]

▓ Extent of Abuse

Regier et al. (1988) used household interviews as a basis for estimating that 2.3 million adults meet the clinical criteria for drug abuse in any given month, 3.4 million over a 6-month period. Surveyors for the Institute of Medicine (1990) estimated that 1.5 million of the 14.5 million U.S. adults who had used drugs at least once in the past 30 days clearly needed drug abuse treatment; 3.1 million had a probable need;

Table 10.1   Use of Illicit Drugs, Alcohol, and Cigarettes: Past Month, Past Year, and Ever[a]

	Past Month	*Past Year*	*Ever*
Anabolic steroids	—[d]	307	1,042
Cocaine	1,892	6,383	23,715
Heroin	—[d]	701	2,886
Inhalants	1,213	2,876	11,270
Marijuana	9,721	19,549	67,689
Nonmedical Use of:			
Analgesics	1,403	5,090	12,337
Psychedelics[b]	693	2,787	16,692
Sedatives	755	2,130	8,684
Stimulants	668	2,709	14,249
Tranquilizers	889	3,408	11,331
Needle users[c]	—[d]	1,083	3,768
Any illicit dug use	12,647	26,062	75,351
Alcohol	103,232	138,238	171,857
Cigarettes	54,805	65,119	147,531

NOTES: a. Estimates are in thousands. Multiply each entry by 1,000 to get actual population figures. For example, 307,000 people admitted using anabolic steroids during the past year.
b. LSD, PCP, and similar substances.
c. Needle use includes use of cocaine, heroin, or amphetamines with a needle.
d. No estimates reported.

2.9 million a possible need; and 6.9 million no need. Hilton (1987) reported that 7% of all alcohol drinkers had experienced moderate levels of dependence symptoms during the preceding year; and Moore et al. (1989) found that 25% of newly admitted adult hospital inpatients met the criteria for alcoholism.

▓ Trends in Use

Between 1985 and 1991, according to the National Household Survey on Drug Abuse (NIDA, 1991), the prevalence rates for current use (past month) of any illicit drug declined from 14.9% to 6.8% among 12- to 17-year-olds, from 25.7% to 15.4% among 18- to 25-year-olds, and from 8.5% to 4.5% among people age 26 and older. During the same time period, rates of alcohol and cigarette use also declined in all three age

Table 10.2 Reported Drug Use Within Last 30 Days Among High School

Question: "On how many occasions, if any, have you used . . . during the last

Type of Drug	Class of 1980	Class of 1981	Class of 1982	Class of 1983	Class of 1984
Marijuana/hashish	33.7	31.6	28.5	27.0	25.2
Inhalants[a]	1.4	1.5	1.5	1.7	1.9
Adjusted[b]	2.7	2.5	2.5	2.5	2.5
Amyl and butyl nitrites[c, d]	1.8	1.4	1.1	1.4	1.4
Hallucinogens	3.7	3.7	3.4	2.8	2.6
Adjusted[e]	4.4	4.5	4.1	3.5	3.2
LSD	2.3	2.5	2.4	1.9	1.5
PCP[c, d]	1.4	1.4	1.0	1.3	1.0
Cocaine	5.2	5.8	5.0	4.9	5.8
"Crack"[f]	NA	NA	NA	NA	NA
Other cocaine[g]	NA	NA	NA	NA	NA
Heroin	0.2	0.2	0.2	0.2	0.3
Other opiates[h]	2.4	2.1	1.8	1.8	1.8
Stimulants[h]	12.1	15.8	13.7	12.4	NA
Adjusted[h, i]	NA	NA	10.7	8.9	8.3
Crystal methamphetamine[j]	NA	NA	NA	NA	NA
Sedatives[h, k]	4.8	4.6	3.4	3.0	2.3
Barbiturates[h]	2.9	2.6	2.0	2.1	1.7
Methaqualone[h, k]	3.3	3.1	2.4	1.8	1.1
Tranquilizers[h]	3.1	2.7	2.4	2.5	2.1
Alcohol	72.0	70.7	69.7	69.4	67.2
Steroids[j]	NA	NA	NA	NA	NA
Cigarettes	30.5	29.4	30.0	30.3	29.3

SOURCE: L. D. Johnston, P. M. O'Malley, & J. G. Backman, *National Survey Results on Drug Use From Monitoring the Future Study, 1975-1992*, U.S. Department of Health and Human Services, National Institute on Drug Abuse (Washington, DC: Government Printing Office, 1993). Table adapted by SOURCEBOOK staff; *Bureau of Justice Statistics Sourcebook of Criminal Justice Statistics 1992. Washington, DC: Hindelang Criminal Justice Research Center.*
NOTES: a. Data based on four questionnaire forms in 1976-1988; N is four fifths of N indicated. Data based on five questionnaire forms in 1986-1992; N is five sixths of N indicated.
b. Adjusted for underreporting of amyl and butyl nitrites.
c. Data based on a single questionnaire form; N is one fifth of N indicated in 1979-1988 and one sixth of N indicated in 1989-1992.
d. Question text changed slightly in 1987.
e. Adjusted for underreporting of PCP.
f. Data based on a single questionnaire form in 1986; N is one fifth of N indicated. Data based on two questionnaire forms in 1987-1989; N is two fifths of N indicated in 1987-1988 and two sixths of N indicated in 1989. Data based on six questionnaire forms in 1990-1992.

Seniors, by Type of Drug, 1980-1992

30 days?" (Percentage who used in last 30 days)

Class of 1985	Class of 1986	Class of 1987	Class of 1988	Class of 1989	Class of 1990	Class of 1991	Class of 1992
25.7	23.4	21.0	18.0	16.7	14.0	13.8	11.9
2.2	2.5	2.8	2.6	2.3	2.7	2.4	2.3
3.0	3.2	3.5	3.0	2.7	2.9	2.6	2.5
1.5	1.3	1.3	0.6	0.6	0.6	0.4	0.3
2.5	2.5	2.5	2.2	2.2	2.2	2.2	2.1
3.8	3.5	2.8	2.3	2.9	2.3	2.4	2.3
1.6	1.7	1.8	1.8	1.8	1.9	1.9	2.0
1.5	1.3	0.6	0.3	1.4	0.4	0.5	0.6
6.7	6.2	4.3	3.4	2.8	1.9	1.4	1.3
NA	NA	1.3	1.6	1.4	0.7	0.7	0.6
NA	NA	4.1	3.2	1.9	1.7	1.2	1.0
0.3	0.2	0.2	0.2	0.3	0.2	0.2	0.3
2.3	2.0	1.8	1.6	1.6	1.5	1.0	1.2
NA	NA	NA	NA	NA	NA	NA	NA
6.8	5.5	5.2	4.6	4.2	3.7	3.2	2.8
NA	NA	NA	NA	NA	0.6	0.6	0.5
2.4	2.2	1.7	1.4	1.6	1.4	1.5	1.2
2.0	1.8	1.4	1.2	1.4	1.3	1.4	1.1
1.0	0.9	0.6	0.5	0.6	0.2	0.2.	0.4
2.1	2.1	2.0	1.5	1.3	1.2	1.4	1.0
65.9	65.3	66.4	63.9	60.0	57.1	54.0	51.3
NA	NA	NA	NA	0.8	1.0	0.8	0.6
30.1	29.6	29.4	28.7	28.6	29.4	28.3	27.8

g. Data based on a single questionnaire form in 1987-1989; N is one fifth of N indicated in 1987-1988 and one sixth of N indicated in 1989. Data based on four questionnaire forms in 1990-1992; N is four sixths of N indicated.

h. Only drug use that was not under a doctor's care is included here.

i. Beginning in 1982 the question about stimulant use (i.e., amphetamines) was revised to get respondents to exclude the inappropriate reporting of non-prescription stimulants. The prevalence rate dropped slightly as a result of this methodological change.

j. Data based on two questionnaire forms; N is two sixths of N indicated. Steroid data based on a single questionnaire form in 1989-1990.

k. Data based on five questionnaire forms in 1975-1988, six questionnaire forms in 1989, and one questionnaire form in 1990-1992. N is one sixth of N indicated in 1990-1992.

Table 10.3 Intercorrelations Between Reported Use of 19 Different Drugs[a]

	1	2	3	4	5	6	7	8	9
1. Alcohol	—								
2. Barbiturates	.15	—							
3. Marijuana	.28	.39	—						
4. Hashish	.20	.38	.77	—					
5. LSD	.05	.50	.55	.57	—				
6. Other psychedelics	.03	.38	.51	.61	.65	—			
7. Opiates	.01	.35	.39	.48	.49	.49	—		
8. Methadone	.05	.19	.18	.19	.14	.12	.32	—	
9. Pain killers	.10	.23	.08	.09	.13	.14	.23	.06	—
10. Antidepressants	.08	.30	.08	.17	.13	.18	.25	.09	.30
11. Tranquilizers	.04	.37	.12	.11	.23	.14	.34	.28	.42
12. Sedatives	.07	.36	.16	.18	.26	.24	.30	.03	.42
13. Cocaine	.05	.44	.58	.55	.66	.57	.51	.19	.15
14. Amphetamine	.13	.44	.44	.48	.47	.42	.44	.13	.15
15. Relaxants	.01	.46	.12	.14	.26	.24	.32	.16	.39
16. Over-the-counter	.00	.09	−.01	−.04	−.08	−.04	−.13	−.01	.00
17. Anti-infectious	.01	.13	−.07	−.02	−.03	.14	.18	.09	.34
18. Diet pills	.00	.21	.14	.25	.20	.27	.30	.07	.16
19. Tobacco	.14	.14	.18	.13	.08	.11	.12	.12	.11

SOURCE: Reprinted from F. Douglass & K. Khavari, "The Drug Use Index: A Measure of the Extent Dekker, Inc.
NOTE: a. r^2 greater than .15 are significant at the .01 level.

groups. Table 10.2 shows trends from 1980 to 1992 in recent use of various drugs by high school seniors. Smart (1991b) reported data on world trends in known legal production and sales of alcohol; between 1970 and 1980, per capita consumption increased 3.6%, with the greatest increase in North America (24.4%).

10	11	12	13	14	15	16	17	18
—								
.40	—							
.20	.41	—						
.19	.17	.26	—					
.22	.16	.27	.47	—				
.32	.48	.38	.26	.20	—			
.00	−.02	.01	−.09	.04	.06	—		
.07	.24	.36	.05	.07	.23	.09	—	
.28	.20	.14	.19	.25	.17	.10	.04	—
.13	.12	.11	.15	.14	.16	.00	−.02	.06

of Polydrug Use," *International Journal of Addiction*, 1978, 13, pp. 981-993, by courtesy of Marcel

�֍ Polydrug Use

The person who takes pills to lose weight, fall asleep, stay awake, or have bowel movements with clocklike regularity, has many traits in common with users of illicit drugs such as cocaine and heroin. College students most willing to use tobacco, alcohol, and caffeine were also most willing to use amphetamines, hallucinogens, and opiates (Brehm & Back, 1968). Use of any of several legal and illegal drugs by adolescents correlated significantly with use of others (Block, Block, & Keyes, 1988). Heroin addicts drink alcohol excessively and misuse sedative-hypnotics (O'Donnell, 1968; Ricjman, Jackson, & Trigg, 1973). Ninety-two percent of alcoholics and 99% of heroin addicts smoke (Russell, 1971a, 1971b); and increases in marijuana use are associated with heavier use of other drugs (Cohen, 1972). From surveys of industrial workers and college students, Douglass and Khavari (1978) computed intercorrelations between different drugs and drug classes. As seen in Table 10.3, many are significant.

⊗ Who Uses

The preceding statistics show that drug use is not restricted to scattered enclaves in Berkeley, Greenwich Village, and Harlem. In fact, LaBarre (1975), Wasson (1968), and Siegel (1989) have suggested that drugs have been used in virtually every culture throughout recorded history. Alcoholic beverages predate even Monday night football. The Bible reports that Noah "planted a vineyard and he drank of the wine, and was drunken." Plato, in 400 B.C., discussed juvenile drunkenness. A Chinese emperor of 2200 B.C. described marijuana use. A grave in Peru dating from A.D. 500 contained several bags of coca leaves among necessities for the afterlife. Another happy corpse was discovered in South America with a snuff tube. A tablet from 4000 B.C. mentioned the "joy plant," almost surely opium. The *Amanita muscaria* mushroom was probably used as far back as 2000 B.C.

Balabanova, Parsche, and Pirsig (1992) used **radioimmunoassay** and **gas chromatography/mass spectrometry** on samples of soft tissue, bone, and hair from three female and six male Egyptian mummies who lived during a period spanning from about 1070 B.C. to A.D. 395. Cocaine and hashish were detected in all nine samples and nicotine in eight.

Extending the boundaries even more, Siegel (1986) explored drug use among animals. We all know about reindeer (see p. 40), but as indicated in Table 10.4, there are many other jungle revelers.

Table 10.4   Wild Animals and the Drugs They Consume

Species	Drug
Pigeons	Cannabis seeds
Horses	Tea leaves
Mongooses	Bufotenine-rich toads
Elephants	Fermented palm fruit
Goats	Coffee plants
Donkeys	Wild tobacco
Cows, water buffalo, antelope	Opium poppies
Squirrels, birds, elephants	Fermenting fruit (alcohol)
Jaguars	A hallucinogenic bark
Boars	A hallucinogenic root
Dogs, cattle	Psilocybin mushrooms

▨ Demographic Characteristics of Users

GENDER

Table 10.5, consistent with the general finding that men commit more crimes of all sorts than do women (Silverman, 1982), indicates that more men than women report using illicit drugs. Interestingly, twice as many women as men were addicted to opioid narcotics until the drugs were made illegal in the United States, and the same trend occurred in England (Erickson & Watson, 1990). Men use more alcohol and tobacco, women more prescription and over-the-counter drugs. Possible reasons for the latter are that women live longer (the elderly are our major drug users—see below), are more likely to survive their spouses and use drugs during the mourning period, have more symptoms from acute and chronic conditions (Verbrugge, 1982), and have major physiological changes—menstrual cycle, pregnancy, childbirth, and menopause—during which times their chances of receiving psychotherapeutic drugs are greater than normal.

RACE

Table 10.5 shows differences in gender, race, and age for self-reporting of drug use. Tables 10.6 and 10.7 are based on surveys of high school seniors over the years 1985-1989 (Bachman et al., 1991). The order of

Table 10.5 Demographic Characteristics of Drug Users

	Illicit Drugs		Cigarettes		Alcohol	
Percentage Using	Past Month	Ever	Past Month	Ever	Past Month	Ever
Gender						
Male	7.5	41.1	28.7	77.3	58.1	90.0
Female	5.0	33.5	25.5	68.5	44.3	80.7
Race						
Black	9.4	39.2	27.9	65.4	43.7	79.0
Hispanic	6.4	31.0	24.7	60.6	47.5	77.4
White	5.8	37.8	27.3	75.8	52.7	86.8
Age						
12-17	6.8	20.1	10.8	37.9	20.3	46.4
18-25	15.4	54.7	32.2	71.2	63.6	90.2
26-34	8.9	61.8	32.9	76.4	61.7	92.4
35+	3.0	27.5	26.6	78.0	49.5	87.5

reported drug use, from high to low, was Native American, White, Latino, African American, and Asian American.

AGE

Table 10.8 shows the grade of first use for 16 types of drugs. Young adults are the group most heavily involved with illicit drugs and alcohol, but the drug problem is also serious among elderly people (65 and older); they comprise about 12% of the U.S. population and use about 33% of prescription drugs (Ellor & Kurz, 1982). Many take several drugs in combination and say they could not otherwise do their daily activities (Guttman, 1977). Lipscomb (1976) criticized physicians for prescribing a drug for each patient complaint, thereby creating a group of "ancient chemical hippies." He called it the "spaced out grandmother syndrome."

The situation is particularly grim in nursing homes. In one three-state survey, investigators found that 8 of the 10 most frequently prescribed drugs were psychoactive (Prentice, 1979). Beers et al. (1992) had a panel of experts evaluate drug prescriptions in nursing homes in the Los Angeles area. They concluded that (a) 40% of 1,106 residents received at least one inappropriate prescription and 10% received two

Table 10.6 Thirty-Day Prevalence of 14 Types of Drugs, 1985-1989 (data combined, by sex and race)

Types of Drugs	Percentage Who Used in Last 30 Days											
	White Male	Black Male	Mex Am Male	PR&LA Male	Asian Male	Nat Am Male	White Female	Black Female	Mex Am Female	PR&LA Female	Asian Female	Nat Am Female
Minimum N =	(28,056)	(3,688)	(1,518)	(680)	(982)	(537)	(29,808)	(4,499)	(1,599)	(712)	(917)	(531)
Marijuana/Hashish	25.0	18.5	22.0	18.9	9.7	27.6	19.8	9.9	13.6	9.6	8.1	23.9
Inhalants[a]	3.4	1.4	2.3	2.0	1.3	5.2	2.0	1.4	2.1	0.8	0.8	0.9
Hallucinogens	3.5	0.9	2.4	3.0	1.5	3.6	1.7	0.3	0.7	0.4	0.3	2.7
LSD	2.8	0.6	1.9	1.6	1.1	3.1	1.1	0.2	0.3	0.2	0.1	2.2
Cocaine	5.6	2.6	8.2	8.1	1.8	7.3	4.1	1.3	3.0	2.9	2.6	9.2
Heroin	0.3	0.5	0.3	0.9	0.1	1.1	0.1	0.3	0.2	0.2	0.0	0.4
Other opiates[b]	2.3	0.9	1.1	1.5	1.6	4.0	1.9	0.6	0.7	0.5	0.7	2.4
Stimulants[b]	5.6	1.9	4.9	3.1	2.1	8.1	6.0	1.3	4.8	1.2	3.6	10.3
Sedatives[b]	2.2	1.1	2.0	1.8	1.9	4.8	1.7	0.5	0.9	1.3	1.3	2.6
Barbiturates[b]	1.8	0.9	1.7	1.3	1.4	3.7	1.5	0.5	0.8	1.2	1.0	2.1
Methaqualone[b]	0.9	0.5	0.6	0.9	0.8	2.5	0.5	0.1	0.2	0.1	0.6	0.9
Tranquilizers[b]	1.9	0.8	0.8	0.6	1.7	3.1	2.0	0.5	0.9	1.5	0.9	2.2
Alcohol	72.3	49.2	65.0	55.4	43.7	69.0	66.6	32.8	50.5	43.0	34.2	60.2
Cigarettes	29.8	15.6	23.8	22.0	16.8	36.8	34.0	13.3	18.7	24.7	14.3	13.6

SOURCE: From "Racial/Ethnic Differences in Smoking, Drinking, and Illicit Drug Use Among American High School Seniors, 1976-1989" by J. Bachman, J. Wallace, P. O'Malley, L. Johnston, C. Kurth, & H. Neighbors, 1991, *American Journal of Public Health, 81*, pp. 372-377. Copyright © 1991 by *American Journal of Public Health*. Used by permission.

NOTES: a. Data based on four questionnaire forms. N is four fifths of N indicated.
b. Only drug use which was not under a doctor's orders is included here.

Table 10.7 Daily Use of Three Types of Drugs in the Last 30 Days, 1965-1989 (data combined, by sex and race)

Types of Drugs	Percentage Who Used in Last 30 Days											
	White Male	Black Male	Mex Am Male	PR&LA Male	Asian Male	Nat Am Male	White Female	Black Female	Mex Am Female	PR&LA Female	Asian Female	Nat Am Female
Minimum N =	(28,056)	(3,688)	(1,518)	(680)	(982)	(537)	(29,808)	(4,499)	(1,599)	(712)	(917)	(531)
Marijuana/ Hashish	5.1	2.8	4.2	3.5	1.7	8.2	2.1	0.9	1.1	0.5	0.5	4.3
Alcohol Daily	7.0	4.2	8.3	4.0	2.3	10.1	2.8	0.7	2.6	0.9	0.9	5.4
5+ drinks in a row/last 2 weeks	48.1	24.0	45.3	31.4	19.4	48.1	31.3	9.3	23.6	14.5	10.7	33.7
Cigarettes	18.8	8.6	11.6	13.3	9.0	26.0	22.5	7.1	8.1	13.3	9.4	33.8
Half-pack or more per day	12.5	3.3	5.2	6.1	4.4	18.4	13.3	2.2	2.5	4.2	4.5	23.4

SOURCE: From "Racial/Ethnic Differences in Smoking, Drinking, and Illicit Drug Use Among American High School Seniors, 1976-1989" by J. Bachman, J. Wallace, P. O'Malley, L. Johnston, C. Kurth, & H. Neighbors, 1991, *American Journal of Public Health, 81*, pp. 372-377. Copyright © 1991 by *American Journal of Public Health*. Used by permission.

Table 10.8 Incidence of Use for Various Types of Drugs, by Grade; Twelfth Graders, 1992 (Entries are percentages)

Grade in Which Drug Was First Used	Marijuana[a]	Inhalants[a]	Amyl/Butyl Nitrates	Hallucinogens[a]	LSD	PCP	Cocaine	Crack	Other Forms of Cocaine	Heroin	Other Opiates	Stimulants[b]	Barbiturates	Methaqualone	Tranquilizers	Alcohol	Been Drunk	Cigarettes	Cigarettes (Daily)	Smokeless Tobacco	Steroids
6th	2.4	2.1	0.1	0.2	0.2	0.3	0.1	0.0	0.1	0.1	0.2	0.7	0.5	0.2	0.2	11.7	3.5	17.6	1.8	9.2	0.1
7th-8th	7.1	4.8	0.2	1.0	10.9	0.4	0.9	0.4	0.6	0.5	1.1	3.0	1.2	0.3	1.2	25.1	14.8	20.0	5.4	8.5	0.2
9th	7.5	2.9	0.5	1.6	1.5	0.7	1.5	0.6	1.5	0.3	1.4	3.5	1.7	0.4	1.4	21.1	16.1	10.0	4.6	4.3	0.2
10th	6.3	2.7	0.1	2.2	2.2	0.3	1.3	0.5	1.1	0.1	1.4	2.7	1.0	0.2	1.4	14.5	13.6	6.1	3.7	4.1	0.4
11th	5.2	2.3	0.2	2.2	1.9	0.4	1.3	0.6	1.1	0.2	1.4	2.2	0.7	0.2	1.0	10.3	10.1	5.1	3.0	4.4	0.6
12th	4.0	1.7	0.3	1.9	1.8	0.3	1.0	0.5	0.9	0.0	0.7	1.7	0.5	0.2	0.8	4.8	6.4	3.0	1.9	1.8	0.5
Never used	67.4	83.4	98.5	90.8	91.4	97.6	93.9	97.4	94.7	98.8	93.9	86.1	94.5	98.4	94.0	12.5	36.2	38.2	79.6	67.6	97.9

SOURCE: L.D. Johnston, P. M. O'Malley, & J. G. Backman, *National Survey Results on Drug Use From Monitoring the Future Study, 1975-1992*, U.S. Department of Health and Human Services, National Institute on Drug Abuse (Washington, DC: Government Printing Office, 1993). Table adapted by SOURCE BOOK staff; *Bureau of Justice Statistics Sourcebook of Criminal Statistics 1992* (Washington, DC: Hindelang Criminal Justice Research Center).
NOTE: Percentages are based on three of the six forms (N = approximately 7,100) except for cocaine and crack which are based on four of the six forms (N = approximately 9,500), inhalants, other forms of cocaine, smokeless tobacco and steroids which are based on two of the six forms (N = approximately 4,700), and PCP and nitrites which are based on one of the six forms (N = approximately 2,400).
a. Unadjusted for known underreporting of certain drugs. See text for details.
b. Based on the data from the revised question, which attempts to exclude the inappropriate reporting of non-prescription stimulants.

201

or more concurrently; (b) 7% of all prescriptions were inappropriate; and (c) more women than men received inappropriate prescriptions.

▓ Antecedents of Use

GENETICS

A huge body of literature has established a genetic component to the development of alcoholism. Until recently, the evidence was much stronger for males than females; but Kendler et al. (1992) reported that genetic factors play a major role in the development of alcoholism in women. The genetic contribution to other forms of drug abuse is also firmly established (cf. Pickens & Svikis, 1988), although not discussed below. Many of the studies on inheritance of alcoholism were summarized in the Seventh Special Report to the U.S. Congress on Alcohol and Health [Seventh Special Report] (1990) and are cited below without original references. (References are given to studies not cited in the Seventh Special Report.)

Studies of Families

More than half the people treated for alcoholism or other drug abuse have a family history of alcoholism or drug abuse (Cotton, 1979; Goodwin, 1985). Of course, family members usually have environments as well as genes in common.

Twin and Adoption Studies

A much higher proportion of identical than fraternal twins of alcoholics are themselves alcoholic. Until recently thought true only of men, this applies to women too (Kendler et al., 1992). Genetic factors contribute to the effects of alcohol on body sway, hand steadiness, arithmetic ability, and pulse rate. Among adult twin brothers, they play a significant role in frequency, quantity, and density of drinking episodes.

Studies of children adopted at birth have led to characterization of two subgroups of alcoholics. All sons of alcoholic parents are at greater risk for alcoholism than sons of nonalcoholics, even if adopted at birth and raised by nonalcoholics. However, for only about 25% are genetic factors generally sufficient for development of the disease; these 25%

typically begin drinking heavily at an early age, deteriorate rapidly, and become involved with the police. For the other 75% of male alcoholics, a complex interplay of genetic and environmental influences is required.

Animal Studies

Selective breeding has produced genetic lines that differ in several alcohol-related traits. Alcohol-preferring (AP) rats voluntarily consume and work for alcohol even when water and other nutrients are available. Alcohol-nonpreferring rats (NP) do not. AP rats work for alcohol even if it is delivered directly to the stomach, suggesting that their payoff is in psychic effects rather than taste. Even prior to alcohol exposure, AP rats have lower levels than NPs of serotonin and dopamine in several brain regions. Drugs that increase brain serotonin or dopamine reduce the drinking of APs.

Genetic Markers

A brain wave, called the P3 wave, normally appears in people performing **cognitive** tasks. Even before ever drinking alcohol, sons of alcoholics have smaller P3 waves than sons of nonalcoholics. Sons of alcoholics report smaller subjective effects of alcohol, and they experience less motor impairment and have smaller alcohol-induced changes in secretion of several hormones (see Schuckit et al. [1991] for references).

Pihl, Peterson, and Finn (1990) observed no differences between daughters of alcoholics and nonalcoholics. But the sons of alcoholics, compared with the sons of nonalcoholics, were hyperreactive to a variety of stimuli.

Acetaldehyde, a toxic metabolic product of alcohol, is normally rapidly metabolized to acetic acid by aldehyde dehydrogenase. Many Asians have an inactive form of aldehyde dehydrogenase; as a result, levels of acetaldehyde accumulate and cause an unpleasant flush reaction that may deter further drinking. The frequency of this inactive enzyme is much lower among Japanese alcoholics than in the general Japanese population.

PARENTAL ANTECEDENTS

In a book edited by Kandel (1978), several authors presented survey data on early environmental precursors of later drug abuse. Four parental correlates were lack of closeness between parents and children, lack of or inconsistent discipline, parents who frequently used drugs (both legal and illegal), and low parental educational aspirations for children. Marital conflict was shown to be an important factor (Simcha-Fagan, Gersten, & Langner, 1986). Baumrind (1985), while reporting similar findings, added two points. First, parental characteristics that promoted abstention tended to be unoptimal in other respects; for example, boys of restrictive parents were unlikely to try drugs in adolescence but tended to be socially unassertive. Second, the most socially mature and competent children, especially girls, were most likely to experiment with drugs a few years later.

Block et al. (1988) worked with a sample of children for more than 15 years, starting when the children were 3 or 4 years old. They gave a variety of personality tests and assessed family life. Early family environment related to adolescent drug usage in girls but not boys. The findings are presented in Table 10.9.

Nyberg and colleagues (Jacobson et al., 1990; Nyberg, Allebeck, Eklund, & Jacobson, 1992) reported intriguing findings on the effects of an extremely early parental antecedent. They compared birth records of opiate addicts, amphetamine addicts, and their nonaddicted siblings. Mothers had received significantly more opiates, barbiturates, and nitrous oxide within 10 hours of birth of the future addicts than of their siblings.

EARLY PERSONALITY CORRELATES

In the Block et al. study, personality traits of nursery school girls that predicted adolescent drug use included the following: not neat, eager to please, doesn't share, unconcerned with moral issues, immature in behavior when under stress, sulky, emotionally labile, doesn't recognize the feelings of others, inconsiderate, transfers blame to others, not calm, dominating, unprotective of others, doesn't get along well with and teases other children, feels deprived, less likely to yield in conflictful situations, cries easily, and jealous and envious of others.

Among the nursery school boys, the predictive traits included: unable to recoup after stress, cries readily, openly expresses negative feelings, not shy, not helpful or cooperative, inattentive and unable to concentrate, energetic and lively, not calm, aggressive, competitive, incautious, emotionally labile, not obedient, not planful, not inhibited, physically active, behaves immaturely under stress, teases, rapid in

Table 10.9 Age 6 Environmental Q-Set Spearman Correlates of Drug Use at Age 14: Girls

EQS Item	r With Marijuana Use	r With Hard Drug Use
Hazards around the house	.51**	.37*
House is crowded and cramped	.43**	.47**
Home a center for the child's activities	.43**	.31*
House appears messy, dirty, and unkempt	.40**	.42**
Congenial, informal family atmosphere	.38**	.32*
Mother-child communication is direct and open	.36*	.20
Noise level of house is high	.32*	.35*
Mother indulgent of child	.30*	.28
Home a productive center of projects	.30*	.23
Home and grounds are well tended	−.48**	−.49**
Home environment emphasizes manners and propriety	−.46**	−.39**
Home environment is orderly and predictable	−.40**	−.48**
Mother pressures child to achieve	−.39**	−.30*
Religion important in the family	−.33*	−.37*
Family politics and philosophy conservative	−.30*	−.32*
Child subject to discrimination	−.28	−.31*

SOURCE: From "Longitudinally Foretelling Drug Usage in Adolescence: Early Childhood Personality and Environmental Precursors" by J. Block, J. Block, & S. Keyes, 1988, *Child Development, 59,* pp. 336-355. Copyright © 1988 by *Child Development.* Used by permission.
NOTES: $N = 45$-48.
* $p < .05$; ** $p < .01$.

tempo, not dependable, overreacts to frustrations, less likely to day-dream, less likely to yield in conflictful situations, emotionally expressive, dislikes solitariness, unable to delay gratification, stretches limits, dominating, talkative, agile, exaggerates mishaps, and restless.

Kellam and Brown (1982) found the combination of aggression and shyness in first graders highly predictive of later drug abuse. Emsinger, Kellam, and Rubin (1983) reported that aggressive, antisocial grade school children are most at risk for growing up to abuse drugs, and many other investigators confirmed a strong association between early antisocial behavior and later drug abuse (cf. Helzer, 1985).

▩ Current Environments

Environments in which peers actually use and are perceived to use drugs promote drug use (Kandel, 1982). So do stressful environments. Nurses in stressful specialties, such as psychiatry and casualty, were more likely to smoke than those in pediatrics; and more likely to smoke while on night duty, which they considered stressful (Hawkins, White, & Morris, 1982). Heavy smokers reported more stress than nonsmokers (Mitic, McGuire, & Neumann, 1985); and negative life events correlated strongly with both smoking and heavy use of alcohol (Baer et al., 1987; Wills, 1986). Svarstad (1983) found a strong relationship between psychological distress and nonprescription drug use. School is often stressful, and many adolescents attempt to cope by abusing drugs (Johnston & O'Malley, 1986). People raised under conditions of severe deprivation are at much greater risk than others for abusing drugs (Hawkins, Lishner, Jenson, & Catalano, 1987). Many additional studies relate subjective stress to drug abuse (cf. Wills, 1990).

Surveys demonstrate a relationship, but not necessarily a causal one, between stress and drug abuse. For that, experiments are necessary. Laboratory animals deprived of food increased both oral and intravenous self-administration of a variety of drugs (Carroll, France, & Meisch, 1979; Oei, Singer, & Jefferys, 1980; Smith & Lang, 1980). Monkeys reared under stressful conditions drank more alcohol than controls, as did monkeys temporarily separated from their cage mates (Higley, Hasert, Suomi, & Linnoila, 1991).

An extensive series of experiments, with exciting and far-reaching implications, shows that stressful environments elicit many excessive behaviors including drug abuse (see Falk [1983] for review). In the first set of experiments, Falk fed food-deprived rats small food pellets at approximately one-minute intervals during daily 3-hour test sessions. The rats stayed healthy but drank enormous quantities of water during the 3-hour periods. Although water was always available in their home cages, they averaged 10 times the normal 24-hour intake during those 3-hour periods. Then Falk placed rats under the same reinforcement schedule after depriving them of sawdust or access to running wheels. (A reinforcement schedule is a rule for delivering rewards, in this case one food pellet or opportunity to roll in sawdust or access to the activity wheel per minute.) The rats drank excessively. In addition, they behaved excessively in other ways (wheel running, pecking, and attacks against a second animal) when water was unavailable. The phenomenon occurred in many other species including humans.

The same pattern emerged when, instead of water, drugs were made available to hungry rats fed on intermittent schedules. Intakes varied, but alcohol, amphetamine, cocaine, chlordiazepoxide, heroin, methadone, marijuana, and nicotine all were taken in much greater than normal amounts.

Falk (in press) used a similar schedule to induce excessive water drinking. Then he offered the rats water in one bottle and a solution of alcohol in a second. He shined a light over the bottle containing alcohol. Next he substituted, in turn, cocaine, nicotine, caffeine, and lidocaine for the alcohol. All but lidocaine are drugs that rats self-administer when given the opportunity. Falk always shined a light over the bottle containing drug. In all cases, the rats preferred the drug solution to water. Then he switched the light to the water bottle, and the rats' preferences switched to water. Switching the light back restored their preference for drug.

Falk concluded that the initial preference for lidocaine, a drug not normally abused by humans or self-administered by rats, must have been caused by a nonpharmacological factor—the light. But naive rats given choices between fluids with and without light showed no preferences. The light became a reinforcing stimulus only because of its prior association with reinforcing drugs. Furthermore, the light eventually controlled the rats' behavior to a greater extent than did any of the drugs. In humans as well, stimuli previously associated with drug-taking may play an important role in maintaining drug habits and evoking strong craving. Falk emphasized that the stimuli are not limited to those that occur during or immediately before taking drug.

▓ Personality Correlates of Use and Abuse

Not surprisingly, given that political, educational, and religious leaders publicly denounce users of illicit drugs and laws make them criminals, many are rebellious, impulsive, and have extreme disregard for social and moral norms (Sutker & Archer, 1979). Surveys of college users in the late 1960s and 1970s, but not in 1989, showed that many felt alienated from U.S. society; perhaps the change indicates that drug use has become mainstream (Pope, Ionescu-Pioggia, Aizley, & Varma, 1990). Pope et al. reported that, through two decades of surveys, two features consistently distinguished users from nonusers: Users reported more visits to a psychiatrist and were more sexually active.

Personality characteristics of drug abusers are assessed primarily from standardized tests and surveys of people in custody or therapy. The results do not distinguish between characteristics that predate the abuse and those caused by it. Also, people in custody are not representative of the wider drug-using population. Comparisons between different types of drug abusers are especially problematic, as they come to the attention of researchers in different ways. Alcoholics are more likely to be identified because of absenteeism from work, cocaine and heroin abusers following arrest for a crime. Alcoholics tend to be older than cocaine or heroin abusers at the time of identification (Ciotola & Peterson, 1976). So, comparisons can be misleading.

Spotts and Shontz (1991) administered a personality test, the 16PF, to non-drug users and nonhospitalized, unincarcerated, heavy, chronic users of either cocaine, amphetamine, opiates, or barbiturates. The nonusers described themselves as more outgoing, stable, enthusiastic, self-assured, relaxed, stubborn, and competitive than any of the user groups. All user groups described themselves as more easily affected by feelings, anxious, and concerned with self-sufficiency. Andrucci, Archer, Pancoast, and Gordon (1989) reported that the Sensation Seeking Scales, which measure "the need for varied, novel, and complex sensations and experiences and the willingness to take physical and social risks for the sake of such experience," were the best predictors of adolescent drug use.

Many psychiatric patients abuse both illicit drugs (cf. Dixon et al., 1991; El-Guebaly, 1990) and licit ones (Hughes, Hatsukami, Mitchell, & Dahlgren, 1986; Kushner, Sher, & Beitman, 1990); and many drug abusers have additional psychiatric disorders (cf. Mirin, Weiss, Griffin, & Michael, 1991). Mirin et al. assessed the personalities of opioid, cocaine, and sedative-hypnotic drug abusers in a hospital for treating drug dependence. The researchers used both psychological tests and psychiatric interviews. As shown in Table 10.10, more than half the patients had other disorders. Major depression was the most common additional diagnosis for both opioid and cocaine abusers, panic disorder for sedative-hypnotic abusers.

Table 10.10 Percentage Distribution of DSM-III Diagnoses in 350 Drug Abusers

Diagnosis (%)	Drug of Choice			
	Opioids (n = 186)	Cocaine (n = 120)	Sedative-Hypnotics (n = 44)	Total Sample (N = 350)
Alcohol abuse/ dependence	51.6	55.8	45.5	52.3
Major depression	12.4	9.2	13.6	11.4
Bipolar disorder	3.8	5.0	2.3	4.0
Cyclothymic disorder *	1.6	12.5	4.5	5.7
Panic disorder †	2.2	0.0	15.9	3.1
Generalized anxiety disorder ‡	0.5	0.8	9.1	1.7
Attention deficit disorder, residual types §	0.0	4.2	0.0	1.4
Other axis 1 diagnoses	11.8	13.3	38.6	15.7
All non-drug axis 1 diagnoses ¶	29.6	40.0	59.1	36.9
Antisocial personality disorder ‖	29.6	16.7	6.8	22.3

SOURCE: From "Psychopathology in Drug Abusers and Their Families" by S. Mirin, R. Weiss, M. Griffin, & J. Michael, 1991, *Comprehensive Psychiatry, 32*, pp. 36-51. Copyright © *Comprehensive Psychiatry*, 1991. Used with permission.
NOTES: * $\chi^2 = 16.17$, df = 2, $p < .0005$.
† $\chi^2 = 16.29$, df = 2, $p < .001$.
‡ $\chi^2 = 16.29$, df = 2, $p < .001$.
§ $\chi^2 = 9.72$, df = 2, $p < .01$.
¶ $\chi^2 = 14.10$, df = 2, $p < .001$.
‖ $\chi^2 = 13.96$, df = 2, $p < .001$.

The mental health of the abusers' first-degree relatives was also assessed. Thirty-five percent had had at least one psychiatric diagnosis during their lifetime. Male relatives had greater overall psychopathology, and higher rates of alcoholism and other drug abuse than did female relatives. The females had more depressive and anxiety/panic disorders. The results support the view that genetic factors contribute to drug abuse.

Cigarette smokers are more likely than nonsmokers to suffer from depression, anxiety, schizophrenia, and alcoholism (Glassman, 1993). So, differences between psychiatric patients and normal comparison subjects in such measures as sleep patterns and cerebrospinal fluid composition may be due primarily to the greater likelihood that psychiatric patients smoke. The mortality rate is higher for depressed than nondepressed people, even after suicide is accounted for. Smoking may be a major reason.

Unlike researchers who study drug abusers only after they come to the attention of authorities, some study them prospectively. Wilsnack, Klassen, Schur, and Wilsnack (1991) interviewed the same group of women in 1981 and 1986; the most consistent predictor of problem drinking in 1986 was sexual dysfunction in 1981. Block et al. (1988) tested people repeatedly over a period of more than a decade. Their subjects were only 3 or 4 years of age at the start, and of course none had used drugs. Shedler and Block's (1990) findings on the personality characteristics of the children at age 18 are presented in Table 10.11. At age 18, frequent drug users were judged more alienated, deficient in impulse control, and distressed than occasional users. But abstainers were also judged psychologically less healthy: anxious, emotionally constricted, and lacking in social skills. Ambrose Bierce may have anticipated the results more than 100 years ago; in his *The Devil's Dictionary*, he offered the following definition:

> ABSTAINER, n. A weak person who yields to the temptation of denying himself a pleasure. A total abstainer is one who abstains from everything but abstention, and especially from inactivity in the affairs of others.

▩ Motivations for Use

SURVEY DATA

The reasons for drug use vary with individuals, drugs, and circumstances. Understanding the reasons might help in developing programs for preventing and treating abuse. The following list, based on self-reports, has been compiled from Dembo and LaGrand (1978), Johnston and O'Malley (1986), and Dixon et al. (1991):

- To produce positive feelings or reduce anxiety or depression
- To relax
- To increase energy
- To work and study better
- To mask causes of psychic distress such as fears, impulses, and wishes to escape from responsibility

Table 10.11 Mean Scores for Age 18 California Adult Q-Sort (CAQ) Items

Group CAQ Item	Abstainers	Experimenters	Frequent Users
1. Is critical, skeptical, not easily impressed.	4.9	4.6	5.6***
2. Is a genuinely dependable and responsible person.	7.7	7.5	5.9***
5. Behaves in a giving way with others.	6.4	6.5	5.5***
6. Is fastidious.	5.3**	4.9	4.2**
7. Favors conservative values in a variety of areas.	5.6**	5.0	3.6***
13. Thin-skinned; sensitive to anything that can be construed as criticism.	4.2	4.0	4.7**
17. Behaves in a sympathetic or considerate manner.	7.2	7.3	6.2***
18. Initiates humor.	5.3*	5.7	5.3
19. Seeks reassurance from others.	5.0	4.9	4.3*
21. Arouses nurturant feelings in others.	5.1*	5.4	4.7***
22. Feels a lack of personal meaning in life.	2.6	2.7	3.8***
23. Extrapunitive; tends to transfer or project blame.	3.7*	3.4	4.0**
24. Prides self on being "objective," rational.	6.2***	5.5	5.1
25. Overcontrols needs and impulses; delays gratification unnecessarily.	4.8***	3.9	3.3**
26. Is productive; gets things done.	7.1*	6.7	5.6***
27. Shows condescending behavior to others.	2.5	2.2	3.0***
28. Tends to arouse liking and acceptance in people.	7.0***	7.6	6.2***
29. Is turned to for advice and reassurance.	5.0	5.0	4.3***
30. Gives up and withdraws in face of frustration, adversity.	3.6	4.0	4.7*

(Continued)

Table 10.11 Continued

Group CAQ Item	Abstainers	Experimenters	Frequent Users
31. Regards self as physically attractive.	5.4**	5.8	5.4
34. Overreactive to minor frustrations; irritable.	3.5	3.4	4.4***
35. Has warmth, capacity for close relationships.	7.2	7.5	6.7***
36. Is subtly negativistic; tends to undermine, sabotage.	2.9	2.5	4.0***
37. Is guileful and deceitful, manipulative, opportunistic.	1.7	1.6	2.4***
38. Has hostility toward others.	3.5	3.3	4.4***
39. Thinks and associates to ideas in unusual ways.	4.2	4.3	5.0**
41. Is moralistic.	4.6***	4.2	3.9
42. Delays or avoids action.	3.4*	3.8	4.1
43. Is facially and/or gesturally expressive.	5.2***	5.9	5.5
45. Has a brittle ego-defense system; maladaptive under stress.	3.0	2.9	3.6**
48. Keeps people at a distance; avoids close interpersonal relationships.	3.7**	3.0	3.9**
49. Is basically distrustful of people in general.	3.4	3.1	4.2***
50. Is unpredictable and changeable in behavior, attitudes.	3.7**	4.0	4.9***
51. Genuinely values intellectual and cognitive matters.	7.0*	6.5	6.0
53. Undercontrols needs and impulses; unable to delay gratification.	2.9***	3.7	4.4***
54. Emphasizes being with others; gregarious.	5.6**	6.2	5.3***
55. Is self-defeating.	3.2	3.0	4.1***
56. Responds to humor.	6.8*	7.2	6.8
58. Enjoys sensuous experiences (touch, taste, smell, physical contact).	5.3***	5.7	6.0**

Table 10.11 Continued

Group CAQ Item	Abstainers	Experimenters	Frequent Users
62. Tends to be rebellious and nonconforming.	3.5	3.8	5.8***
63. Judges self and others in conventional terms (e.g., "popularity").	5.4	5.2	4.4***
65. Characteristically pushes and tries to stretch limits.	3.6	3.7	5.2***
67. Is self-indulgent.	4.1	4.2	4.9***
68. Is basically anxious.	4.3**	3.8	4.3
69. Is sensitive to anything that can be construed as a demand.	4.7	4.4	5.1**
70. Behaves in an ethically consistent manner.	6.8	6.5	6.0**
71. Has high aspiration level for self.	7.0	6.4	5.4***
72. Concerned with own adequacy as a person.	5.4	5.0	6.0***
73. Tends to perceive many different contexts in sexual terms.	3.9***	4.3	4.7*
74. Subjectively unaware of self-concern, satisfied with self.	5.1	5.5	4.9*
75. Has clear-cut, internally consistent personality.	6.7	6.6	5.9***
76. Tends to project own feelings and motivations onto others.	4.5	4.5	4.9**
77. Appears straightforward, forthright, candid with others.	7.1***	7.6	6.0***
78. Feels cheated and victimized by life; self-pitying.	2.2	2.1	3.0***
80. Interested in members of the opposite sex.	6.1***	6.6	6.6
81. Is physically attractive; good-looking.	5.9***	6.6	6.1*
82. Has fluctuating moods.	4.8	4.9	5.5***
84. Is cheerful.	6.9*	7.6	5.7***
86. Handles anxiety and conflict by denial, repression.	4.5	4.2	4.7*

(Continued)

Table 10.11 Continued

Group CAQ Item	Abstainers	Experimenters	Frequent Users
88. Is personally charming.	5.9**	6.5	5.5***
92. Has social poise and presence; is socially at ease.	6.3**	6.9	5.6***
93. Is sex-typed (masculine/ feminine).	6.8	7.0	6.4**
94. Expresses hostile feelings directly	3.8	3.9	4.3**
96. Values own independence and autonomy.	7.0	7.1	7.8***

SOURCE: "Adolescent Drug Use and Psychological Health: A Longitudinal Inquiry," by J. Shedler & J. Block, *American Psychologist, 45*, 1990, pp. 612-630. Copyright © *American Psychologist*, 1990. Used by permission.
NOTES: * Differs from experimenters, $p < .10$; ** Differs from experimenters, $p < .05$; *** Differs from experimenters, $p < .01$.

- To allow the acting out of a role or behavior pattern that might not otherwise be part of the user's lifestyle and that the user might normally find unacceptable
- To help gain attention, acceptance, and affection
- To help express feelings
- As a guide in searching for meaning and independence
- As a way of showing rebellion and defiance against authority or society in general
- To help find a deeper meaning in life; to expand consciousness and be creative
- For risk and excitement, both in procuring and using drugs
- To evidence adulthood
- To have a good time with friends
- Out of curiosity
- To relieve boredom
- Peer pressure

Newcomb, Chou, Bentler, and Huba (1988) noted that most studies on reasons focused primarily on alcohol and did not indicate whether the stated reasons predicted actual drug use. From questionnaire data with high school students, Newcomb et al. extracted four factors (not including enhancement of sexual functioning, which they felt was too sensitive a topic for teenagers) that reflected 15 reasons for using alcohol or marijuana:

I. Reduce Negative Affect: stop boredom; get rid of anxiety or tension; overcome sad, blue, or depressed feelings
II. Enhance Positive Affect and Creativity: know myself better; be more creative and original; enjoy what I am doing more; understand things differently; feel better about myself
III. Social Cohesion: feel good around people; friends pressure me into using it; everybody else uses it; get along better with friends
IV. Addiction: helps me get through the day; feel bad when I don't use it; helps me with problems

The factors were highly intercorrelated. Boys were more likely than girls to report using drugs for social cohesion and to enhance positive affect. The more reasons a subject listed, the more likely the subject actually was to use alcohol, marijuana, cocaine, or a variety of other drugs including sedatives, barbiturates, LSD, heroin, and PCP.

Jurich and Polson (1984) identified 24 adolescent drug abusers and matched them on gender, age, place of residence, socioeconomic status, and marital status with 24 people who had recently used but did not abuse drugs. Open-ended interviews revealed some similarities and several differences between the groups in motivations for use. Both groups used drugs to cope with problems, seek a sense of self-definition and identity, and rebel against adult norms and values. Users more than abusers used drugs recreationally. Abusers used more to relieve personal stress, to improve self-concept, and because of feelings of disillusionment, hopelessness, and powerlessness.

THE SELF-MEDICATION HYPOTHESIS

One major motivation for drug use, according to the current dominant theory, is **self-medication.** Hall (1980) speculated that psychiatric patients smoke a great deal because they have norepinephrine deficiencies that are reduced by smoking. Many agoraphobics say they began drinking alcohol to control anxiety symptoms (Bibb & Chambless, 1986). Khantzian (1985) concluded that opiates help addicts cope with rage and aggression. Weiss and Mirin (1986) described five types of cocaine abusers, with self-medication as a major factor for each of the first four:

(a) depressed patients who value its mood elevating effects; (b) patients with bipolar disorder who use it to relieve depression or augment manic or hypomanic symptoms; (c) adults with attention-deficit disorder; who use it to increase attention span; (d) narcissistic patients who use cocaine to bolster their self-esteem; and (e) patients with antisocial personality disorder who use it as part of an overall pattern of antisocial behavior. Schizophrenic drug-abusing patients told Dixon et al. (1991) that various drugs decreased their depression and anxiety while increasing energy.

Woody, McLellan, and O'Brien (1990) support the self-medication hypothesis. According to them, clinicians frequently observe the following pattern: A patient with no serious psychiatric problem other than opiate abuse, who has been maintained on methadone for months or years, is detoxified. Within a few hours or days of the last methadone dose, a full-blown schizophrenic disorder emerges requiring hospitalization and antipsychotic drugs. They speculated that the methadone had protected against the symptoms.

Summary

Workers in the drug field often assign people to one of two categories: abstainers and abusers. The dichotomy ignores important differences between users and abusers.

Data on use and abuse come from several imperfect sources. Surveyors fail to reach groups of people, such as the homeless, prisoners, and school dropouts, who use more drugs than the norm. Respondents typically underreport use. Data from prescriptions, coroner's reports, emergency room admissions, and treatment facilities permit other use estimates.

Drug use has occurred throughout human history and extends to the animal kingdom. People who use any one drug are likely to use others.

Men use more illicit drugs, alcohol, and tobacco than women. Women use more over-the-counter and prescription drugs.

Several sources of evidence point to a strong genetic component to drug use.

Parental correlates associated with subsequent drug use are lack of closeness between parents and children, lack of or inconsistent discipline, parents who frequently used drugs, and low parental educational aspirations for children. Parental characteristics that promoted abstention tended to be unoptimal in other respects.

The combination of aggression and shyness in first graders was highly predictive of later drug abuse.

Both surveys and experiments point to a relationship between stressful current environments and likelihood of drug abuse.

Users of illicit drugs tend to reject many of society's values. Drug abusers score high on a scale that measures rebelliousness, impulsiveness, and extreme disregard for social and moral norms. Score on a scale that measures the need for varied experiences is a good predictor of adolescent drug use.

A high proportion of drug abusers have coexisting psychiatric disorders, and many appear to use drugs to self-medicate.

Adolescents who used drugs moderately were judged psychologically healthier than either abusers or abstainers.

Four factors reflect 15 reasons for using drugs: reduction of negative affect; enhancement of positive affect and creativity; social cohesion; and addiction.

▨ NOTE

1. Barone and Roberts (1984) estimated caffeine amounts in various drinks as follows:

5 ounce cup of coffee	
ground, roasted	85 mg
instant	60
decaffeinated	3
5 ounce cup of tea	
leaf or bag	40
instant	30
6 ounce cola drinks	18
5 ounce cocoa	
or hot chocolate	4
8 ounce	
chocolate milk	5

Mini-Quiz: Users and Abusers

Survey estimates of drug use are too low. Why?

a. **People who refuse or aren't given the opportunity to respond to surveys have higher rates of drug abuse than the general population.**
b. **People sometimes give false answers to survey questions, and they probably minimize their drug use.**

T/F: A higher proportion of men than women use illicit drugs.

true

Women use more _____ drugs than men do.

prescription and over-the-counter

T/F: Genetics plays an insignificant role in the development of drug abuse.

false

Many Asians have an inactive form of the enzyme _____, which metabolizes alcohol.

aldehyde dehydrogenase

T/F: Parental characteristics that promote abstinence in their children tend to be optimal in most other respects as well.

false

The combination of _____ and _____ in first graders was highly predictive of later drug abuse.

aggression; shyness

T/F: Both surveys and laboratory experiments demonstrate a relationship between stress and drug use.

true

Describe the reinforcement schedule that led laboratory rats to excessive use of a variety of drugs.

The rats were fed at approximately 1-minute intervals for 3 hours per day.

Interpretations of personality characteristics of drug abusers are rarely unambiguous. Why?

Personalities are assessed from people who have been abusing; their characteristics may have predisposed them to use or been caused by drug use.

The most frequent psychiatric diagnosis, in addition to drug abuse, for both opioid and cocaine abusers, is ____.

depression

The best predictor of future problem drinking in women was ____.

current sexual dysfunction

What is the self-medication hypothesis of drug abuse?

People use drugs to help them overcome emotional problems.

By the time you finish reading this chapter, you should be able to answer the following questions:

What are the different types of preventive interventions?

How convincing is the evidence on effectiveness of various interventions?

Prevention of Drug Abuse

A Short and Depressing Chapter

Contents

The rationales for most prevention and treatment programs seem plausible, and both participants and administrators have generally expressed satisfaction with outcomes. But until recently, critics found extensive and almost universal methodological deficiencies that seriously compromised conclusions from the programs. Schaps et al. (1981) reviewed 127 drug abuse prevention programs and reported that only 4 measured drug use. Other problems included no or inappropriate control groups, improper statistical analyses, high dropout rates, and inability to replicate successful programs because of insufficient documentation on how they were run. In addition, broad generalizations

221

were made from programs for preventing alcohol and tobacco use by white middle-class students. For details, see Bell and Battjes (1985), Goodstadt (1981), Leukefeld and Bukoski (1991), Moskowitz (1989), and OSAP (1989). Methodology has improved in the past few years, but problems remain including disagreements over basic goals. Some programs encourage total abstinence, others strive to reduce negative consequences, delay onset of drug use, or interrupt possible progression from so-called gateway drugs like tobacco and alcohol to cocaine or heroin.

Moskowitz (1989), writing about alcohol, listed four preventive interventions: (a) enactment of policies that affect the physical, economic, and social availability of alcohol; (b) formal social controls (legal sanctions); (c) environmental safety measures; and (d) primary prevention. Factors that affect alcohol availability include its price, the number of retail outlets and their hours of operation, and the minimum legal drinking age. Moskowitz concluded that reductions in availability have impacted favorably on measures of abuse (see pp. 176-179 for further discussion of effects of availability on abuse). Formal social controls, primarily programs that increase the likelihood of punishment for drinking-driving offenders, have not been effective. Enactment of environmental safety measures, such as instituting higher standards for vehicle and highway construction, has substantially reduced injuries and deaths caused by drunken drivers.

Government funding for prevention has increased significantly during the past dozen years—see Table 11.1—and especially for primary prevention. The NIDA *Prevention Planning Workbook* (1981) described four types of primary prevention: information, education, alternatives, and interventions. Programs need not be restricted to a single type.

▓ Information

The goal of information programs, as stated in the 1981 workbook, was to disseminate accurate, objective information about drugs and their effects on human systems. Strategies included media campaigns, flyers, posters, brochures, and seminars for youth, parents, and the general public. The emphasis has changed: Bukoski (1991) gave the purpose of information programs as specifying "the harmful physical and psychological consequences of drug consumption." Possibly because many people in positions of authority give precedence to fear-provoking

Table 11.1 National Drug Control Budget—Prevention

Budget Authority $ Millions	1981	1982	1983	1984	1985	1986	1987	1988	1989	1990	1991	1992	1993
DAPA	2.5	6.8	6.9	6.8	6.9	6.9	7.8	5.9	10.1	10.5	12.5	12.3	13.4
AID	0.0	0.0	0.0	0.0	1.2	1.9	5.2	4.5	3.1	5.4	7.1	10.2	5.3
DoD	21.2	36.2	46.4	49.8	63.0	63.4	77.8	83.8	69.7	66.8	71.5	77.3	78.5
DoE	2.9	2.9	2.9	2.9	3.0	2.9	203.0	220.8	354.5	541.7	608.9	626.8	656.9
ACF	0.0	0.0	0.0	0.0	0.0	0.0	0.0	0.0	0.0	0.0	74.6	79.4	89.0
ADAMHA	16.1	30.0	32.5	32.1	34.1	32.6	98.4	85.2	150.7	329.7	420.1	431.6	455.0
CDC	0.0	0.0	0.0	0.0	0.0	0.0	0.0	0.0	20.0	25.2	29.3	28.8	31.5
FSA	0.0	0.0	0.0	0.0	0.0	0.0	0.0	0.0	3.0	2.0	0.0	0.0	0.0
HDS	0.0	0.0	0.0	0.0	0.0	0.0	0.0	0.0	43.9	57.1	0.0	0.0	0.0
IHS	0.0	0.0	0.0	0.0	0.0	0.0	0.0	0.0	0.0	2.7	0.0	0.0	0.0
HUD	0.0	0.0	0.0	0.0	0.0	0.0	0.0	0.0	8.2	98.3	150.0	165.0	165.0
BIA	0.0	0.0	0.0	0.0	0.0	0.0	3.5	0.8	2.6	2.2	3.1	3.6	3.6
BLM	0.0	0.0	0.0	0.0	0.0	0.0	0.0	0.0	0.1	0.3	0.3	0.4	0.4
NPS	0.0	0.0	0.0	0.0	0.0	0.0	0.0	0.0	0.2	0.4	0.4	0.3	0.7
OTIA	0.0	0.0	0.0	0.0	0.0	0.0	0.0	0.0	0.0	0.1	0.4	0.7	0.5
DEA	0.0	0.0	0.0	0.1	0.1	0.4	0.9	1.9	2.2	2.2	2.2	2.2	2.2
OJP	0.0	0.0	0.0	0.0	0.0	3.3	3.7	7.4	13.0	34.2	21.6	21.3	19.9
DoL	43.4	25.9	35.8	36.0	37.3	33.1	41.1	37.5	38.6	46.0	67.6	73.2	72.6

Table 11.1 Continued

Budget Authority $ Millions	1981	1982	1983	1984	1985	1986	1987	1988	1989	1990	1991	1992	1993
ONDCP	0.0	0.0	0.0	0.0	0.0	0.0	0.0	0.0	1.2	4.0	5.6	6.1	6.1
SBA	0.0	0.0	0.0	0.0	0.0	0.0	0.0	0.0	0.0	0.0	0.1	0.1	0.2
FAA	0.4	0.2	0.4	0.5	0.4	0.5	0.9	5.5	4.3	9.1	7.3	9.8	11.2
DVA	0.0	0.0	0.0	0.0	0.0	0.0	0.0	0.0	0.0	0.0	0.0	0.7	0.7
Weed & Seed	0.0	0.0	0.0	0.0	0.0	0.0	0.0	0.0	0.0	0.0	0.0	0.0	4.4
White House Conference	0.0	0.0	0.0	0.0	0.0	0.0	2.0	2.5	0.0	0.0	0.0	0.0	0.0
	86.4	101.9	124.9	128.1	146.0	145.0	444.3	464.7	725.4	1,238.0	1,482.7	1,549.8	1,617.0

SOURCE: Executive Office of the President, Office of National Drug Control Policy. *National Drug Control Strategy: Budget Summary,* January 1992.

materials over accurate and objective information, young adults often discount the warnings of parents, school personnel, police officers, and clergy (Fejer, Smart, Whitehead, & LaForest, 1971; Hanneman, 1972).

Both school-based and mass media information campaigns increase students' knowledge, but often with negligible or even negative effects on attitudes toward and use of drugs (Bry, 1978; Goodstadt, 1980). The authors of OSAP (1989) wrote:

> The tobacco experience gives reason for caution about the limits of even the least ambiguous health education. Despite virtually universal awareness of the deadly health risk and addictive nature of smoking, 60 million Americans still smoke tobacco cigarettes, and the rate of daily tobacco smoking among high school seniors not only remains high (just under 20 percent of the class) but has not fallen in the past 3 years.

The failure of information campaigns should not be too surprising; well-informed physicians use illicit drugs at a higher rate than does the general population (Aach et al., 1992; Domenighetti et al., 1991). Also relevant is a quote attributed to Henry Strauss (cited in Cohen & Cohen, 1980): "I have every sympathy with the American who was so horrified by what he had read of the effects of smoking that he gave up reading."

One information approach seems promising. Warning people about impending challenges to their attitudes strengthens their resistance to the challenges (McGuire, 1985). Many adolescents finishing primary school have negative attitudes toward smoking, but the attitudes soften soon after. So Pfau, Van Bockern, and Kang (1992) asked adolescents to watch two short videos. The first cautioned that many of them would succumb to peer pressure and begin smoking. The second raised and then refuted specific challenges to their attitudes, for example, that experimental smoking is unlikely to lead to regular smoking. Control subjects did not watch the videos. The manipulation succeeded with low-esteem adolescents; those exposed to the videos subsequently showed increased resistance to smoking.

▨ Education

Activities are designed, usually in schools, to encourage students to explore their values and develop skills in decision making, coping with stress, problem solving, communicating, and resisting peer pressure.

They are made aware of different career opportunities and helped with career planning. The rationale is that students deficient in such skills are at greatest risk for abusing drugs. Several positive results have been reported. Moskowitz (1989), however, stressing the importance of proper methodology and citing more than 10 reviews of the prevention literature, concluded that, "educational programs have been largely ineffective in preventing substance use or abuse."

▒ Alternatives

Opportunities are provided to allow young people to increase their range of experiences, learn craft skills like carpentry or masonry, and work with peers on meaningful tasks that meet community needs. But some alternatives may increase drug use. In one study, about 14,000 Pennsylvania students in Grades 7 through 12 filled out questionnaires on both drug use and alternative activities. The researchers, Swisher and Hu (1983), concluded the following:

1. Involvement in academic or religious activities was associated with less use of most drugs.
2. Participation in sports was associated with less use of most drugs, more of beer.
3. Active hobbies were associated with less use of beer and stimulants.
4. Participation in entertainment, social, extracurricular, or vocational activities was associated with more use of most drugs.

Hu, Swisher, McDonnell, and Stein (1982), Schaps et al. (1981), and Stein, Swisher, Hu, and McDonnell (1984) found little impact of programs that provided alternatives.

▒ Intervention

People with current or potential drug abuse problems can avail themselves of many forms of assistance. These include crisis intervention and drug hot lines, peer counseling, peer leadership programs, parent peer groups, and psychological counseling at the individual and family level. Some useful, toll-free hot-line phone numbers are:

1-800-4-CANCER: for tips on quitting smoking and materials on health consequences of smoking

1-800-COCAINE: provides confidential help in finding services for treating problems associated with cocaine

1-800-662-HELP: provides confidential discussion and referrals to programs for any type of drug abuse

1-800-356-9996: support groups for people with an alcoholic family member

1-800-333-1606: addresses special needs of women alcoholics

1-800-234-0420: for parents of adult children abusing drugs

1-800-222-LINK: self-help and referral line

▩ Early and Minimal Intervention for Alcohol Problems

People at high risk for becoming alcoholic can be identified in health care settings and worksites, as a result of arrests for driving while intoxicated, and through mass media recruitment campaigns. Evidence is accumulating that subsequent health, work performance, and personal happiness are improved when they are provided with brief counseling, advice, or moderation training (Seventh Special Report, 1990). Similar early, inexpensive interventions would almost certainly help with other forms of drug abuse.

▩ Notes on Targeting

Best et al. (1988) wrote, "smoking prevention researchers have focused very heavily on program content considerations, and paid virtually no attention to the other potentially equally powerful, and conceptually critical, determinants of program impact." The other determinants can indeed be critical, and people who promote drugs are well aware of them.

Ackoff and Emshoff (1975) worked for a major brewery with the goal of increasing consumption. They developed personality tests that discriminated between four types of alcoholics. They speculated that each type drinks to produce short-run changes that parallel normal changes due to aging. For example, introverts become more introverted both as they age and after drinking, whereas both aging and drinking increase extroversion in extroverts. Ackoff and Emshoff found that beer commercials work best when **targeted** to the specific needs of each type. Prevention workers should try to tailor programs to specific characteristics of their target populations (cf. Kumpfer [1987] for discussion).

▩ Environments

Recall from pages 206-207 that sparse reinforcement schedules elicit high levels of drug-taking in several animal species. The phenomenon occurs reliably in normally reared animals with no genetic anomalies or disreputable ancestors. Two related findings have important implications for prevention and treatment specialists.

1. If drugs are unavailable, other maladaptive behaviors including aggression occur at abnormally high levels.
2. Physical dependence can develop under such schedules. Without the drug, severe withdrawal symptoms occur and even death. Yet physically dependent rats stop taking freely accessible drug when the sparse schedules are discontinued.

Bry (1983) observed that many people's lives are characterized by schedules that generate excessive behavior—holding nonchallenging jobs, sitting through boring classes, waiting for buses, waiting for the next small allowance or paycheck, being lonely. Preventive approaches that fail to alter such schedules are unlikely to produce lasting effects.

Summary

Few prevention programs have been rigorously conducted or evaluated.

Programs differ greatly in their goals.

The four accepted primary prevention modalities are information, education, alternatives, and interventions. Little evidence testifies to the effectiveness of any of them.

Preventive approaches that ignore environments characterized by sparse reinforcement schedules are unlikely to produce lasting benefits.

Mini-Quiz: Prevention

T/F: Methodology for testing the success of prevention programs has varied enormously.

true, and until recently the methodology has been largely inadequate

T/F: There is general consensus about the aims of prevention programs.

false

Moskowitz listed four prevention interventions. What are they?

1. **enactment of policies that affect availability**
2. **legal sanctions**
3. **environmental safety measures**
4. **primary prevention**

Which of the above four interventions has had the most favorable impact on alcohol abuse?

enactment of policies that affect availability

Low-esteem adolescents were better able to resist pressure to start smoking if they had been exposed to a video that _____.

challenged their negative attitudes toward smoking, then refuted the challenges

T/F: Providing adolescents with alternatives to drugs reduces drug use.

only partly true—some alternatives increase use

T/F: Various interventions administered in the early stages of alcohol abuse have proven very helpful.

true

CHAPTER

12

By the time you finish reading this chapter, you should be able to answer the following:

Why is it important for therapists to recognize the particular model(s) they have about causes of drug abuse?

Adherents of which model believe that abusers are physically, not mentally, ill?

According to which model is drug abuse a symptom of an underlying psychopathology?

Why is it recommended that therapists use more than one model?

What factors make it difficult to do methodologically sound studies on treatment effectiveness?

What famous person created the first known cocaine addict?

What was the original medical use for heroin?

Give examples of drugs that have been used as substitutes, antagonists, and deterrents for drugs of abuse.

What are the advantages of methadone over heroin?

Name some behavioral treatment methods for treating drug abuse.

What strategies have been developed for preventing relapse?

What is contingency management?

What is the relevance of schedule-induced drinking research to development of treatments for abuse?

Treatment of Drug Abuse

Contents

Table 12.1 gives the Federal budget for drug abuse treatment for the years 1981-1993. Treatment is clearly a growth enterprise.

The goals of treatment programs vary even more than those in the prevention field. Goals should be clearly stated, as changes in addicts' drug habits, general health, work, crime, and social and psychological well-being occur relatively independently (Jaffe, 1984). The following is adapted from the Institute of Medicine's (1990) list of goals, whose authors noted that clients, clinicians, program managers, third-party reimbursers (health insurers and public health bureaus), regulatory agencies, politicians, and other interested parties often have conflicting interests:

Table 12.1 National Drug Control Budget—Treatment

Budget Authority $ Millions	1981	1982	1983	1984	1985	1986	1987	1988	1989	1990	1991	1992	1993
Drug Abuse Treatment													
DoD	12.4	21.4	23.3	24.1	18.5	19.6	20.9	22.1	12.4	16.6	15.0	14.6	14.7
Department of Education	6.8	7.3	9.1	11.3	12.7	15.9	20.0	24.9	22.6	61.2	74.1	88.7	94.0
Administration for Children and Families	0.0	0.0	0.0	0.0	0.0	0.0	0.0	0.0	0.0	0.0	31.7	31.7	32.5
ADAMHA	156.1	120.0	130.1	126.5	136.5	130.7	263.3	261.0	463.9	727.9	800.6	819.1	962.1
Health Care Financing Administration	70.0	70.0	80.0	90.0	100.0	110.0	120.0	130.0	140.0	170.0	190.5	201.5	231.5
Human Development Services	0.0	0.0	0.0	0.0	0.0	0.0	0.0	0.0	0.0	4.9	0.0	0.0	0.0
Indian Health Service	1.5	1.6	2.1	2.3	2.4	2.4	21.7	16.2	18.7	30.1	35.3	35.2	37.0
Judiciary	4.2	4.9	5.3	6.6	8.3	10.8	15.9	21.2	23.3	31.9	34.6	35.2	44.4
Bureau of Prisons	2.9	2.9	2.8	2.7	3.1	3.3	3.8	4.3	4.1	8.0	10.7	22.5	27.7
Office of Justice Programs	0.0	0.0	0.0	0.0	0.0	1.2	19.6	8.1	34.4	88.9	83.1	80.1	86.0
ONDCP	0.0	0.0	0.0	0.0	0.0	0.0	0.0	0.0	1.2	4.0	5.6	6.1	6.1
DVA	192.1	210.6	234.0	251.5	272.6	287.0	336.3	355.3	356.2	429.5	470.9	541.3	587.5
	448.0	438.7	486.7	517.0	554.1	580.8	821.5	863.1	1,076.8	1,573.0	1,752.0	1,876.1	2,123.6

SOURCE: Executive Office of the President, Office of National Drug Control Policy, *National Drug Control Strategy: Budget Summary,* January 1992.

- Reduce or eliminate the use by treated individuals of illicit drugs
- Reduce or eliminate their crimes against others
- Reduce or eliminate their use of legal psychoactive drugs
- Reduce or eliminate their specific educational or vocational deficits
- Help them find jobs
- Change their personal values to approximate more closely mainstream commitments regarding work, family, and the law
- Improve their health, longevity, and psychological well-being
- Reduce specific behaviors such as sharing of needles and multiple unprotected sexual encounters that help spread the AIDS virus
- Reduce the size, violence, seductiveness, and profitability of the market for illicit drugs
- Reduce the number of infants born with drug dependence symptoms or other impairments owing to intrauterine exposure to illicit drugs

Prospective clients are almost always ambivalent about seeking treatment and invariably have one or more serious problems—illness, chronic depression, a felony case, an angry spouse, the threat of imprisonment or assault—in addition to drug use (Institute of Medicine, 1990). They must choose from an imposing array of therapeutic modalities, each requiring specialists. Many apply essentially the same treatment to everybody regardless of specific problems and needs. Yet McLellan and Alterman (1991) cited many studies in which careful matching of clients to modalities improved therapeutic outcomes.

The conceptions of drug abuse held by therapists and clients influence treatment. Brower, Blow, and Beresford (1989) analyzed the implications of five basic models, each with unique advantages and disadvantages.

▧ Moral Model

The moral model attributes drug abuse to moral weakness or lack of willpower. Abusers are regarded as evil or weak, and the therapist's role is to foster goodness and strength. Two treatment strategies are teaching reliance on God and punishing drug use.

ADVANTAGES

1. Moral concerns are a powerful incentive for some drug abusers.

2. Holding people responsible for their actions helps overcome denial and reduces resistance to change.

3. Therapists who subscribe to other models sometimes find themselves feeling angry with and blaming clients. This signals that they have shifted to the moral model. By monitoring their own attitudes and behaviors, therapists can gain important diagnostic information and clues to treatment.

DISADVANTAGES

1. The therapist, by being blaming and punitive, develops an adversarial relationship with the client.

2. Most people come for treatment only after having failed to quit on their own, so emphasizing willpower reduces their self-esteem.

▨ Learning Model

According to the learning model, addictive behaviors are learned and can be unlearned. The goal is to increase self-control, so addicts are taught new coping skills and cognitive restructuring.

ADVANTAGES

1. There is no punishment or blame.

2. Clients are held responsible for obtaining and implementing the learning.

DISADVANTAGE

The model's emphasis on control undermines the therapeutic value for many drug abusers in admitting their loss of control.

▨ Disease Model

According to the disease model, drug abusers are physically, not mentally, ill. There is no known cure for their condition, so the goal of treatment must be complete abstinence. The major treatment strategy is to focus on the disease as the primary problem rather than lack of willpower, self-control, or mental health.

ADVANTAGES

1. There is no punishment, and blame can be directed toward the disease rather than the afflicted person.

2. People are given responsibility for seeking treatment, and treatment services are encouraged as with any other disease.

3. Drug abuse is recognized as the problem rather than something secondary to improper learning, psychopathology, or other factors.

DISADVANTAGES

1. Many alcoholics return to **asymptomatic drinking**. The model cannot explain that or the occasional return of abusers of other drugs to moderate use. The belief is false that one dose invariably triggers a chain reaction leading to uncontrollable use. For example, alcoholics given either vodka or placebo in a mix did not differ in post-drinking craving scores (Merry, 1966; see Mello [1975] for further discussion).

2. Coexisting psychopathology is minimized and often untreated.

▓ Self-Medication Model

According to this model, drug abuse is a method of self-treatment by people who have another primary mental disorder or psychological deficit. The therapist's goal is to treat the underlying psychopathology. The treatment strategies include psychotherapy and pharmacotherapy.

ADVANTAGES

1. There is no punishment or blame.

2. Stress is placed on diagnosing and treating coexisting psychiatric problems.

DISADVANTAGES

1. The model is factually incorrect; psychopathology is not the sole cause of drug abuse.

2. Factors that perpetuate abuse may differ from those that cause it.

3. Focusing on underlying psychological factors makes it easy for clients to deny that drug dependency is a problem.

▨ Social Model

In this model, drug abuse results from environmental, cultural, social, peer, or family influences. The goal of treatment is to alter abusers' social environments or their coping responses to environmental stressors. The strategies for changing environments include family and couples therapy, self-help groups, and residential treatment. The strategies for changing coping responses include group and interpersonal therapy, social skills and assertiveness training, and stress management.

ADVANTAGES

1. Interpersonal functioning, social supports, environmental stressors, social pressures, and cultural factors are recognized as critical elements that treatment should address.

2. The social model is compatible with and easily integrated into other models.

DISADVANTAGES

1. The drug abuser may come to feel victimized by unchangeable circumstances and thus renounce responsibility for solutions.

2. Focusing on social factors may tempt both therapist and abuser to minimize the seriousness of the drug dependency problem.

Brower et al. (1989) recommended that therapists use integrative models that exploit the advantages and avoid the disadvantages of the basic models. For example, a depressed drug abuser who accepted either the self-medication or social model might insist that therapy focus on the depression. Therapist agreement would mean denial by both parties—countertherapeutically—that drug abuse is important. By contrast, a therapist who believed in the disease model would interpret statements about depression as rationalizations and try to break through the denial. Mutual antagonism would be likely. Treatment benefits are optimized if the beliefs of all parties are assessed and addressed at an early stage. Brower et al. (1989) gave an example of what an integrative therapist might say to a depressed drug abuser:

> I agree that you appear depressed and this is certainly a problem for you. We need to address that. It is also true from what you have told me that you have a diagnosis of chemical dependency. We need to address that too and let me tell you why. Any attempt I make to determine the type of depression you have will be confounded by further chemical use. Also, any treatment that I can give you for your depression will be sabotaged by further chemical use. This is because we know that regardless of which came first (the depression or the chemicals) and regardless of why you use, chemicals make depression worse over long periods of time. In short, you have two problems, they both require treatment, and the best way I can treat your depression right now is to give you treatment for chemical dependency. After that treatment is begun, we will be better able to see if other treatments for your depression are needed.

🌣 Treatment Modalities

METHODOLOGICAL ISSUES

For obvious ethical reasons, drug abuse clients have rarely been randomly assigned to treatment and control groups. But then the interpretation, should improvements be shown, is problematic. Some drug abusers quit on their own, possibly as a natural consequence of aging or changes in social, economic, or personal well-being. Cigarette smokers who wanted to quit did about equally well whether or not they attended treatment programs (Cohen et al., 1989). Heavy amphetamine abuse is generally self-limited to about 10 years, probably because it causes central nervous system toxicity (Woody et al., 1990). And cocaine use declined markedly among cocaine abusers while they waited to enter a residential treatment center (Brown et al., 1988). Perhaps the best-supported conclusions are that treating someone who does not want to quit rarely succeeds, and treating someone who does is often unnecessary.

Both therapists and clients prefer favorable treatment outcomes. Ineffective therapists may lose their jobs, and clients who revert to drugs may lose jobs, spouses, and freedom. So, to minimize the risk that biases will exaggerate treatment effectiveness, all evaluations should be double-blind (see p. 267). Yet double-blind studies have been rare. Compounding the problem, most evaluations have been supervised by program administrators. Compounding it further, evaluations depend almost entirely on clients' self-reports of drug use and criminal activity, often about details of events that occurred months or years previously (Apsler, 1991). Some clients falsely and systematically deny both drug use and other criminality, leading to a false correlation between the two (Magura et al., 1987).

According to two large-scale independent evaluations (Hubbard et al., 1989; Simpson & Sells, 1982), the major treatment modalities are equally and substantially effective in reducing drug abuse and related problems. But the primary type of evidence, that people who stay in treatment longer tend to do better, is not compelling. For one thing, improvements may be due to the special attention enrollees receive rather than specific program components. Second, all programs require considerable commitment. In a study of disulfiram treatment for alcoholism (Fuller et al., 1986), potential clients were so carefully screened that only 24% met the criteria for inclusion; yet 62% of those refused to participate. Fewer than 50% of eligible heroin abusers enroll in methadone programs (Woody, O'Brien, & Greenstein, 1978), and about 5% accept treatment with a narcotic antagonist (Greenstein et al., 1983). Fifty-five million U.S. citizens smoke cigarettes despite an abundance of inexpensive cessation programs. So, successes may be due to the strong motivations of enrollees rather than unique program qualities. In any event, treatments that work with highly motivated clients may fail with others.

Third, dropout rates are high and often due to drug use: Leon (1991) reported that 10-month dropout rates from drug-free residential therapeutic communities are rarely less than 75%, and only 10% to 15% of clients complete the necessary 2 years. One-year retention rates for enrollees in methadone clinics range from 34% to 85% (Hubbard et al., 1989; O'Brien, 1987); and most clients fail to complete alcohol outpatient treatment programs (Polich, Armor, & Braiker, 1979). Of the few heroin addicts willing to be treated with the narcotic antagonist naltrexone, far fewer remain long in treatment (Zweben & Payte, 1990).

Kleinman, Lukoff, and Kail (1977) evaluated a typical, large-scale methadone program. Estimated heroin use by people who remained in the program declined from a high of 38% toward the end of the first year to 21% at the end of the fourth. It would appear that treatment was effective. But Kleinman et al. noted that 1,042 of the original 1,774 enrollees dropped out during the first 2 years, and each year's dropouts were among the worst offenders the previous year. As an analogy, imagine a program for increasing people's height. If the shortest 25% were dismissed each year, the remaining participants would on average be taller. In the methadone program, estimated heroin use by specific individuals *increased* with each year in the program.

Enrollees who remained in the program the longest showed the greatest gains in employment status, but 25% never worked during more than 3 years of treatment. Criminal activity declined, but primarily in drug-related charges; rate of assaultive charges was highest after 2 years of treatment—and was higher than the rate for the entire period from onset of addiction to entry into the program.

▩ Pharmacological Treatments

The appealingly simple strategy of using a drug to cure a drug habit is not without hazards: Sigmund Freud prescribed cocaine to treat a friend's morphine addiction, thereby creating the first known cocaine addict (Ritchie, Cohen, & Dripps, 1965). *Heroin* derives from *hero* and was so-named because of its alleged heroic powers in curing both morphine and opium addiction (Cohen, 1969). FASE Reports (1989-1990) juxtaposed four quotes spanning almost a century:

> The use of morphine in the place of alcohol is but a choice of evils, and by far the lesser. (*Cincinnati Lancet-Clinic*, 1889)

> Heroin will take the place of morphine without its disagreeable qualities. (*New York Medical Journal*, 1901)

> Some [heroin] addicts readily admit that they prefer methadone as their drug of abuse. (*International Journal of Pharmacology*, 1975)

> Clonidine has recently gained prominence as a chemotherapeutic agent for the detoxification of individuals dependent upon . . . methadone. (*NIDA Treatment Research Monograph*, 1983)

Drug treatment alone rarely improves the well-being of addicts. In fact, treatment that successfully reduces the rewarding properties of drugs leaves voids for people who previously depended on them. Unless they learn skills for coping with the problems that caused the abuse, addicts' lives may deteriorate. Many people withdrawing from opiates begin abusing alcohol, marijuana, or other drugs (Kolb, 1962; NIDA, 1974; Simpson & Sells, 1982). Extreme irritability is a trademark of nicotine withdrawal (Schachter et al., 1977). And many abstaining alcoholics develop marriage, work, and health problems (Gerard, Saenger, & Wile, 1952).

Drugs for treating drug abuse are of several types. Benzodiazepines, clonidine, doxepin, and desipramine relieve specific symptoms of withdrawal such as anxiety, depression, insomnia, and craving. Antidepressants and antianxiety drugs reduce coexisting psychiatric pathology. (Alcoholics metabolize antidepressants more rapidly than do nonalcoholics, so they need larger doses [Ciraulo et al., 1982]. Interactions occur between other psychiatric drugs and drugs of abuse [Fischman, Foltin, Nestadt, & Pearlson, 1990; O'Brien et al., 1988]).

Jarvik and Henningfield (1988) listed several beneficial effects of nicotine—anxiety and appetite reduction, mood regulation, and improvement of performance on measures of cognitive function—and suggested that nicotine-dependent people be treated with safer drugs that confer one or more of the same benefits. All drugs of abuse confer some benefits, so the same rationale applies.

Several serotoninergic drugs decrease alcohol consumption in both rats and people (Naranjo et al., 1984; Naranjo et al., 1987). Lithium markedly reduced the number of disabling drinking episodes of depressed alcoholics although, interestingly, without affecting their depressions (Kline & Cooper, 1975). Dackis and Gold (1985) speculated that chronic use of cocaine, by depleting brain dopamine, eventually leads to craving. The dopamine-like drug bromocriptine blocks craving (Dackis et al., 1987). The serotonergic drug mazindol reduced cocaine self-administration by rhesus monkeys (Balster, Mansbach, Gold, & Harris, 1992) and, in an uncontrolled study, reduced cocaine craving and abuse in seven people (Berger, Gawin, & Kosten, 1989).

Tables 12.2-12.4 list substitute, antagonist, and deterrent drugs for treating abuse of alcohol, heroin and other opioids, and nicotine.

SUBSTITUTES FOR DRUGS OF ABUSE

Most drugs of abuse have congeners (closely related drugs; see Table 12.2) that produce qualitatively similar but weaker responses. Follow-

Table 12.2 Substitutes for Drugs of Abuse

Alcohol	Heroin	Nicotine
none	methadone	nicotine gum
	buprenorphine	nicotine patch
	LAAM	

ing cessation of the drug of abuse, short-term administration of the right congener suppresses craving and other withdrawal symptoms. Maintenance doses may prevent relapse although some congeners, mildly satisfying and with fewer negative effects, are abused themselves.

Substitutes for Opioids

Methadone is a synthetic opioid with two important advantages over heroin: (a) It can be taken orally whereas heroin must be injected, often with contaminated needles; and (b) it is effective for 24 to 36 hours in preventing withdrawal symptoms and craving for opiates, whereas heroin must be administered several times a day. Once stabilized, methadone recipients experience neither euphoria nor sedation. More than 80,000 are currently in treatment (Institute of Medicine, 1990). Zweben and Payte (1990) expressed concern that, for political reasons, the maximal dose allowed in some settings is considerably less than optimal.

Several reviewers (Dole, 1988; Sells, 1977; Zweben & Payte, 1990) have concluded that addicts maintained on methadone fare better than they had previously in terms of health, criminality, and opioid use. On the other hand, *The Houston Chronicle* (1992) reported that methadone killed more Houston-area residents in 1991 than the combined number of deaths from overdoses of heroin, morphine, and other opioids. Woody et al. (1978) pointed to additional problems:

- There is little evidence that methadone produces long-term cures.
- Programs either require daily attendance, which is inconvenient and often incompatible with full-time employment, or permit take-home doses that may be accidentally ingested by children or sold to other drug abusers.
- Daily dosing entails handling, storage, and bookkeeping expenses that might otherwise be spent for rehabilitation of clients.

Methadone program successes, whether actual or artifactual, have been reported. The successful programs have had well-trained, enthusiastic staff. The others had low standards for staff, as indicated by a "Help Wanted" advertisement in a 1988 *Philadelphia Inquirer* (from Woody et al., 1990):

COUNSELOR for D/A Prog.
Full Time. No Experience
Necessary. $12,000. Send
resume to: XXX XXXXX XX
Phila., PA.

Woody et al. found that the addition of psychotherapy or counseling to methadone programs generally improved outcomes, but some therapists had little effect and some made patients worse. The strongest predictor of favorable outcome was patients' ratings, after the third session, of the extent to which they thought they were being helped.

Buprenorphine and levo-alpha acetylmethadol (LAAM) also reduce heroin withdrawal symptoms and may help with addiction. Buprenorphine, with both heroin agonist and antagonistic effects, reduces heroin self-administration by heroin-dependent men and cocaine self-administration by men with dual cocaine and heroin dependence (Mello, 1992). LAAM has a longer duration of action than methadone, so patients need not come to the clinic every day. But LAAM is no longer patentable, so pharmaceutical companies have little incentive to produce it.

Substitutes for Cigarette Smoking

Nicotine chewing gum is prescribed in the United States in 2 mg. pieces, each piece roughly equivalent to half a cigarette in producing nicotine-related effects. It poses health risks, but fewer than from cigarettes. Patients must limit their swallowing while chewing nicotine gum and avoid acidic beverages such as coffee and soft drinks that reduce absorption of nicotine from the gum (Jarvik & Henningfield, 1988).

Schwartz (1987) reviewed 28 studies and concluded that nicotine gum can help people quit smoking—especially if they are strongly physically dependent and receive support, counseling, or therapy. But the relapse rate is high when patients stop taking the gum, and it increases greatly from 6 months to 1 year. Schwartz noted that many investiga-

Table 12.3 Antagonists of Drugs of Abuse

Alcohol	Heroin	Nicotine
Ro15-4513	naltrexone naloxone	mecamylamine

tors reported follow-ups of less than 1 year, despite counting the first day of treatment as day 1 of follow-up. So, at 6-month follow-ups, patients who had used gum for 6 months were counted as successful quitters though they had never been both gum- and cigarette-free. One-year successes included everybody who discontinued the gum at any point during the year and were still not smoking.

Recently developed methods for administering nicotine safely include a nasal nicotine spray and a transdermal patch. Both are effective (cf. Daughton et al., 1991; Sutherland et al., 1992; Tonnesen, Norregaard, Simonsen, & Sawe, 1991).

ANTAGONISTS

Antagonists block the pharmacological effects of the abused drug (see Table 12.3). They are not addicting and have no abuse potential. Only highly motivated people volunteer for treatment with an antagonist.

Antagonism of Alcohol Effects

The drug Ro15-4513 interacts with brain receptors that mediate the effects of alcohol (Ticku & Kulkarnisk, 1988). Ro15-4513 reduces alcohol consumption by rats and weakens its intoxicating and antianxiety effects (McBride, Murphy, Lumeng, & Li, 1988; Suzdak et al., 1986). But Ro15-4513 has little clinical potential, because it does not reduce alcohol toxicity; people pretreated with Ro15-4513 might try to overcome its effects by drinking much more than usual; they might die.

Antagonism of Heroin Effects

Naloxone is a short-acting opioid antagonist. Used to treat heroin overdose, naloxone quickly reverses the effects. Naltrexone is longer acting and, given daily, prevents heroin users from experiencing positive effects.

Table 12.4   Deterrents of Drugs of Abuse

Alcohol	*Heroin*	*Nicotine*
disulfiram		silver acetate
calcium carbimide		

Antagonism of Nicotine Effects

Mecamylamine impairs ability to discriminate nicotine from placebo (Henningfield & Goldberg, 1983). In an uncontrolled study of heavy smokers, it reduced both craving for tobacco and smoking (Tennant, Tarver, & Rawson, 1984). Jarvik and Henningfield (1988) listed three obstacles to use: (a) Mecamylamine lowers blood pressure; (b) compliance is likely to be poor; (c) people smoke for reasons other than the pharmacological effects of nicotine.

DETERRENTS

Deterrent drugs cause unpleasantness when combined with the drug of abuse (see Table 12.4). They are not addicting and have no abuse potential. Only highly motivated people need apply. In addition, as noted by Jarvik and Henningfield (1988), unreliable deterrents or those with long-delayed consequences are minimally effective. Despite overwhelming evidence that cigarette smoking causes lung cancer (but years later and not in all people), smoking has not been eliminated.

Deterrents for Alcohol

Alcohol is normally metabolized to acetaldehyde, which in turn is metabolized by the enzyme aldehyde dehydrogenase to carbon dioxide and water. Substances that inhibit aldehyde dehydrogenase cause acetaldehyde to accumulate, which produces several unpleasant effects. Disulfiram inhibits aldehyde dehydrogenase for up to 2 weeks, so is used to promote sobriety. But evidence on its effectiveness is meager. Fuller et al. (1986) found that men who complied with their treatment regimen, whether given disulfiram or placebo, had higher one-year abstinence rates. (Most men who received disulfiram did not comply.) Disulfiram treatment did not make one-year abstinence more likely although, of the men who returned to drinking, those on disulfiram drank on fewer days.

Banys (1988) claimed that disulfiram, as one component of a structured treatment program, helps some patients. He listed the following selection criteria:

- Patients who can tolerate a treatment relationship: According to Banys, many alcoholics are reluctant to become dependent upon anybody including a therapist
- Patients who are relapse-prone but remain in treatment: Only patients who have previously relapsed may be willing to acknowledge that their other abstinence strategies are failing
- People who have failed with less structured approaches
- Patients in early abstinence who experience stress or crises: When facing divorce, dismissal, detention, or debt, patients can't afford even a brief relapse
- Patients who need support while receiving psychotherapy: People in psychotherapy often become distressed as a result of exploring painful personal histories; their familiar method for dealing with distress is drinking
- By request

Calcium carbimide inhibits aldehyde dehydrogenase for about 24 hours. It has fewer side effects than disulfiram and may be an effective alternative (Peachey & Annis, 1984).

Deterrents for Nicotine

Silver acetate gum has been marketed as a deterrent to smoking (Malcolm, Currey, Mitchell, & Keil, 1986). When silver acetate contacts the sulfides in cigarette smoke, sulfide salts are produced that most people find highly distasteful. But the effect is short-lived, so the gum must be chewed throughout the day.

▩ Nonpharmacological Treatments

THERAPEUTIC COMMUNITIES AND
CHEMICAL DEPENDENCY PROGRAMS

Although there are many differences between therapeutic communities (TCs), De Leon's (1988) remarks apply to most or all of them:

The principal aim of the TC is a global change in lifestyle: abstinence from illicit substances, elimination of antisocial activity, employability, and prosocial attitudes and values. A critical assumption for the TC is that stable recovery depends upon a successful integration of both social and psychological goals. Rehabilitation, therefore, requires multidimensional influences and training, which for most can occur only in a 24-hour, long-term residential setting.

TCs are distinguished from other major drug treatment modalities in two fundamental ways. First, the primary "therapist" and teacher in TCs is the community itself: peers and staff. As role models of successful personal change, they guide the recovery process. The community provides a 24-hour learning experience in which individual changes in conduct, attitudes, and emotions are monitored and mutually reinforced in the daily regime. Second, TCs are guided by an explicit perspective on the drug use disorder, the client, and recovery.

Most TCs are run by ex-addicts. They give residents, who generally stay for 9 to 15 months, highly structured rules for behavior and rewards and punishments based on adherence to the rules. A typical day begins with a 7 a.m. wake-up and ends at 11 p.m. Because they believe that the problem is within the person, not the drug, TCs offer many services: individual psychotherapy, group psychotherapy, and training in vocational, educational, and social skills. Although the dropout rate is very high, people who complete at least 6 months in residence show dramatic, positive personality changes (Kennard & Wilson, 1979). Graduates are more likely than untreated addicts to find and keep jobs, and they commit fewer crimes. Even those who revert to crime don't do so while residents, so TCs benefit society independent of their rehabilitative value.

Most chemical dependency programs are residential, providing 3 to 6 weeks of family services, medical attention, and psychotherapy. Operating on the premise that dependence is permanent but controllable, they demand total abstinence. After leaving the program, clients are expected to attend Alcoholics or Cocaine or Narcotics Anonymous meetings for at least 2 years. The authors of the Institute of Medicine (1990) review of drug abuse treatments noted that chemical dependency programs have not been adequately evaluated.

PEER SUPPORT SELF-HELP GROUPS

Participants in self-help groups share experiences and support each other in remaining drug-free. The various groups are modeled after the best-known, Alcoholics Anonymous (AA). Others include Al-Anon and Alateen for relatives of alcoholics, and Narcotics Anonymous and Cocaine Anonymous. (Some self-help groups, such as Gamblers Anonymous and Overeaters Anonymous, focus on compulsions unrelated to drugs.)

Members are taught that they are helpless against their compulsion and urged to find faith in a higher power—God, some other spiritual power, or the organization itself. They are encouraged to seek insights into the causes of their abuse and to share their understanding with others in the group. They are asked to atone for the grief they have caused, partly by helping people with the same compulsion.

People motivated enough to attend self-help groups probably derive many benefits. The groups are free and available worldwide for life, which must be very reassuring. Beyond that, their effectiveness is uncertain. Tournier (1979) noted that the tradition of anonymity precludes accurate counts of either current membership or dropouts. Many active members suffer relapses (Fingarette, 1988). In addition, already-abstinent abusers may attend meetings to sustain their recoveries or for fellowship (Bateman & Peterson, 1971).

The AA Central Office in New York surveys individual chapters every 3 years to get an approximate membership count. Mann, Smart, Anglin, and Adlaf (1991) obtained the data for all 50 U.S. states and the District of Columbia for the years 1974 through 1983. They also collected data on deaths from liver cirrhosis in each state during the same time period. They calculated that a 1% increase in AA membership was associated with a 0.06% decrease in cirrhosis mortality, whereas the number of patients receiving various treatment services for alcoholism was not significantly correlated with cirrhosis mortality. The data, although correlational, suggest that AA membership reduces drinking in people who might otherwise die from liver cirrhosis.

PSYCHOTHERAPY

Limited research exists on the effects of psychotherapy on drug abuse. Onken (1991) organized the available data into three categories: therapy, therapist, and patient variables. Her conclusions follow.

Therapy

Psychotherapy is inadvisable until after abstinence is achieved. Different types of therapy—individual behavioral, supportive, psychodynamic, and family—are all useful independent and concurrent with other treatments. None is convincingly better than others.

Therapist

Both therapists and drug counselors differ strikingly in success rates. In fact, therapist differences overshadow the types of therapy administered. Therapist characteristics associated with positive outcomes include ability to establish an early, positive alliance with the patient, consistent adherence to a particular method, and documentation of relatively complete treatment plans and records.

Patient

As discussed in Chapter 10, many drug abusers have coexisting mental disorders. They improve most when psychotherapy is a component of a drug treatment program. But antisocial personality disorder, commonly found among drug abusers, does not respond well to psychotherapy. Patients classified as low in severity of psychiatric problems do just as well with paraprofessional drug counseling.

BEHAVIORAL THERAPY

Both human and nonhuman animals vigorously self-administer many drugs. Their responses, if repeatedly followed by drug reinforcement, become difficult to eliminate. Stitzer, Bigelow, and Gross (1989) noted that both the behavioral processes leading to dependence, and treatment techniques, are similar for different species and across a range of drugs. Stitzer et al. described four behavioral treatment methods: behavioral counseling, relapse prevention skills training, stimulus counterconditioning, and contingency management.

Behavioral Counseling

Therapists try to identify conditions that precipitate drug use, then teach clients to avoid or cope with them. For example, a client who uses drugs following marital conflicts is taught how to handle conflicts. If drug-abusing friends or dealers promote use, the client is encouraged to seek new friendships and change telephone numbers. Therapists help clients find pleasurable nondrug activities and teach them to reward themselves for periods of abstinence with self-praise or material purchases.

Relapse Prevention Skills Training

At one time, detoxification was believed the key to drug abuse treatment. But most long-term users have detoxified (gone through withdrawal) at least once. Newly arrested heroin addicts and alcoholics do so in prison. People who require a morning cup of coffee to function properly often detoxify on weekends. Many cigarette smokers initiate the process at the start of each new year, and smoking cessation treatments produce abstinence in 90% to 100% of clients (Brandon, Tiffany, & Baker, 1986). But most resume use. Some addicts deliberately self-induce withdrawal to regain the euphoric highs that preceded onset of tolerance (Scher, 1961). Clearly, and despite movie and newspaper dramatizations that suggest otherwise, physical dependence and fear of withdrawal are relatively minor aspects of addiction. A much more serious problem is proneness to relapse, as summed up in Mark Twain's remark that quitting smoking is easy . . . "I've done it many times."

Of 72 cigarette smokers who successfully completed an abstinence program, 54 relapsed within 2 years (Brandon et al., 1986). The first relapse episode occurred an average of 58 days after completion of treatment and was followed about 50% of the time by a second cigarette on the same day. Forty-nine of the 54 people who smoked a single cigarette returned to daily smoking, with an average of 42 days between the two events. Hall, Wasserman, and Havassy (1991) reported a comparable pattern with opiate abusers—90% of treated addicts who relapsed once returned to using at least 4 days a week by the end of 12 weeks. For both alcohol and nicotine, relapse is more likely for women than men (U.S. Public Health Service, 1980).

Table 12.5, based on interviews with 2,280 clients who had completed one of four types of program, gives drug use patterns one year after treatment (Hubbard & Marsden, 1986). For example, line 2 shows that 5.1% of heroin abusers were using heroin and other narcotics, 38.7% heroin alone, 2.8% other narcotics, 10.6% nonnarcotics, and 42.8% had not relapsed. A trend can be observed toward use of drugs with less serious legal consequences than what the relapsers had used previously. The times to relapse are shown in Table 12.6. Thus 15.3% of relapsers to heroin did so at termination of treatment, 28.9% within one week of termination, and so forth.

Table 12.5 Relapse Rates to Different Drug Use Patterns in the Year After
              Treatment for Clients With Five Pretreatment Use Patterns

Pretreatment Drug Use Pattern	Posttreatment Drug Use Pattern				
	Heroin-Other Narcotics %	Heroin %	Other Narcotics %	Non-narcotics %	Non-relapsers* %
Heroin-other narcotics (n = 225)	20.4	7.6	16.4	12.7	44.9
Heroin (n = 643)	5.1	38.7	2.8	10.6	42.8
Other narcotics (n = 295)	8.1	2.0	24.4	18.3	47.1
Nonnarcotics (n = 508)	2.4	4.7	6.1	27.8	59.0
Alcohol/marijuana minimal (n = 609)	2.8	3.8	4.9	12.8	75.7

SOURCE: From "Relapse to Use of Heroin, Cocaine, and Other Drugs in the First Year After Treatment," by R. Hubbard & M. Marsden, in *Relapse and Recovery in Drug Abuse*, edited by F. Tims & C. Leukefeld, *NIDA Research Monograph No. 72*, 1986.
NOTE: * Includes all clients not classified as relapsing during the year of posttreatment. Some of these may have had alcohol, marijuana, or infrequent other drug use.

Table 12.6 Time Until First Use in the First Year After Treatment Among
              Clients Who Reported Posttreatment Use of Each of Four Drug
              Types

Weeks After Termination	Drug Used Posttreatment			
	Heroin %	Other Narcotics %	Cocaine %	Other Nonnarcotics %
Used at termination	15.3	14.4	10.7	15.2
Within 1 week	28.9	22.8	21.6	24.3
2-4 weeks	21.4	24.1	24.6	24.5
5-13 weeks	15.8	13.9	17.6	16.0
14 or more weeks	18.6	24.8	25.5	20.0
Total	100.0	100.0	100.0	100.0
Number of posttreatment users	720	626	984	1,026
Mean days to relapse among those who used posttreatment	55.0	68.3	71.9	58.8

SOURCE: From "Relapse to Use of Heroin, Cocaine, and Other Drugs in the First Year After Treatment," by R. Hubbard & M. Marsden, in *Relapse and Recovery in Drug Abuse*, edited by F. Tims & C. Leukefeld, *NIDA Research Monograph No. 72*, 1986.

Treated heroin, cigarette, and alcohol abusers cited negative emotional states, interpersonal conflict, and social pressure to use as the major precipitating events for relapse (Marlatt & Gordon, 1980). Similarly, Brandon et al. (1986) reported that most relapses followed a period of depression, anxiety, or other negative emotions. Relapses typically led to feelings of guilt and helplessness. So Marlatt and Gordon (1980), Hall, Rugg, Tunstall, and Jones (1984), Hawkins, Catalano, Gilmore, and Wells (1989), and others taught clients various skills for coping with high-risk situations; if relapses occurred, the clients were reassured and told to consider them natural but temporary setbacks. Outcomes from coping-skills training programs have been mixed (cf. Hall et al., 1991).

Stimulus Counterconditioning and Extinction

Hungry dogs salivate at the sight and smell of food. When Pavlov repeatedly rang a bell just prior to offering food, the dogs eventually began salivating to the bell alone. In the same way, stimuli associated with addiction and withdrawal condition physiological responses. These may be interpreted as drug cravings and lead to re-addiction. For example, Goldberg and Schuster (1967) repeatedly sounded a buzzer, then injected morphine-dependent monkeys with the narcotic antagonist nalorphine. The nalorphine-induced withdrawal symptoms soon occurred to the buzzer alone. Similarly, O'Brien et al. (1977) injected heroin addicts with the narcotic antagonist naloxone; each time withdrawal symptoms intensified, they increased the loudness of a background tone and the strength of a piped-in peppermint odor. Then, with tone and peppermint odor present, saline was injected and withdrawal symptoms appeared. The results show the importance of conditioning in addiction—and that people are as smart as dogs and monkeys. They confirm Wikler's (1948) observation that withdrawal symptoms often appear in postdependent addicts when they discuss drugs. O'Brien (1976) gave an example. A 28-year old man with a 10-year history of addiction went through withdrawal and began to feel well. He decided to be through with drugs. Then,

> On the way home after release from prison, he began thinking of drugs and feeling nauseated. As the subway approached his stop, he began sweating, tearing from his eyes and gagging. This was an area where he had frequently experienced narcotic withdrawal symptoms while trying to acquire drugs. As he got off the subway, he vomited onto the tracks. He soon

bought drugs, and was relieved. The following day he again experienced craving and withdrawal symptoms in his neighborhood, and he again relieved them by injecting heroin. The cycle repeated itself over the next few days and soon he became readdicted.

O'Brien and Ternes (1977) met many patients who claimed to be heroin addicts and had needle marks. But their urinalyses tested negative for heroin, and naloxone precipitated weak or no withdrawal symptoms. The patients, methadone maintenance applicants, were not heroin-dependent. They had been injecting weak heroin diluted with quinine. O'Brien and Ternes speculated that many addicts are unwitting "needle freaks," with no pharmacological dependence. Yet they have been conditioned to regard the acquisition, administration, and experiencing of drug effects as rewarding and drug absence as painful.

Counterconditioning. Two counterconditioning procedures are relaxation training and aversive conditioning. In the first, patients are taught to relax in the presence of stimuli that normally elicit anxiety or craving. Unfortunately, such training has little impact on relapse rate (Stitzer et al., 1989). The goal of aversive conditioning is to break the connection between drug use locations, rituals, paraphernalia, and effects, on the one hand, and drug-seeking on the other. So, stimuli that normally lead to drug-seeking are presented repeatedly and always followed by something unpleasant. For example:

- Patients are encouraged to administer their favored drug and repeatedly shocked while doing so.
- Patients take their favored drug along with another that causes them to throw up.
- Patients smoke rapidly while a machine blows hot smoke at them.
- Patients carry a special cigarette case that delivers shock when opened.

Aversive conditioning for drug abuse can be traced back to ancient Rome, where spiders placed at the bottom of wine glasses discouraged excessive drinking. The strong motivation of participants to such procedures may account for scattered positive findings. Patients who refused aversive conditioning had much lower abstinence rates than those willing but unable to take it (Voetglin, Broz, & O'Hollaren, 1941). A second problem is that aversive conditioning is acquired under well-defined circumstances, for example, the therapist's office. Rats can discriminate between environments that offer different schedules of reinforcement, and humans are no less capable. People who receive electric shocks while drinking with their therapists will probably stop drinking with their therapists, but they may drink just as much elsewhere. So, aversive conditioning is probably not effective for treating drug abuse.

Extinction. When Pavlov sounded the bell several days in a row but did not follow it with food, his dogs eventually stopped salivating to the bell. Their responses were extinguished. Drug-abusing responses can also be extinguished. Blakey and Baker (1980) reviewed drinking histories of alcoholics to identify the cues that triggered craving (which were different for each patient); then they presented those cues without allowing the patients to drink. Cues presented repeatedly and not followed by drugs eventually lost their power to elicit craving. The same technique reduced conditioned craving in heroin and cocaine abusers (Childress, McLellan, Ehrman, & O'Brien, 1988; O'Brien, McLellan, Alterman, & Childress, 1992).

Contingency Management

Contingency management provides incentives that make abstinence attractive and drug use unattractive. Rewards and punishments are administered, depending on cooperation with clinic rules, results of urinalyses, employment status, and so forth. Stitzer et al. (1989) listed some reinforcers that have been successful components of contingency management programs:

- Continued treatment availability
- Take-home doses of methadone
- Patient-controlled dose alteration
- Reduced (or increased) counseling requirements
- Reduced (or increased) clinic fee requirements
- Provision of methadone for vacations away from the clinic
- Notification of employer that the patient has used drugs
- Praise from parents or spouse
- Leaving the house or locking patients out who have used drugs
- Reduced (or increased) parole-probation requirements and sentence time
- Loss of money left as security deposit

QUITTING ON ONE'S OWN

In a survey of 278 polydrug abusers, nicotine was rated above heroin, methadone, amphetamine, barbiturates, LSD, marijuana, alcohol, and caffeine as the drug they could least do without (Russell, 1971c). Yet about 3 million Americans stop smoking each year, most without help (National Cancer Institute, 1991; Schwartz, 1987). The methods listed below, modified from a National Cancer Institute booklet (available free, by calling 1-800-4-CANCER), may help with many types of drug abuse.

Prepare to Quit

- Try not thinking about how difficult quitting will be.
- List the reasons for quitting and repeat one of the reasons each night before going to bed.
- Set a target date for quitting and don't let anything change it.

Know What to Expect

- The goal is possible. Whatever the abused drug, many people quit each year.
- Withdrawal symptoms are only temporary.
- Relapses may occur but are not fatal. Many people quit for good only after several attempts.

Involve Someone Else

- Bet a friend you can quit on the target date.
- Ask your spouse or a friend to quit with you.
- Tell friends and family that you're quitting and when.

Cut Down

- Use less each day. Postpone taking your first dose.
- Set an upper limit for each day. Every time you exceed the limit, donate a dollar to a cause you intensely dislike.
- Cutting down can help you quit but does not substitute for quitting. Once you've stabilized at a low level, set a target quit date and stick to it.

Make Drug Use Unpleasant

- If you like using with others, use alone.
- Use only while sitting in an uncomfortable chair or a dark or noisy room.

On the Day You Quit

- Throw away all your drug paraphernalia.
- Remind your family and friends that this is your quit date and ask them to help you over the rough spots.
- Do something special to celebrate.

Avoid Temptations

- Avoid situations you associate with the pleasurable aspects of the drug.
- Until you're confident of your ability to refuse, avoid situations where you might be offered the drug.

Keep Your Guard Up

Remind yourself that you've quit and are a nonuser. Recognize that the urge to use again will probably recur many times. Dampen the urge in the following ways:

- Review your list of reasons for wanting to quit, especially when you're tempted to re-use.
- Anticipate situations, people, and feelings likely to tempt you; either avoid those triggers or practice ways to cope with them.
- Each time you get through a day without using, reward yourself. Buy a record or go to a movie or concert.
- Breathing exercises and meditation relieve tension that might otherwise lead to drug use.
- Talk about your nonuse with friends and relatives and enlist their support.

CHANGING ENVIRONMENTS

In most lay and professional conceptions of drug abuse, environments act primarily to facilitate interactions between vulnerable people and addictive substances. The interactions provide momentary ecstasy that impels further drug use. Before long, physical dependence and the threat of agonizing withdrawal bar escape from addiction. At that point, environments become irrelevant. The view is wrong.

One type of evidence is that stimuli associated with drug use often become powerful reinforcers themselves. Second, environments in which desired commodities are sparsely rationed lead to various excessive behaviors including drug ingestion (see pp. 206-207). Falk and Tang (1988) wrote:

> The prototypical animal experiments using schedule-induction seem most akin to those conditions characterizing a human subcultural niche (e.g., unemployed ghetto resident) predisposing to alcoholism and other drug abuse. Like the food-limitation condition of the animal experiments, the static niche of the economically marginal ghetto is also impoverished of reinforcing opportunities that could serve as alternatives to drugs. This is not to imply that only economic marginality is the relevant condition modelled by schedule-induction conditions. There are hosts of ways lives can be marginal and impoverished. Drug abuse appears overrepresented in groups whose work subjects them to schedules of reinforcement with intermediate intermittency rates. These are life situations where problematic consequentiality is faced almost continually: e.g., market speculators, prospectors, high-construction workers, test pilots, a variety of hustling jobs, such as commission salesmen and promoters, performing jobs, such as politicians, actors, sports performers, and a variety of small-time criminals who must continually engage in streetwise action. The continuous facing of small events which are of critical consequence at an intermediate reinforcement rate describes just the sort of environmental situation that generates adjunctive behavior excesses such as alcoholism and drug abuse.

Falk and Tang's speculations that their rat experiments are relevant to understanding human drug abuse are supported by Robins's work. Robins (1973) investigated the fates of returning war veterans who had become addicted to pure heroin and opium in Vietnam. Despite dire predictions about their fates, 92% stopped using regularly within a year. Offsetting the 8% who continued to use were an approximately equal number who had been using prior to entering the service but stopped upon returning home. Goldstein (cited in Fort & Cory, 1975) commented, "If we could send most of our addicts 'home' to somewhere else, a lot of them would be cured too." Ross (1973), Frykholm (1979), and Maddux and Desmond (1982) all reported that residence relocation was a major factor in achieving abstinence.

Falk and colleagues (Tang, Ahrendsen, & Falk, 1981; Tang, Brown, & Falk, 1982) extended the work on schedule-induced drinking and reported remarkable findings:

- Rats fed at one-minute intervals for 3 hours per day drank more than twice as much alcohol as control rats given their food all at one time. The experiment continued for 130 days, and drinking remained stable throughout. Every 10th day the rats received food all at one time, and on those days they drank only as much as controls. Neither a history of alcohol drinking nor physical dependence affected drinking; what counted was the current feeding schedule—the environment.
- Rats fed at one-minute intervals for 3 hours per day became physically dependent on phenobarbital, exhibiting withdrawal signs when the drug was removed. Nevertheless, despite the constant availability of phenobarbital solution during their 21 hours per day in the home cages, they drank very little there. They were phenobarbital addicts—but only in a specific environment.

Falk and Tang (1988) sounded an optimistic note for therapy. Their comments were about alcohol but apply to all forms of drug abuse.

If the drinking of even severely alcoholic animals is driven mainly by the schedule of availability of the important things in life, then correspondingly simple changes in the schedule or range of availability of commodities and/or activities could have profound effects on human drinking. One of the therapist's tasks is perhaps to identify and, if possible, change the schedules in the life of the alcoholic that may be generating the excessive behavior. Some forms of therapy may only require appropriate alternatives to ethanol. For example, even in the presence of severe dependence, with schedule-induced animals having had a long history of choosing ethanol in preference to water, a glucose or saccharin solution that is concentrated enough alleviates the indulgence.

Summary

Conceptions of drug abuse vary greatly among both therapists and clients, and these affect treatment. Therapists should analyze their conceptual models and use integrative ones when possible.

Evaluating treatment programs for drug abuse requires knowing the programs' goals. These vary greatly. Several methodological problems make evaluations difficult.

1. Clients are rarely randomly assigned to experimental and control groups.
2. Both clients and therapists have a strong bias toward favorable outcomes.
3. Only a small proportion of eligible candidates agree to participate in programs.
4. The dropout rate from most programs is very high.

Pharmacological treatments for drug abuse should be supplemented with some form of therapy. Pharmacological treatments may be used to relieve specific symptoms of withdrawal, reduce coexisting psychiatric pathology, or reduce craving. Drugs are available that substitute for, antagonize, and deter use of drugs of abuse.

Therapeutic communities, usually run by ex-addicts, try to change the entire lifestyle of residents. They offer psychotherapy, occupational therapy, and education. The dropout rate is high, but completers show strong, positive changes and commit fewer crimes.

Self-help groups, of which Alcoholics Anonymous is the model, teach members that they are powerless against their addiction. Members are encouraged to seek and share with others in the group insights into the causes of their abuse. Although evaluation is difficult, correlational evidence suggests that AA membership reduces drinking in people who might otherwise die from liver cirrhosis.

Psychotherapy has so far proved of limited value in treating drug abusers.

A high proportion of drug abusers stop using for varying periods of time but then have relapses. So, behavior therapists try to identify situations that precipitate relapse and teach clients to cope with them.

Aversive conditioning is not effective for treating drug abuse.

A promising technique involves identifying the cues that trigger craving, then presenting the cues but denying access to the drug. After repeated presentations of cues not followed by drug reinforcement, the cues stop eliciting craving.

Contingency management techniques offer rewards and punishments for appropriate behaviors with respect to drugs.

Many abusers quit on their own. Several techniques are available that help.

Certain environments promote drug abuse. Recognizing and changing key environmental features may have a significant impact.

Mini-Quiz: Treatment

List the five basic models of drug abuse.

moral, learning, disease, self-medication, social

Which model, according to Brower, is best?

None is invariably best. Brower suggested using integrative models.

T/F: Many cigarette smokers quit on their own, but abusers of heroin, amphetamine, and cocaine rarely do.

false

T/F: The text suggests that evaluations of programs for treating drug abuse probably overestimate their successes.

true

There is a positive correlation between time spent in drug abuse treatment programs and success in staying off drugs of abuse. Why does that not prove that the programs work?

a. **People who enroll in programs are highly committed to succeed, and they might succeed even without the program.**
b. **The less committed people tend to drop out of programs.**

What is the role of drugs like benzodiazepines and antidepressants in drug abuse programs?

They relieve symptoms of withdrawal.

According to a theory discussed in the text, chronic use of cocaine depletes brain stores of _____; the drug _____ restores activity of the depleted NT and blocks craving for cocaine.

dopamine; bromocriptine

Alcohol intake is reduced by drugs that increase levels of the NT _____.

serotonin

A synthetic opioid that is widely used to reduce withdrawal symptoms from heroin is _____.

methadone

Why do many people prefer that heroin addicts get methadone rather than heroin?

methadone can be taken orally and is long-acting

Methadone substitutes for heroin as _____ substitutes for cigarette smoking.

nicotine chewing gum

Name an antagonist for alcohol. For heroin. For nicotine.

RO15-4513; naloxone; mecamylamine

Name a deterrent for alcohol. For nicotine.

disulfiram; silver acetate gum

Which type of treatment tries to effect a global change in the abuser's lifestyle?

therapeutic community

Which type of program is run primarily by ex-abusers?

therapeutic community

What is the best known peer-support self-help group?

Alcoholics Anonymous

Why is it so difficult to evaluate the effectiveness of AA?

Because of the tradition of anonymity, there are no accurate counts of members or dropouts.

T/F: Psychoanalysis is better than other forms of psychotherapy for treating drug abusers.

false; no form of psychotherapy has been shown more effective than other forms

A trait common to many drug abusers that does not respond well to psychotherapy is _____.

antisocial personality disorder

The four behavioral treatment methods discussed in the text are _____.

behavioral counseling, relapse prevention skills training, stimulus counter-conditioning, and contingency management

T/F: Most therapists believe that the key to drug abuse treatment is detoxification.

false

T/F: Aversive conditioning has not been shown to be very effective in treating drug abuse.

true

T/F: Falk showed that a light that had been associated with a drug eventually became a more powerful reinforcer than the drug itself.

true

By the time you finish reading this chapter, you should be able to answer the following questions:

What clear-cut behavioral effect is observed when high doses of antipsychotic drugs are administered to animals?

What are the most commonly used drugs in nursing homes? Why are they popular?

What are the two key features of experiments?

What is a double-blind study?

What are active placebos?

Why should evaluations of drug effectiveness not focus on elimination of negative symptoms?

What factors work against the observation of positive drug effects?

Why are psychiatrists biased toward prescribing psychiatric drugs?

Do reasonable alternatives exist to psychiatric drugs?

T/F: Psychiatrists generally agree that drugs are very helpful for treating the different types of mental illness.

T/F: Double-blind studies ensure that neither researchers nor patients can figure out who has received which treatment.

T/F: To study drug effects properly, therapists should not show enthusiasm toward patients.

Psychopharmacotherapy

Methodological Issues

Contents

In the 1974 edition of *Drugs and Behavior,* the psychopharmacotherapy chapter opened with a ringing endorsement by Kline (1959) on the use of drugs to treat mental illness.

> In the 175-year history of public mental hospitals in the United States there had always been (until 1956) more patients in the hospitals at the end of any single year than there were at the beginning. This total had then reached the staggering number of 750,000, i.e., three-quarters of a million patients with an estimated cost to our economy of some four billion dollars a year.

Kline went on to say that more patients were discharged than admitted in 1956, and the reversed trend has continued. The reason, according to him, was the discovery and subsequent widespread use of a few magical drugs.

By the 1982 edition, the picture had become considerably murkier and the following words from Jarvik, Flinn, and West (1976) were judged more apt:

Many thousands of schizophrenics have been thrust back into their communities under dubious conditions solely because psychotropic drugs have rendered them manageable. There they often stagnate in board and care homes or wander harmlessly through the streets dazed by drugs, each patient wrapped in a chemical cocoon. Thus modern drugs make it possible for large numbers of mental patients—most of them schizophrenics—to be managed in the community at relatively low cost. However, this may mean denying them opportunities for other forms of treatment (psychotherapy, group therapy, occupational and recreational therapies, vocational rehabilitation, etc.) that a truly good psychiatric hospital provides.

Debate continues. Since the last edition, several authors have argued that drugs be given a greatly diminished role in managing psychiatric illnesses (cf. Breggin, 1983; Fisher & Greenberg, 1989b). They urge greater emphasis on alternative treatments. However, critics are in the minority. (For the majority view, cf. Kane, 1987; Rickels & Schweizer, 1990; Baldessarini, 1990a; Teboul & Chouinard, 1991.) Because the drugs cause side effects, cost money, and are often aversive to patients, the burden of proof should be with the drug proponents.

A focal point of the debate, especially as applied to antipsychotic drugs, is that the drugs sedate. When high doses of antipsychotics are injected into laboratory animals, the animals can be molded into bizarre positions and will remain there. The duration of the immobility is correlated with antipsychotic efficacy in humans. The following passage from Delay and Deniker (cited in Marholin & Phillips, 1976) indicates that people respond similarly. Their last sentence makes clear Delay and Deniker's belief that chlorpromazine is beneficial.

> Sitting or lying, the patient is motionless in his bed, often pale and with eyelids lowered. He remains silent most of the time. If he is questioned, he answers slowly and deliberately in a monotonous, indifferent voice; he expresses himself in a few words and becomes silent. Without exception the response is fairly appropriate and adaptable, showing that the subject is capable of attention and of thought. But he rarely initiates a question and he does not express his anxieties, desires, or preferences. He is usually aware of the improvement induced by the treatment but does not show euphoria.

The prevailing view, that antipsychotic drugs "generally have a dramatic effect on the symptoms of schizophrenia (e.g., delusions, hallucinations, and thought disorder)" (Kane, 1987) seems at odds with their use in nursing homes, prisons, and institutions for the mentally retarded. The incidence of schizophrenia in such places is not substantially higher than in the population at large. Yet in one three-state survey, investigators found that 8 of the 10 most frequently prescribed drugs in nursing homes were psychoactive, with major tranquilizers being first and third on the list (Prentice, 1979). More recently, Avorn, Dreyer, Connelly, and Soumerai (1989) surveyed 55 rest homes in Massachusetts and found that psychoactive drugs had been prescribed for almost half the residents; 40% were receiving antipsychotic drugs, and 18%, two or more antipsychotics. Clements (cited in Breggin, 1983) reported that 70% of 750 inmates in one penal institution were taking antipsychotics. Psychotropic drug use in institutions for the mentally retarded ranges from 19% to 86%, with more prescribed in larger facilities with the most restrictive environments (Singh & Winton, 1989). Bates, Smeltzer, and Arnoczky (1986) estimated that only 45% of the prescriptions were appropriate, and Singh and Winton (1989) argued that there is no acceptable reason for using antipsychotic drugs with the mentally retarded. Plotkin and Rigling (1979) also reported extensive use of the drugs in long-term facilities for the mentally retarded. They wrote, "Phenothiazines satisfy the institution's need to reduce objectionable behavior by reducing virtually all behavior."

So critics charge that psychiatric drugs are prescribed exclusively for their sedating effects, and advocates respond that sedation has nothing to do with it. Perhaps both sides should acknowledge that hospital staff in charge of the mentally ill and parents of hyperactive children are often beleaguered. Their charges disrupt, demand attention, and interfere with the care of others. Sedation, although not an adequate solution, compares favorably with many alternatives.

There have been literally tens of thousands of studies with psychiatric drugs, and reports of outcome range from dismal to spectacular. A set of statistical techniques called meta-analysis enables investigators to combine results from groups of studies to answer questions such as, "What is the average effect of a treatment?" and "Under what conditions is a treatment particularly effective or ineffective?" One noteworthy finding is the inverse relationship between rigor of research design and strength of reported effect. On average, the smallest improvements due to drug have been reported from the most carefully conducted studies (Smith, Traganza, & Harrison, 1969). On the other hand, many well-designed studies have demonstrated clear-cut, beneficial drug effects. Researchers are working diligently to identify the special matches of patient, drug, and context that augur therapeutic success.

▓ Evidence for the Effectiveness of Drugs Used in Psychiatry

A FEW METHODOLOGICAL PRINCIPLES

Experimentation, the best method for evaluating treatment effectiveness, has two key features. First, each subject must either be assigned randomly to one of the treatment groups or exposed to all treatments in random order. Second, except for the specific treatments, all subjects must be handled identically.

Random Assignment

Random assignment, which helps prevent researchers' biases from influencing data collection, requires using a chance procedure such as a random number table. No other basis for assignment, including order of arrival, severity of symptoms, financial need, or geographical location, is acceptable. Assigning all subjects to receive the same treatment, that is, not having a control group, is a cardinal methodological sin that inflates the likelihood of false positive results. Uncontrolled drug studies were common in the not-too-distant past. Despite their shortcomings, they helped shape opinion on the efficacy of the drugs (cf. reviews by Foulds, 1963; Smith et al., 1969; Smith & Lang, 1980; Wechsler, Grosser, & Greenblatt, 1965).

Treatment of Experimental and Control Groups

Random assignment makes it highly probable that experimental and control groups start out approximately equal. If both groups are then treated identically in all respects but one, researchers can justifiably attribute subsequent differences to that one factor. Groups treated differently in more than one way may differ for more than one reason. For example, the finding that rats injected with a drug show more stress than uninjected controls would not conclusively demonstrate that the drug increases stress. A plausible alternative would be that needle insertion was the stress inducer. So researchers use placebo control groups; even then, both nonpharmacological and nonspecific pharmacological factors may contribute to differences between drugged and control subjects.

Researchers who believe in a treatment's efficacy and know who have and have not received it may (not necessarily intentionally) influence outcomes by conveying their expectations (cf. Rosenthal & Rosnow, 1969; Smith & Lang, 1980). So psychopharmacologists do double-blind studies, in which neither experimenters nor subjects know who has received what until all the data are in. But if drug and placebo preparations look different (they often do—cf. Hill, Nunn, & Fox, 1976), or if the drug produces side effects such as dry mouth, nausea, or changes in heart rate, respiration, pupil size, appetite, frequency of urination, sleep patterns, and so forth, either experimenters or subjects or both may deduce who has received the drug. Rabkin et al. (1986) asked both patients and physicians in a double-blind study to guess whether the patients had received placebo or active drug. Patients guessed correctly 79% and physicians 87% of the time; even when patients were judged not to have responded to the drug, physicians correctly guessed 84% of the time. Similarly, Margraf et al. (1991) found that the great majority of panic disorder patients and their physicians guessed correctly whether active drug (alprazolam or imipramine) or placebo had been given; the physicians even distinguished between the two active drugs and did so halfway through treatment.

The solution currently regarded as optimal is to give active placebos—drugs with discriminable side effects but neutral with respect to the condition being treated. Greenberg and Fisher (1989) cited studies showing that the apparent advantage of antidepressant drugs over placebos is reduced when the placebos are active. On the other hand, active placebos sometimes produce negative effects; so patients who receive an ineffective drug are comparatively better, and researchers might conclude incorrectly that the drug is therapeutic (Lipman et al., 1966).

In recent years, experimenters have routinely initiated drug studies by giving placebos for 7 to 10 days to all potential subjects. Those who markedly improve—generally about 20% (Rabkin et al., 1987)—would subsequently be expected to show the smallest drug/placebo differences but are disqualified from further participation. So, although they constitute a significant portion of the psychiatric population, findings do not apply to them.

Measurement Issues

Neither psychiatrists nor psychologists have achieved consensus on the criteria for clinical improvement. In drug studies, psychiatrists often use a single measure—global assessment of patients with a scale that the psychiatrist has privately developed. Such scales have unknown validity and reliability and are susceptible to bias. Murray (1989) urged researchers to use more than one measure and pointed out that exclusive use of psychiatrists' ratings devalues the perspective of patients and their families. (Reserpine, one of the first drugs for treating schizophrenia, reduced the incidence of hallucinations and disordered thought. So, from the standpoint of the therapist, reserpine was successful. But the patients often felt worse. Jarvik (1965) wrote, "administration has been associated with depression severe enough to cause suicide by some patients.")

Murray compared the Hamilton Rating Scale for Depression (HAM-D), an interview measure, with the Beck Depression Inventory (BDI), a self-report measure. The (HAM-D) is less reliable and valid but more widely used. Reports of antidepressant drug effects have generally been larger following use of the HAM-D.

Whether data are gathered by clinical interview, self-report, or both, antipsychotic drug effectiveness should not be judged primarily by the extent to which the drugs reduce negative symptoms. Patients sitting motionless in bed display few symptoms, nor would patients cracked over the head with baseball bats. But the goal of therapy should be to replace negative symptoms with positive ones.

Statistical Issues

Halperin (1989) analyzed 49 studies on antianxiety and antidepressant drugs, and he concluded that three important statistical issues compromise interpretations. First, at least one subject in each study dropped out before the end. None of the authors used statistical techniques for coping with attrition.

Second, many authors used a battery of physiological and psychological tests; some probably appeared significant by chance. Suppose, for example, that a coin came up heads five out of five times. The probability of that happening with a fair coin is .03, so an observer could justifiably conclude that either the coin was biased or somebody cheated. But the probability is almost .80 that if 50 unbiased coins are all flipped fairly, at least one will turn up heads five times out of five. By the same reasoning, a researcher who tests 50 variables at the .03 level has a .80 chance of finding at least one spuriously significant result.

Third, Halperin reported that several authors used incorrect statistical procedures or violated the assumptions required of the tests they used. A special statistical problem arises with meta-analysis (combining results from several studies): Reports of positive drug effects are more likely to be published than those in which a drug has been ineffective. So, if only published studies are analyzed, the size of the effect is likely to appear greater than it actually is. See page 101 for further discussion.

Cost-Benefit Analysis

For many medical conditions, most patients respond to proper treatment with complete and permanent remission of symptoms. But many victims of mental disease are not helped by psychiatric drugs; virtually none have symptoms eliminated completely; and most are at serious risk for relapse if their drugs are discontinued. Table 13.1 summarizes relapse data from several studies on a variety of conditions.

So the costs of pharmacotherapy must be weighed against possibly small, short-lived improvements. Fisher and Greenberg (1989b) wrote:

What if the true difference in efficacy between placebo and tricyclic is somewhere between 20% and 30%? Does such an advantage outweigh the potential threat of a side effect like drug-induced psychosis? If there is a potential 5%-6% probability of being rendered psychotic (albeit temporarily) by an antidepressant drug, should one seriously hesitate about accepting it as a reasonable treatment? Incidentally, we do not know what long-term effects a tricyclic-induced delirium has upon individuals. Do such individuals, as a result, suffer persistent elevations in anxiety about their future stability (e.g., "I am crazy" or "I am a person who can become crazy")? How much of a risk of psychosis is it worth taking to gain relief from moderate or even severe depression, which typically has a fairly self-limiting course? Related questions arise for each therapeutic drug in relation to its own peculiar side effects. What is the impact upon a schizophrenic man who becomes impotent as the result of taking an antipsychotic drug? How devastating is such an episode of impotence upon long-term sexual self-regard? Does it introduce permanent doubts about one's sexual functioning? Does this, in turn, feed back and increase the likelihood of future psychotic disruptions? Analogous questions come to mind

Table 13.1 Results of Drug Discontinuation

Psychiatric Illness	Main Finding	Reference
Schizophrenia	Drug holidays or reduction in dose led to a worse psychosis than the original one in 22% of patients.	Chouinard et al. (1986)
	Among successfully maintained schizophrenic out-patients, nearly one third were judged too ill to risk drug discontinuation; of the remainder, two thirds relapsed following withdrawal.	Hogarty (1976)
Depression	About 50% of depressed patients relapse within 2 years of recovery.	Belsher & Costello (1988)
	Of patients who had been symptom free for at least 16 weeks, about 20% relapsed within 8 weeks when switched from drug to placebo. Of patients who had been symptom free for fewer than 16 weeks, 59% relapsed.	Prien & Kupfer (1986)
Obsessive-Compulsive disorder	16 of 18 patients switched from drug to placebo experienced severe worsening of symptoms within 4 weeks.	Pato et al. (1988)
Panic attacks	In a study involving 3 different drugs, when the drug was stopped after a year of treatment, between 71% and 92% had a recurrence of symptoms within 3 months	Sheehan (cited in Kahn, 1990)
Generalized anxiety disorder	The rate of relapse in the year following treatment was 63%	Rickels et al. (1986)
	Rebound anxiety following withdrawal ranged from 25% for drugs with a long half-life to 70% for drugs with a short half-life.	Teboul & Chouinard (1991)
	After receiving long-term therapy with even modest doses of benzodiazepines, more than 50% of patients are physically dependent and experience withdrawal symptoms upon discontinuation.	Rickels et al. (1991)

for an agent like clomipramine that gives improvement rates (30%-40%) significantly greater than placebo for obsessive-compulsive behavior, but which apparently in most instances also leads to partial or total anorgasmia.

Dewan and Koss (1989) reported that side effects from psychiatric drugs lead to drug discontinuation in about 5% to 10% of patients. For many, the side effects are worse than the original sickness, and figures on their incidence are probably too low. Of patients taking an antihypertensive drug, 10% volunteered that they had become impotent; when asked directly, the figure was 26%; and 47% admitted it when they filled out a questionnaire in private (DeLeo & Magni, 1983).

FACTORS WORKING AGAINST THE OBSERVATION OF POSITIVE DRUG EFFECTS

Double-blind studies, especially with active placebos, minimize the likelihood that an ineffective treatment will appear useful. But they may also make useful treatments appear ineffective. Two lines of evidence are relevant. First, in both blind and nonblind studies, enthusiastic therapists are more likely than unenthusiastic ones to get positive results (Fisher et al., 1964; Sheard, 1963; Uhlenhuth, 1966; Uhlenhuth, Canter, Neustadt, & Payson, 1959; Wheatley, 1968). Second, the response to an active drug may be weakened if recipients are uncertain about its effectiveness (Volgyesi, 1954; Wilson & Abrams, 1977).

Coolness toward patients is not a methodological commandment, but disciplined scientists probably display considerably less enthusiasm than do true believers. As to patients, ethical concerns dictate that they be told they may receive placebo. Then, perhaps especially because they suffer psychiatric illness, they may be wary about stating that a possibly inactive medication has helped them.

Several other factors conspire against psychiatric researchers. Laboratory scientists typically restrict their experiments to homogeneous subjects, such as college sophomore women or male rats of the same strain, age, weight, and prior experiences; but psychiatric patients are heterogeneous in demographic characteristics, length and severity of their illnesses, and pre- and post-treatment life situations. Only rarely do they all receive medication at the same time from the same therapist. Because of the great variability, only very strong effects reach statistical significance.

WHY ARE THE DRUGS PRESCRIBED?

Despite evidence that psychiatric drugs are often ineffective and may cause pain and physical damage, psychiatrists prescribe them in large quantities. Breggin (1983) offered two explanations. First, as discussed in Chapter 6, the drugs are heavily promoted by the pharmaceutical industry. Not only do drug manufacturers offer gifts and misleading product information to prescribers and potential prescribers but, according to Schrag (1978):

> Most of the major figures in drug research serve as consultants to drug firms and, at the same time, to NIMH and the Food and Drug Administration, which licenses the drugs. They review each other's grant proposals, sit on the same committees, work on the same studies, write for each other's journals. NIMH employees collaborate with drug-company consultants in mental health research; NIMH consultants appear before FDA review committees on behalf of drug companies; editors of journals heavily supported by drug-company advertising serve on "impartial" FDA committees reviewing the safety and efficacy of medication produced by their advertisers.

Kleinman and Cohen (1991) observed that drug advertisements ignore the role of social factors in causing mental illness. By implying that treatment requires only transformation of the individual, they undermine competing therapies such as vocational rehabilitation and occupational therapy; and they fully ignore remedies such as improvements in housing, job opportunities, education, economic equality, and organization of family domestic life.

Pam (1990) noted that research grant money is readily accessible to drug-oriented psychiatrists from drug companies and the government. Research leads to professional recognition and prestigious academic posts. Eminent academics influence incoming residents: They often receive government posts and become responsible for offering grants to medical schools. Pam wrote, "Fundamentally, the pharmaceutical industry is a lobby within psychiatry, pushing for biological findings in etiological research and thus justifying biological treatments."

Breggin's second reason is that the capacity to prescribe drugs distinguishes psychiatrists from other psychotherapists. This enhances their identity with the medical profession, as it enables them to offer therapy beyond mere talking. It also increases their earning power. Breggin (1983) quoted Weiss and Tanner (1981), "Physicians who do *procedures*—

surgery, radiotherapy, even electroshock or prescribing pills—can earn as much in ten minutes as a psychiatrist or family doctors doing psychotherapy or counseling can in an hour." Of course, the same factors that cause psychiatrists to favor drugs promote an antidrug bias among psychologists. Patients cured by drugs don't pay for extended psychotherapy. Breggin is a psychiatrist, but most of the contributors to Fisher and Greenberg's book are not.

ALTERNATIVES TO DRUGS

Given the questions about psychiatric drugs, they ought to be a last rather than first resort for treating the mentally ill. In some cases, effective alternatives reduce or eliminate the need for drugs. In others, combined drug/alternative therapy is superior to either alone. In contrast to the often health-impairing side effects of drugs, the alternatives typically promote physical as well as mental health.

Koranyi (1980) reported that about 50% of 2,000 psychiatric outpatients had major medical illnesses undiagnosed by their referring clinicians; and Bartels (1989) summarized evidence showing that physical illness is the sole cause of symptoms in about 20%, and makes symptoms worse in about 67%, of psychiatric patients. Gold (1987) stated that nearly 40% of diagnoses of depression are misdiagnoses of physical illnesses. Drugs used to treat medical illnesses may cause depression, anxiety, or psychosis, particularly in the elderly (Salzman & Shader, 1978). These include digitalis, reserpine, guanethidine, clonidine, L-dopa, bronchodilators, and cortisones. Caffeine, a mild antidepressant for most people, induces depression in some (Christensen & Burrows, 1990). Identifying and treating the cause of symptoms in such cases is clearly preferable to administering a psychiatric drug.

Certain foods and environmental toxins like lead and aluminum sometimes cause or exacerbate emotional disorders. Dohan (1979) reported that symptoms improved among schizophrenics placed on a wheat- and dairy-free diet, whereas King and Mandell (1978) provoked psychiatric symptoms by exposing adults to common allergens. DeFreitas and Schwartz (1979) surreptitiously switched the coffee on a psychiatric ward to a decaffeinated brand; the mostly schizophrenic patients improved significantly, then reverted when regular coffee was reintroduced.

Egger et al. (1985) put children diagnosed with attention-deficit disorder on diets restricted to one type of meat, carbohydrate, and vegetable, plus water, calcium, and vitamins. Some children showed rapid positive behavioral changes, and others responded when subsequently tried with other, equally restrictive diets. Foods were introduced one by one to the diets over the following few months, and if symptoms worsened, were listed as potential causative agents. Double-blind testing confirmed or disconfirmed the suspicions. Additives, colorings, and 43 naturally occurring foods all induced symptoms in at least one child.

Pfeiffer (1987), along with other orthomolecular psychiatrists, blames emotional disturbances on dietary inadequacies. He attributed many cures (mostly from nonblind studies) to vitamin supplements. Godfrey et al. (1990) noted that anemia caused by folate (vitamin B_{12}) deficiency is associated with psychiatric complications in about two-thirds of patients, and almost one-quarter of psychiatric patients have depressed folate levels. They gave methylfolate or placebo, plus standard psychotropic drugs, to 123 depressed or schizophrenic patients with low folate levels. At both 3- and 6-month follow-ups, both schizophrenic and depressed methylfolate-treated patients did better than their counterparts who received placebo.

In certain parts of the world, selenium levels in food are so low that people may experience a subclinical deficiency leading to depression. Benton and Cook (1991) administered selenium or placebo to subjects for 5 weeks; then, after a 6-month washout period, they gave the subjects the alternate treatment. At several key points, the subjects completed a standardized test for evaluating mood. During the period of selenium intake, the moods of subjects and especially those who had been relatively selenium-deficient, improved significantly.

In many cases, thyroid hormone relieves depression and other psychiatric illnesses (Prange, Garbutt, & Loosen, 1987). Depressed people often have disordered biological rhythms, and some become worse each winter when days grow short. Daily exposure to bright light during normal dark hours often helps, especially among victims of seasonal affective depression (Lewy et al., 1988).

Studies on both clinical and nonclinical subjects show that regular physical exercise is therapeutic (Johnsgaard, 1989; Plante & Rodin, 1990). Exercise improves mood and well-being and reduces anxiety, depression, and stress.

Last but not least is psychotherapy. Yeats (1989), commenting on a study in which antidepressants failed to successfully treat depressed women with marital problems, wrote, "Trying to treat depression without treating the marital distress is like trying to treat hayfever when the patient works in a flower shop." In the volume edited by

Fisher and Greenberg (1989a), studies were analyzed in which drugs were compared with psychotherapy for depression (Greenberg & Fisher, 1989b), anxiety disorders (Lipman, 1989), and schizophrenia (Karon, 1989). In general, psychotherapy-treated patients did at least as well.

Hollon and Beck (1987) noted that efficacy is not the only criterion by which to compare treatments. Others include changes in specific symptoms, acceptability, safety, cost-effectiveness, and range of applicability. Hughes and Pierattini (1992) pointed out that pharmacotherapists often use symptom relief as their criterion of success, whereas psychotherapists use functional criteria such as return to work.

Summary

Mental health workers disagree among themselves about the value of psychiatric drugs. Critics argue that the drugs are used because they make patients manageable. Proponents point to several studies that, they claim, conclusively establish the value of the drugs. But much of the evidence is unsatisfactory, based on research lacking methodological rigor. Concerns include the following:

1. *Lack of Double-Blindness.* Even when placebo controls have been used, both therapists and patients have guessed with considerably better than chance accuracy which patients received which treatments.

2. *Measurement of Improvement.* Therapists have assessed improvement primarily from their perspectives, not from patients'.

3. *Statistical Issues.* Therapists have violated several statistical principles in analyzing data.

Drug advertisements, and prominent researchers with financial ties to pharmaceutical companies, have had undue influence on prescribing practices of psychiatrists. Another factor that leads to overprescribing is that psychiatrists distinguish themselves from other psychotherapists by their capacity to prescribe drugs.

Several alternatives to psychiatric drugs are available: identifying and correcting problems associated with physical illnesses, environmental toxins, and vitamin deficiencies that cause or contribute to psychiatric symptoms; physical exercise; and psychotherapy.

Mini-Quiz: Psychopharmacotherapy: Methodology

T/F: The incidence of schizophrenia is far greater in nursing homes and homes for the retarded than in the population at large.

false

T/F: Antipsychotic drugs are prescribed at much higher rates in nursing homes and homes for the retarded than in the population at large.

true

A set of statistical techniques that lets researchers combine results from groups of studies is called _____.

meta-analysis

What are the two key features of experiments?

    a. Each subject must either be assigned randomly to one of the treatment groups or exposed to all treatments in random order.

    b. Except for the specific treatments, all subjects must be handled identically.

In a _____ study, neither experiments nor subjects know which subjects get which treatments until the end of the study.

double-blind

Control subjects may be given a drug with discriminable side effects but neutral with respect to the condition being treated. The drug is called a(n) _____.

active placebo

If an active placebo produces negative effects, an ineffective drug that is compared with it may seem _____.

beneficial

T/F: According to the text, the best measure of the effectiveness of antipsychotic drugs is the extent to which they reduce negative symptoms.

false

T/F: The incidence of side effects from psychiatric drugs is probably considerably more than what is reported.

true

T/F: In double-blind studies, enthusiastic therapists are more likely than nonenthusiastic ones to get positive results.

true

Why, according to critics, are psychiatric drugs so overprescribed?

    a. **The drugs are heavily promoted by the pharmaceutical industry.**

    b. **Psychiatrists gain status over other therapists because of their ability to prescribe drugs, and they make more money doing so.**

The text lists several alternatives to drugs for treating psychiatric conditions. Name six.

    a. **Diagnose and treat physical illness.**

    b. **Eliminate a drug or environmental toxin that is causing mental symptoms.**

    c. **Check for a vitamin deficiency and correct as needed.**

    d. **Expose depressed people to bright light.**

    e. **Put people on an exercise regimen.**

    f. **Offer psychotherapy.**

By the time you finish reading this chapter, you should be able to answer the following questions:

About what percentage of American adults use a drug for emotional problems at least once per year?

The best evidence points to an excess of the neurotransmitter ___ in schizophrenics.

Which neurotransmitter is most associated with anxiety disorders?

Which neurotransmitters are most associated with depression?

What major side effect is observed in about 40% of patients maintained on antipsychotic drugs?

Critics charge that antipsychotic drugs are administered primarily because of their ___ effects.

What type of drugs are most frequently prescribed to children with attention-deficit disorder (hyperactivity)?

What rationale motivated psychiatrists to administer LSD and related drugs to emotionally disturbed patients?

Psychopharmacotherapy

Contents

K lerman (1986) estimated that 10% to 12% of U.S. adults use a drug for emotional problems at least once per year; and about 2 million U.S. children are treated annually for emotional disorders (Links, Boyle, & Offord, 1989).

Clinical psychologists, even if they don't prescribe drugs, should familiarize themselves with **pharmacotherapy**. Hughes and Pierattini (1992) offered several reasons:

1. Many of their patients will be taking psychoactive drugs, and the drugs can influence both assessment and treatment. Cessation of the drugs can induce new symptoms.
2. For some conditions, drugs are important primary or adjunctive treatments.

3. Familiarity with pharmacotherapy may help psychologists recognize inappropriate treatments.
4. Psychologists are sometimes asked by patients, families, or social systems to render an opinion about pharmacotherapy for a particular set of symptoms.

Hughes and Pierattini (1992) offered several general principles of rational prescribing:

1. Most drugs within a class have similar efficacy, so specific drugs should be chosen for side effect profile, rapidity and duration of action, route of administration, and so forth.
2. Because responsiveness to drugs varies tremendously (see Chapter 5), dosage should be determined for each patient individually. Hughes and Pierattini claimed that many psychiatrists use inadequate doses for inadequate periods of time.
3. Target symptoms should be clearly defined and monitored.
4. A drug that produces significant side effects (which often precede therapeutic effects) may nevertheless be the best treatment for a particular condition. Patients should be informed about potential side effects.
5. Drug prescribers should be sensitive to the needs of special populations: Patterns of psychiatric symptoms may differ in children and adults; elderly people taking drugs for medical conditions have increased risk of interactions; women taking psychoactive drugs may become pregnant.

This chapter reviews drugs for treating schizophrenia, depression, bipolar disorder (manic depression), anxiety disorders, and attention-deficit disorder (ADD). For other problems or detailed discussions of specific drugs and dosages, see Ellison (1989) or Gitlin (1990). For additional pediatric problems, see Gadow (1986) or Brumback and Weinberg (1990).

▧ Antipsychotics

Between 1% and 2% of U.S. citizens have had or will have at least one schizophrenic episode, and 25% of all patients in hospitals are schizophrenic (Robins et al., 1984). The term *schizophrenia* applies to a group of disorders with certain common factors. The most frequent problems are of five types:

Perceptual disorders: Physical sensations are distorted and patients may hallucinate.

Emotional disorders: Patients seemingly lack emotional responsiveness and often laugh inappropriately.

Thought and speech disorders: Patients do not put thoughts together in a comprehensible way; they coin words and use sequences of unrelated words.

Delusions: The most common are delusions of persecution, of being controlled by outside forces, and of grandeur.

Motor disorders: Patients may become inactive or frenetically, apparently purposelessly, active.

In 1949, the French surgeon Laborit speculated that inhibition of the ANS would reduce surgical shock. Histamine was believed involved in ANS effects, so he administered the antihistaminic drug promethazine as a preoperative procedure. Although his rationale was incorrect, promethazine-pretreated patients experienced less suffering than others. They also became drowsy and sedated. Laborit initially regarded the side effects as undesirable, then later reasoned that similar drugs with stronger sedating properties might be clinically useful. A search began, and the next year Charpentier synthesized chlorpromazine (CPZ). CPZ, one of thousands of derivatives of phenothiazine, has little antihistaminic but strong antiadrenergic and anticholinergic properties. It soon became the treatment of choice for schizophrenia and remains the standard against which other antipsychotic drugs are judged. (According to Baldessarini [1990a], the antipsychotics benefit virtually all classes of psychotic illness, not just schizophrenia. The discussion below, however, is restricted to schizophrenia.)

Phenothiazines block dopamine (DA) receptors whereas amphetamine, which worsens clinical symptoms in most schizophrenics, increases DA levels. These and related observations led to the hypothesis that schizophrenia is caused by excessive DA activity. The hypothesis was refined to focus on activity of a subset of DA receptors (D2 receptors) within limbic and cortical areas of the brain. High correlations were found between both therapeutic effectiveness and potency of the antipsychotic drugs and their ability to block the D2 receptors (Peroutka & Snyder, 1980; Seeman & Lee, 1975). Post-mortem analyses demonstrated higher concentrations in schizophrenics than normals of certain D2 receptors (Reynolds, 1983).

Although the dopamine hypothesis is promising, other NTs are almost surely also involved in schizophrenia. In addition, there is some conflicting evidence: Amphetamine does not worsen symptoms in all schizophrenics (Van Kammen et al., 1982); there is little direct evidence that schizophrenics have excessive DA activity (Martin, Owen, & Morisha, 1987); and some schizophrenics improve upon administration of drugs that increase level of DA (Crow, Ferrier, & Johnstone, 1986). Finally, the atypical antipsychotic clozapine blocks D2 receptors weakly but D4, alpha-adrenergic, and serotonin (5-HT2) receptors strongly.

ACUTE SCHIZOPHRENIA

Karon (1989), whose strong antidrug position is presented below, conceded that antipsychotics can help during acute episodes.

Patients usually become less frightened and frightening. They also generally become less angry. They may lose some of their dramatic "positive" symptoms, like hallucinations, which were generated to cope with their terror. In other cases, hallucinations and delusions remain, but the patients are not as troubled by them. They take orders better, and comply with other people's demands better. They tend not to frighten ward staff, relatives, and others. Violent patients usually become manageable, although sometimes only by dosage levels that leave the patient barely awake. The ward staff, treating physician, and family do not feel powerless. Patients are spared some of the destructive things that other people, out of fear, often used to do to schizophrenic patients, both in and out of hospitals.

CHRONIC SCHIZOPHRENIA

The Dominant View Concerning
Effectiveness of Antipsychotic Drugs

Kane (1987) wrote: "Maintenance antipsychotic drug treatment has proved to be of enormous value in reducing the risk of psychotic relapse and rehospitalization. Numerous double-blind, placebo-controlled clinical trials can be cited to support this conclusion." Baldessarini (1990a) wrote that antipsychotics are especially effective against specific symptoms including tension, hyperactivity, combativeness, hostility, hallucinations, acute delusions, insomnia, anorexia, poor self-care, and negativism.

Table 14.1 Expenditures for Psychotropic Medications in the United States in 1985

Drug or Drug Class	Expenditure in Thousands of Dollars
Antianxiety and sedative-hypnotic	867,272
Antidepressant	239,755
tricyclic	175,806
second generation antidepressant	57,967
monoamine oxidase inhibitor	5,755
Antipsychotic	262,616
phenothiazine	146,845
haloperidol	64,777

SOURCE: Adapted from Zorc et al. (1991).

Kane (1987) presented a table listing 21 positive studies of antipsychotic drugs, and they have convinced most psychiatrists. In fact, 98% of newly hospitalized schizophrenics receive drugs, and 95% of the drugs are antipsychotics (Zito, Craig, Wanderling, & Siegel, 1987). Retail pharmacies dispensed 21.3 million prescriptions for antipsychotic drugs in 1976 and 18.6 million in 1985 (Wysowski & Baum, 1989). Six drugs—thioridazine, haloperidol, chlorpromazine, trifluoperazine, thiothixene, and fluphenazine—accounted for 90% to 91% of the total. The most notable change during the period was a dramatic increase in prescriptions for haloperidol.

Zorc, Larson, Lyons, and Beardsley (1991) surveyed pharmacies across the United States. Table 14.1, adapted from their work, gives figures on expenditures for antipsychotics and various other drugs and drug classes.

Kane (1987) wrote, "there are at present no convincing data that among medications currently marketed in the United States any one is more effective either in schizophrenia in general or in specific subtypes of the disorder." Ban (1990), however, argued that drug effectiveness varies considerably with the different subtypes. Baldessarini (1990a) advised that drugs be picked according to their side effects. He added that combinations of antipsychotics probably offer no special advantage.

PREDICTORS OF RESPONSIVENESS

Researchers search for reliable, inexpensive tests to distinguish between people who will respond well and poorly to specific drugs. A test may be useful even if its link to a clinical condition is obscure. Three examples of promising **psychophysiological measures** are described below. See Tueting (1991) for a review.

- In schizophrenics who rapidly relapsed when their antipsychotic drug was withdrawn, the stimulant drug methylphenidate increased heart rate only slightly. But spontaneous rate of blinking was greatly increased.
- The greater the blink rate decrease after haloperidol administration, the more favorable was the clinical outcome.
- When treated with antipsychotics, nonresponsive patients showed EEG changes more characteristic of those produced by a stimulant than an antipsychotic.

Voices of Dissent

All but two of the studies Kane cited covered time periods of a year or less, and the difference between drug and placebo groups decreased with time (Karon, 1989). Moreover, whereas a high proportion of drug-free schizophrenics show long-term trends toward improvement (Harding, Zubin, & Strauss, 1987), those maintained on medication do not. Lipton and Burnett (1979) concluded that, despite continued medication, 30% were rehospitalized within a year; and only 30% of the 60% considered socially recovered at the end of 5 years were employed at any time during those years.

Karon analyzed the six major American studies published since 1960 that compared drug treatment with psychotherapy for schizophrenia. Only two of the six (Grinspoon, Ewalt, & Shader, 1972; May, 1968) favored drugs, and several of Karon's insights cast doubt on their validity.

1. The psychotherapists were either generally inexperienced or inexperienced in treating chronic schizophrenics, and some believed that psychotherapy was inappropriate with such patients.
2. For May's project, evaluators rated patients globally from records written by personnel whose main concern was ward adjustment. Drugs improve ward adjustment by making patients more docile, but ward adjustment does not accurately predict long-term successful functioning outside the hospital. Improvement in thought disorder, the best predictor of long-

term success, favored psychotherapy.

Breggin (1983), responding to Klerman's (1970) assertion that antipsychotic drugs act specifically on the target symptoms of schizophrenia, made some interesting observations. Klerman's data show that combativeness, hyperactivity, tension, and hostility were markedly or moderately reduced in two thirds or more of patients. These changes earned patients high ratings for ward adjustment. But hallucinations and delusions, the major symptoms of schizophrenia, were markedly or moderately reduced in only 58% and 48%, respectively, of Klerman's patients. Most of his patients showed no improvement in insight or judgment.

3. The personnel (nurses, therapists, and social workers) in May's study knew which treatment each patient had received.

4. May's 4-year follow-up data included less than half the original sample. One likely reason is that patients find the drugs aversive (see below), so they lie to or avoid hospital personnel who might schedule them for further treatments.

5. May evaluated patients on the day of discharge, which biases against psychotherapy. The day of termination of psychotherapy, especially if the patient has found it meaningful, is a time of crisis.

The debate on effectiveness of antipsychotic drugs would be less urgent except for two facts: The drugs cause serious side effects, and many patients dislike them.

Side Effects. As many as 40% of patients treated with phenothiazines or other antipsychotics (except clozapine—see below) experience movement disorders (Engelhardt, 1974). These may be grouped into three categories.

- Parkinsonism is a condition with symptoms closely resembling those of Parkinson's disease. Limbs stiffen, head and hands shake, and facial expression is reduced. Accompanying Parkinsonism is a slowing of volitional movement, often to the point of immobility.

- The patient cannot keep still, fidgeting compulsively, rocking backwards and forwards, or shuffling up and down. Kalinowsky (1958) said that the movements can be "more difficult to endure than any of the symptoms for which (the patient) was originally treated." Van Putten (1974) added that it can preclude sitting through a movie, let alone a sedentary job.

- Acute reactions often involve muscles of the eyes. One patient complained, "I'm telling you I can't take this medicine. It makes my eyes flip to the top of my head. The other day on the freeway I almost got into an accident.

It's embarrassing. When I'm around my friends and my eyes flip up I just rub my eyes so they won't notice" (Van Putten, 1974). The reactions sometimes involve stressful writhing movements of other parts of the body.

Tardive dyskinesia is a neurological syndrome characterized by slow rhythmic head movements, smacking of the lips, and fly catching dartings of the tongue. Other parts of the body may be involved. The condition appears months or years after the start of medication and continues unchanged even after discontinuation. Estimates of prevalence vary but may be as high as 60% in hospitalized adult schizophrenics (Engelhardt, 1974). It is more likely to appear in patients who have experienced rapidly increasing doses over a few days' time (Beresford & Hall, 1990). Some evidence suggests that high doses of vitamin E reduce the incidence of tardive dyskinesia (Elkashef, Ruskin, Bacher, & Barrett, 1990).

Low potency antipsychotics like chlorpromazine and thioridazine cause dry mouth, constipation, blurred vision, and other anticholinergic effects. High potency antipsychotics such as haloperidol and thiothixene are more likely to produce motor side effects. Other side effects of antipsychotics that occur with measurable frequency include heart complications, retinitis leading to blindness, purplish skin pigmentation, difficulty waking in the morning, hypotension, weight gain, a fall in total white cell count, jaundice, and impotence.

Antipsychotic drugs have *caused* psychotic symptoms. Gelenberg and Mandel (1977) described catatonia resulting from excessive antipsychotic drug use in eight schizophrenic patients; and Van Putten and Multalipassi (1975) reported clinical deterioration in others. Some patients improve when given 30-day drug holidays (Marder et al., 1979).

Antipsychotics block DA receptors in two key brain areas: the limbic system, which plays a major role in emotional responsiveness, and the extrapyramidal system, which controls motor functions. Both systems show rebound hyperactivity when medication is withdrawn. Rebound hyperactivity within the extrapyramidal system may be a cause of tardive dyskinesia and Parkinsonism. Rebound limbic hyperactivity may, by a parallel mechanism, cause supersensitivity psychosis. Chouinard and Jones (1980) described several patients whose condition deteriorated upon withdrawal of antipsychotic drugs. Chouinard and Jones's solution was to readminister the drugs to mask the symptoms and to continue them permanently. Till death do they part.

Pain Caused by the Drugs. Breggin (1983), an uncompromising critic of psychiatric drugs, entitled a chapter, "Physical Pain, Mental Anguish, and Psychosis Induced by the Major Tranquilizers." He quoted Lehmann (1970), a drug advocate, on the reaction of one patient:

> He refuses to take any medication by mouth and resists fiercely any attempt to give it to him against his will—for instance, by injection. Eventually one succeeds, but only after a severe struggle. For this type of patient, one or two injections of the long-acting preparations are often enough to get the patient under control in a few days and produce in him a more cooperative attitude which will allow his physicians and nurses to give him necessary treatment without encountering undue resistance.

Van Putten (1974) asked schizophrenics in a small teaching hospital (not a giant, understaffed state hospital where preservation of order is a dominant concern) about their attitudes toward antipsychotics. Despite having received relatively low doses, 38% habitually complained about the drug effect, felt miserable, and pleaded to have the drug stopped or the dosage reduced. Breggin presented evidence that many patients secretly dispose of their drugs, so 38% was probably an underestimate of the proportion of unhappy users. He wrote,

> Time and again in my clinical experience I have witnessed patients driven to extreme anguish and outrage by having major tranquilizers forced on them. The problem is so great in routine hospital practice that a large percentage of patients have to be threatened with forced intramuscular injection before they will take their drugs.

Breggin argued that treatment with antipsychotic drugs is comparable to lobotomy. One of several lines of evidence is that both procedures produce indifference to bodily pain.

Kotin et al. (1976) reported that 60% of their male patients on thioridazine developed sexual problems. Few had complained until actively questioned, which suggests that the incidence of side effects is much greater than indicated in the literature. About 15 million patients had received thioridazine in the 16 years preceding publication of the Kotin et al. paper, yet only 31 cases of ejaculatory problems had been reported by the manufacturer.

DOSAGE

Within the therapeutic community, Karon (1989) and Breggin (1983) are in the minority in contending that antipsychotic drugs do not effectively treat chronic schizophrenia. But because even staunch advocates acknowledge that the drugs produce severe side effects, administration should be at the smallest possible doses. Zito et al. (1987; Zito, Craig, Wanderling, Siegel, & Green, 1988) analyzed treatments of hospitalized schizophrenics. Higher doses added 16.3% to the costs of drugs but were not associated with better outcomes. The optimal daily dose is generally below 2,000 mg chlorpromazine or its equivalent (Shader & Jackson, 1975), and clinical symptoms worsen when patients get more than 1,500 to 2,000 mg/day (Hansen et al., 1987). Yet Zito et al. (1987) found that some patients were receiving as much as 10,000 mg per day. Boutin (1979) cited 12 studies in which lower doses were at least as effective as higher ones. In one case, patients did as well on 60 mg/day of trifluoperazine as on 600 mg; and in another, 30 mg/day of fluphenazine was associated with better outcomes than 1,200 mg/day (Baldessarini, Gelenberg, & Lipinski, 1976). But the matter is complex: nonresponders often have much lower levels than responders following a given dose of antipsychotic drug (Verghese, Kessel, & Simpson, 1991).

Crane (1973) noted that fewer than 50% of long-term schizophrenics improve in response to antipsychotic drugs, yet 85% of hospitalized schizophrenics receive the drugs at any one time. Patients who present management problems get the largest doses for the longest periods of time, even though the persistence of their psychoses suggests the ineffectiveness of the drugs. Schroeder, Caffey, and Lorlei (1977) reported that 17% of patients in VA hospitals were receiving dosages above the maximum published levels. Reardon et al. (1989) reviewed charts of 206 schizophrenics from a general hospital, a community mental health center, and a state hospital. Over a 10-year period in all three centers, drug potencies had increased and dosages had doubled.

Carpenter et al. (1990) explored two strategies for decreasing total drug dosage: (a) a continuous low dose that is increased only upon appearance of the symptoms that usually precede a psychotic episode; and (b) intermittent doses given only when psychotic symptoms appear. Patients followed for 2 years on one or the other regimen suffered few adverse effects.

CLOZAPINE

Clozapine has been available for more than 30 years but only recently gained acceptance for treating schizophrenics. Several double-blind comparisons with standard antipsychotic drugs gave an edge to clozapine 79% of the time (from a review by Baldessarini & Frankenburg, 1991). Extrapyramidal side effects are rare, which contributes to the patients' well-being. On the negative side, there is a significant risk of seizure (Haller & Binder, 1990). The major problem is that about 2% of chronic users develop a potentially fatal blood abnormality. If the white blood cell count is monitored and abnormalities occur, the drug can be discontinued in time. The manufacturer (Sandoz) initially required that patients be monitored by its subsidiary company, which charged about $9,000 annually. Antitrust suits forced Sandoz to change its policy (Cotton, 1991), but the cost in early 1991 was still more than $4,000 annually.

In light of Baldessarini's strong advocacy of the use of traditional antipsychotic drugs (cf. Baldessarini & Cohen, 1986; Baldessarini, Cohen, & Teicher, 1988), his comment about clozapine in the review with Frankenburg is interesting: "Its reappearance 30 years after it was patented underscores the substantial lack of progress in the development of more effective and safer antipsychotic drugs."

▓ Antidepressants

A former president of the American Psychological Association said, "Depression has been called the common cold of psychological disturbances . . . which underscores its prevalence, but trivializes its impact" (Strickland, cited in Lefton, 1991). From 1% to 2% of men and 4% of women suffer from major depression (Myers et al., 1984).

Several diagnostic subgroups of depressive illness have been described and several drug types used in treatment. Until just a few years ago, many researchers believed that reduced CNS activity of dopamine (DA), norepinephrine (NE), or serotonin (5-HT) were responsible for depression. More recently, the focus has been on 5-HT alone, although Caldecott-Hazard et al. (1991) noted that cholinergic drugs induce depression and anticholinergics elevate mood. Most known antidepressants enhance 5-HT functioning, and manipulations that inhibit its synthesis reverse the antidepressant effects of several drugs (Delgado, Charney, & Price, 1990; Shopsin, Friedman, & Gershon, 1976).

The main classes of antidepressants are tricyclics (TCAs), which inhibit the neuronal reuptake of NE and 5-HT; serotonin selective reuptake inhibitors (SSRIs); and monoamine oxidase inhibitors (MAOIs), which block the metabolism of NE, epinephrine, DA, and 5-HT. Patients who fail to respond to one type often respond to another or to bupropion, a unique antidepressant that inhibits dopamine reuptake. Lithium, especially in combination with other antidepressants, helps many patients. Stimulants are valuable in certain circumstances.

Preskorn and Burke (1992), considering effectiveness, safety, and tolerability, suggested that physically healthy depressed people be started with either a TCA or SSRI. Most will respond within 4 weeks. TCAs are preferable with patients suffering from insomnia, and SSRIs are safer with potential overdose risks. Preskorn and Burke noted that little data exists on drug-effectiveness against recurrences of depression; and the data are limited to a few TCAs and SSRIs.

Tricyclic Antidepressants (TCAs)

Until recently, tricyclic antidepressants (TCAs) were the most widely prescribed antidepressants. Some of the more common ones are amitriptyline, desipramine, doxepin, imipramine, and nortriptyline. TCAs are structurally similar to phenothiazines. Their long half-lives permit once-a-day dosing. Because of large individual differences in metabolizing TCAs, plasma levels may differ by as much as 20-fold in two people following the same dosage regimen (Glassman & Perel, 1973). TCAs produce many side effects: sedation (so they are usually taken at bedtime), blurred vision, increased appetite leading to weight gain, dry mouth, constipation, cardiac symptoms, and fainting. Some patients find the side effects more unpleasant than the depression. Haddad (1992) claimed that TCA overdose is the leading cause of hospitalization and death due to excessive ingestion of prescription drugs.

Serotonin Selective Reuptake Inhibitors

Fluoxetine (Prozac) selectively blocks 5-HT reuptake, thus making more 5-HT available at postsynaptic sites. Fluoxetine was the first SSRI to reach the market and, despite costing $1.50 daily, rapidly generated annual sales of close to $1 billion ("If at First," 1991). Other SSRIs soon became available, including fluvoxamine, sertraline, zimelidine, and paroxetine. Although similar in onset and efficacy to TCAs, they cause fewer unpleasant side effects. Table 14.2, taken from Rickels and Schweizer (1990), compares frequent side effects in patients treated with any of several SSRIs, placebo, or imipramine in placebo-controlled studies.

Brown and Harrison (1992), working with patients who had discontinued fluoxetine because of side effects, started them on an 8-week course of sertraline. Most of the patients completed the non-double-blind study, and most improved significantly. Brown and Harrison concluded that the SSRIs are not interchangeable.

Teicher, Glod, and Cole (1990) reported that six depressed patients developed obsessive and violent suicidal thoughts, more intense than any they had previously experienced, during fluoxetine treatment. Their states persisted for 3 days to 3 months after drug discontinuation. Similar reports followed, which prompted a special meeting of the FDA's Psychopharmacological Drugs Advisory Committee (*FDA Talk Paper*, 1991). After hearing testimony from several experts and analyzing various forms of data, the Committee agreed unanimously that no credible evidence establishes a causal relationship between the use of any antidepressant drugs and suicidal or homicidal behavior.

Monoamine Oxidase Inhibitors (MAOIs)

The monoamine oxidase inhibitors (MAOIs) were the first antidepressants used in the United States. They inactivate MAO, a major metabolic enzyme of NE, E, DA, and 5-HT, until more is synthesized. The first MAOIs were notorious for interacting with drugs that elevate blood pressure and foods containing tyramine (tyramine-rich foods include aged cheeses, chopped liver, broad beans, schmalz pickled herring, and red wines). The interactions caused severe and even fatal hypertensive crises. As a result, the MAOIs fell out of favor as therapeutic agents.

Two recent developments may lead to an MAOI comeback. First, researchers discovered that MAO occurs in two subforms, MAO-A and MAO-B. MAO-A inhibitors are effective antidepressants, and MAO-B inhibitors are used as an adjunct to L-dopa therapy for Parkinson's disease. Second, reversible MAO-A inhibitors were discovered that are shorter-acting and safer than the classic MAOIs.

Table 14.2 Side Effects With an Incidence of ≥ 19% Reported for Several Serotonin Reuptake Inhibitors*

Side Effect	Sertraline N = 1,568	Placebo N = 851	Fluoxetine N = 1,378	Fluvoxamine N = 222	Paroxetine N = 1,387	Nefazodone N = 529	Buspirone[a] N = 207	Imipramine N = 599
Nausea/vomiting	21%	—	25%	37%	29%	21%	27%	—
Headache	—	20%	—	22%	20%	29%	31%	19%
Dry mouth	—	—	—	26%	20%	19%	—	76%
Sedation	—	—	—	26%	24%	—	—	30%
Nervous/restless/anxiety	—	—	21%	—	—	—	—	—
Dizziness	—	—	—	—	—	—	23%	27%
Insomnia	—	—	19%	—	—	—	—	—
Sweating	—	—	—	—	—	—	—	21%
Constipation	—	—	—	—	—	—	—	—

SOURCE: "Clinical Overview of Serotonin Reuptake Inhibitors," by K. Rickels & E. Schweizer, *The Journal of Clinical Psychiatry*, 51(12, Suppl. B), pp. 9-12, 1990. Copyright 1990, Physicians Postgraduate Press. Used with permission.
NOTE: * Adapted from references 3 and 4.
a. Mean buspirone dosage in treatment of anxiety is half that of the antidepressant dose, and no adverse events with ≥ 19% of frequency were observed in anxiety studies.

Cesura and Pletscher (1992) reviewed the characteristics of moclobemide and brofaromine, the two most studied of the new generation of MAOIs. Similar to TCAs in both effectiveness and incidence and severity of side effects, they can be given without important dietary restrictions.

Bupropion

Preskorn and Burke (1992) reported that bupropion, which enhances functioning of the DA system, is less effective than TCAs and SSRIs and causes more adverse effects. But TCA nonresponders may improve with bupropion.

Lithium

Lithium salt is a naturally occurring mineral that, taken alone or in combination with other antidepressants, helps many otherwise refractory depressives (Kim, Delva, & Lawson, 1990; Kramlinger & Post, 1989). Price, Charney, Delgado, and Heninger (1990) speculated that it improves serotonergic functioning. Lithium is the drug of choice for treating bipolar disorder. It is discussed below under that heading.

Stimulants

Stimulants, once popular for treating depression, fell out of favor when other drugs became available. Because depression has many characteristics of exhaustion, Berger (1960) warned that administration of stimulants "is like flogging a tired horse." But when a patient has had an overwhelming grief reaction and needs relief within 1 or 2 days, amphetamine or methylphenidate may be the drug of choice.

When depression occurs in the medically ill and is manifested by apathy, psychomotor retardation, excessive sleeping, and reduced appetite, healing is likely to be retarded. Frierson, Wey, and Tabler (1991) advocated treating such patients with stimulants. Stimulants cause fewer side effects than TCAs and MAOIs, and they act within 36 hours rather than 2 to 3 weeks. Used in a hospital setting, they are effective, safer than other antidepressants, and have low abuse potential. Frierson et al. presented five illustrative cases and cited several double-blind studies to support their argument.

PREDICTORS OF RESPONSIVENESS

Researchers have tried to identify subsets of patients particularly responsive or refractory to different antidepressants, but positive findings have generally been followed by failures to replicate (Bielski & Friedel, 1979; Joyce & Paykel, 1989). Further study is warranted, as patients often respond to one drug after failing to respond to another (Price, Charney, & Heninger, 1985).

Hale, Hannah, Sandler, and Bridges (1989) administered oral tyramine to depressed patients and measured their excretion of tyramine sulphate; low rates of excretion were associated with favorable responses to TCAs. Friedel (1983) concluded that **psychomotor retardation** is the best predictor of response to TCAs. MAOIs may be preferable when depression is accompanied by symptoms such as anxiety, agitation, or excessive sleeping and eating (Kupfer & Spiker, 1981; Quitkin et al., 1988).

Joyce and Paykel (1989) drew several conclusions from their literature review:

- Depressed, delusional patients respond poorly to TCAs and well to electroconvulsive shock therapy and combined antidepressant-antipsychotic drugs.
- Low urinary levels of the norepinephrine metabolite MHPG predict favorable response to imipramine, nortriptyline, and maprotiline.
- Low cerebrospinal fluid levels of the dopamine metabolite HVA predict favorable response to nomifensine and piribedil.
- Depressed people whose mood brightens following administration of amphetamine or another stimulant are good candidates for treatment with imipramine, desimipramine, and desipramine. Those who do not respond or become **dysphoric** are more likely to improve with nortriptyline or amitriptyline.

Sotsky et al. (1991) conducted a collaborative study at three clinical research sites involving 28 therapists; 239 outpatients suffering from major depressive disorder were randomly assigned to receive one of two types of therapy or clinical management plus either placebo or imipramine. The best predictor of good outcome with imipramine was high work dysfunction; other good predictors were severe depression and endogenous depression (no obvious precipitating cause and symptoms including psychomotor retardation, early morning awakening, and loss of appetite). Unmarried patients and those with severe personality disorder or low expectation of improvement responded poorly. The findings were consistent across samples and measures of outcome.

Tueting (1991) reviewed psychophysiological measures that predict response to antidepressants. Below is a sampling of her findings:

- Elderly patients who become dizzy when they suddenly stand up after sitting or lying for a long time, respond well to imipramine, doxepin, and nortriptyline.
- Long speech pauses predict good response to tricyclics.
- The ability of tricyclics to suppress REM sleep (dreaming) correlates positively with clinical response to the drugs. Amitriptyline and desipramine both shorten onset of REM sleep in patients who respond well.

ENDOGENOUS DEPRESSION
AND REM SLEEP (DREAMING)

Endogenous depressions develop gradually and probably reflect biological causes rather than traumatic experiences. Vogel, Buffenstein, Minter, and Hennessey (1990) hypothesized a connection between antidepressant effectiveness and reductions in REM sleep. Specifically, they predicted that drugs that relieve endogenous depression would (a) reduce REM sleep by more than 50% of pretreatment level; (b) maintain a substantial reduction for several weeks; and (c) after withdrawal, be followed by more REM sleep than was present during pretreatment. A literature review supported their hypothesis: Vogel et al. reported that 13 of 17 drugs that improve endogenous depression and have been tested for properties a-c, have those properties. Of many other addictive and nonaddictive drugs they considered, none with properties a-c failed to improve endogenous depression. The data are correlational; they do not prove that reduced REM is the mechanism by which the drugs work.

EFFECTIVENESS
OF ANTIDEPRESSANTS

Smith et al. (1980) analyzed 75 studies and concluded that antidepressant drugs have a significant but modest effect. Moreover, about 50% of recovered patients relapse within 2 years (Belsher & Costello, 1988). One reason the drugs don't work better, according to Baldessarini

(1990b), is that prescribed dosages are often too low. He asserted that proper dosing would reduce mortality among the depressed.

Kane and Lieberman (1984) reviewed the literature on newer antidepressants, including 16 studies that had both placebo and either imipramine or amitriptyline comparison groups. Because the studies were well designed (clear criteria for depression, accepted standards for dosage levels and treatment duration) and focused on the newer drugs, Greenberg and Fisher (1989) assumed minimal bias toward the older ones. So they reanalyzed the data and found that 59% of imipramine- and amitriptyline-recipients, and only 36% of those on placebo, were rated as improved. They called the effect modest. Others might regard a 23% difference as substantial. I would love a 23% increase in my salary.

Antidepressants don't help all and maybe not even most of those who try them, but they certainly help some. Explanations couched in terms of spontaneous recovery or placebo effects seem far-fetched alongside accounts such as the following from Griffin (1991). She described a 42-year-old woman who, for the previous 12 years, had been constantly tired, felt there was little point to her life, and cried for hours each day. The woman was quoted:

> "I was in constant psychic pain. It's like the feeling when somebody very dear to you dies. But it goes on and on and doesn't end." Three weeks after receiving the TCA nortriptyline, she began feeling better. Reflecting on her life in the ensuing eight years, she said, "Everyday life is richer. I'm not distracted by these terrible thoughts. I don't get yanked down under the waves." (Griffin, 1991)

▓ Drugs for Treating Mania and Bipolar Disorder (Manic Depression)

About 2 million Americans have been diagnosed with bipolar disorder, formerly called manic depression. They experience cycles of elation, hyperactivity, and impulsivity alternating with hopelessness and despair. Lithium is the drug of choice for bipolar disorder and for mania alone. It typically acts within 2 weeks, although the full **prophylactic** effect often takes up to a year to develop (Schou, 1986); and it probably prevents recurrence of manic episodes (Consensus Development Panel, 1985).

Lithium has a small therapeutic window, that is, it produces toxic effects at a dose not much greater than the therapeutic dose. So patients' blood levels must be carefully monitored. Blood levels can be affected by fluid intake, perspiration, diarrhea, and various other conditions, so monitoring must be frequent. Even so, side effects such as dizziness, diarrhea, dry mouth, nausea, weight gain, sedation, and swelling of the feet are common.

The anticonvulsant carbamazepine is an alternative to lithium for treating mania. The two drugs have also been used in combination (Placidi, Lenzi, & Lazzerini, 1986; Post et al., 1990; Stuppaeck et al., 1990).

Breggin (1983) disputed lithium's efficacy, emphasized the harm it does, and claimed that its popularity derives from sedating effects. He described a study by Small et al. (1972), who screened 11 subjects for physical and mental normality before administering lithium for 3 weeks in the low range of therapeutic dose levels. The work and school performance of 3 of the subjects were seriously impaired. A 4th dropped out after a week with "severe muscle weakness, confusion, and depression." A 5th developed a "severe, precipitous toxic delirium on the tenth day of taking lithium." Only 2 subjects reported no ill effects.

Breggin's criticisms are important and should be considered by prospective therapists and patients. Most researchers and many patients, however, believe that lithium is an invaluable therapeutic drug. Actress Patty Duke and Broadway director Joshua Logan both suffered from bipolar disorder, and both testified that lithium improved their lives immensely (Duke & Turan, 1987; Logan, 1978).

▓ Antianxiety Drugs

Anxiety disorders affect between 5% and 10% of the United States population (Robins et al., 1984; Weissman, 1988). For many years starting in the early 1960s, the benzodiazepine derivatives diazepam (Valium) and chlordiazepoxide (Librium) dominated pharmacological treatments. Compared with the drugs they supplanted (barbiturates and meprobamate), diazepam and chlordiazepoxide have stronger antianxiety actions, fewer unpleasant side effects, lower abuse potential, and smaller risk of death from overdose. Recently developed benzodiazepines, differing from the originals primarily in pharmacokinetics, include clorazepate, halazepam, prazepam, clonazepam, lorazepam, oxazepam, etizolam, and alprazolam; nonbenzodiazepines used for treating anxiety include buspirone, beta blockers, and various antidepressants.

The drugs have been terribly mis- and overprescribed. Chambers, White, and Lindquist (1983) asked a random sample of 150 physicians which antianxiety drug they prescribed most often, and 10% named either an antipsychotic or antidepressant. Twelve percent of the physicians did not set duration limits, and many of their patients had been taking antianxiety drugs for more than a year. Sixteen percent had had at least one patient die from overdose. Yet 54% did not want their patients receiving package inserts listing side effects, on the grounds that the patients would misunderstand the information.

It should be noted that the improper administration of some drugs is not a valid reason for curtailing their use. Even the most beneficial treatments can be misused. The implications of the Chambers et al. study relate to drug prescribers, not drugs.

Mellinger, Balter, and Uhlenhuth (1984) reported that 11% of adults in the United States had used antianxiety drugs, primarily benzodiazepines, during the previous year. They are used more by women than men, whites than African Americans, older than younger, and unmarried than married (Swartz et al., 1991). A scene from the movie *Starting Over* provides apt commentary on the prevalence of benzodiazepines in our society. Jill Clayburgh has an anxiety attack in a crowded department store. Burt Reynolds calls out to see if anyone has a Valium, and all shoppers within shouting distance reach into their pockets.

Anxiety, although sometimes disabling, is part of life. Learning to cope with anxiety-provoking situations, as taught by many psychotherapists (cf. Bandura, Jeffery, & Wright, 1974), seems preferable to managing the situations ineffectually but losing concern about them. Experiments show that antianxiety drugs impair behaviors associated with punishment and nonreward. For example, normal rats trained to barpress for food, then shocked as well as fed whenever they press, soon stop pressing. Rats treated with antianxiety drugs still feel pain (they escape rapidly when shock comes on—Gray, 1978); but they do not inhibit responses that bring pain; they continue to bar-press (Miczek, 1973).

Most antianxiety drugs enhance functioning of the neurotransmitter gamma-aminobutyric acid (GABA) (cf. Mohler, 1992). Drugs that inhibit the actions of GABA at receptors elicit symptoms of anxiety in normal volunteers (Dorow & Duka, 1986).

GENERALIZED ANXIETY DISORDER

Generalized anxiety disorder (GAD) is a state of constant anxiety. It usually occurs independently of any obvious precipitating event, although one well-established cause is too much caffeine (Reimann, 1967). Almost immediately after they were marketed, the benzodiazepines became the drugs of choice for GAD. However, they should not be. About 50% of patients relapse by 1- to 5-year follow-up (Rickels et al., 1991), and when a benzodiazepine is discontinued, patients frequently suffer a rebound anxiety more severe than in the original illness. The only treatment is more drug (Chouinard, 1986). Perhaps that explains why an American Psychiatric Association task force (Salzman, 1991) found that, though the therapeutic effectiveness of benzodiazepines is usually limited to 60 days or less, about 1.5% of all U.S. adults take them for more than one year. The potential for toxicity is considerable, especially among elderly patients. The nonbenzodiazepine buspirone, which produces few side effects, is not sedating, and has no abuse potential, is an alternative (Rickels, 1990). However, imipramine and other TCAs are probably superior for treating GAD (Kahn, Stevenson, Topol, & Klein, 1986; Lipman, 1989).

PANIC DISORDER

Victims of panic disorder, a condition that afflicts 1% to 3% of the population (American Psychiatric Association, 1987), suffer sudden, unexpected attacks of overwhelming anxiety. Symptoms include dizziness, trembling, cold sweats, shortness of breath, and fear of dying. Although usually lasting only a few minutes, they are so distressing that more people seek treatment for panic disorder than for any other psychological disorder (Boyd, 1986). Recent literature reviews by Balestrieri, Ruggeri, and Bellantuono (1989), Bowden (1992), and Lipman (1989) concluded that both the benzodiazepine alprazolam and antidepressants relieve symptoms and, in conjunction with behavioral treatments, help control further attacks. Alprazolam acts more rapidly.

In 1989, 11 psychiatrists and psychologists wrote a letter criticizing the favorable reports on alprazolam for panic disorder (Marks et al., 1989). Nine psychiatrists wrote a rebuttal (Klerman et al., 1989). The points of contention included nonblindness of treatment, high placebo dropout rate, frequency and severity of side effects, and difference between short- and long-term efficacy. I recommend the letters to readers interested in methodological issues.

OBSESSIVE-COMPULSIVE DISORDER

Obsessions are persistent recurrent thoughts, and compulsions are repetitive actions that a person feels compelled to perform. The lifetime prevalence of obsessive-compulsive disorder is 1.5% to 2.5% (Karno, Golding, Sorenson, & Burnam, 1988). Although classified with the anxiety disorders, obsessive-compulsive disorder has many similarities with depression. The treatment drug of choice has been clomipramine, a TCA. Improvement begins within about a week and accelerates after about 5 weeks (Katz, DeVeaugh-Geiss, & Landau, 1990). Frequent side effects, similar to those observed with other TCAs, include dry mouth and constipation. Because clomipramine powerfully inhibits serotonin reuptake, researchers tried other serotonergic antidepressants. Fluvoxamine and fluoxetine are equally effective; but sertraline, despite even more highly specific serotonergic actions, is less so (Fontaine & Chouinard, 1986; Jenike et al., 1990).

STAGE FRIGHT

Many actors and musicians experience stage fright: racing heart, hand tremor, palpitations, and other symptoms of sympathetic nervous system overactivity. By diminishing sympathetic influence, **beta-blocking drugs** such as propranolol alleviate the symptoms; this explains why 27% of 2,122 members of the International Conference of Symphony and Opera Musicians admitted using propranol, and 19% of those said they use it daily (Lockwood, 1989). Nube (1991) reviewed several studies corroborating that propranolol and related drugs block symptoms associated with stage fright; but she cited other studies indicating that the drugs sedate, impair reaction time and eye-hand coordination, and lower interest level. She questioned whether the negatives outweigh the positives. On the other hand, professional golfer Mac O'Grady stated that several high ranking golf professionals take propranolol to calm them and prevent them from jerking their putting stroke (*Augusta Chronicle*, April 5, 1994).

▓ Drugs for Treating Attention-Deficit Disorder

Attention-deficit disorder (ADD), characterized by severe problems in attention coupled with severe overactivity, is a new diagnostic label for what had previously been called hyperkinetic syndrome and then minimal brain dysfunction. The treatment drug of choice has been methylphenidate, which can be taken orally and has both a rapid onset and a rapid offset of action. Thus, parents can give children drug holidays when their behavior is unlikely to be disruptive. Amphetamine and other stimulants structurally similar to methylphenidate are also used.

Wender (1988) estimated that 3% to 10% of children have ADD, with the diagnosis four times as likely to be applied to boys as girls. Two large surveys, by Goldstein (1987) and Satin, Winsberg, Monetti, Sverd, and Foss (1985), put the incidence for boys at about 33%. The implication, because ADD is considered a psychiatric disorder, is that about one-third of U.S. boys are not normal. McGuiness (1989) put forth the provocative alternative view that ADD does not exist as a meaningful diagnostic entity. She argued as follows:

1. Neurological problems frequently cause inattentive, disruptive behaviors that can be treated with stimulants.

2. Normal children, especially boys, are often inattentive, fidgety, and disruptive. The behaviors are sometimes so disturbing that parents or teachers seek help.

3. Stimulants reduce fidgeting in most children and make them temporarily more manageable. Parents and teachers see immediate benefits. The drugs, however, are disliked by the children, do not improve their social skills or academic performance, and have many side effects.

4. Prescription of drugs requires a diagnosis and a diagnosis implies a disease; so, many childhood behavioral problems are assumed to be organically based and diagnosed as ADD. The problems are viewed as originating within the child. But most can be traced to poor family dynamics, lack of discipline, or academic difficulties. (Recently, however, Hauser et al. [1993] studied relatives of children diagnosed with ADD. Relatives with generalized resistance to thyroid hormone were more likely than those without generalized resistance to meet the criteria for ADD. The authors speculated that many ADD patients have less overt behavioral problems.)

McGuiness discussed Points 3 and 4, the two most contentious ones, in detail. Point 4 concerns the adequacy of diagnosis. Whereas other medical syndromes are comprised of well-defined sets of symptoms, behavioral problems such as hyperactivity, attention deficits, aggressiveness, anxiety, academic problems, social withdrawal, and so forth come in many combinations (Hinshaw, 1987). The impetus for testing a child for ADD typically arises because of classroom difficulties. Experiments conducted outside of classrooms show that ADD children differ only slightly from normal controls in attentiveness, primarily because they do not persist at uninteresting tasks. The major scale for diagnosing ADD measures conduct problems, learning disabilities, and hyperactivity—not attention. Reliabilities of all the diagnostic scales are low.

As to Point 3, children on stimulant drugs persevere at tasks they don't enjoy, which advocates attribute to enhanced attentional control. McGuiness acknowledged the effect but not the explanation, arguing that drugs increase compliance by sapping children's energy to exert willpower against adults. She reviewed studies showing that the drug-induced changes do not result in better academic performance.

Robbins, Jones, and Sahakian (1989) analyzed previously published data. For normal and hyperactive children and normal adults, amphetamine doses that stimulated inactive people had little effect on moderately active ones and calmed the hyperactive. Because ADD children are generally hyperactive, stimulants reduce their activity and may help them focus on simple tasks requiring concentration. But stimulants promote repetitiveness (cf. Randrup & Munkvad, 1967). For example, amphetamine increases performance of dull, well-learned tasks such as naming colors, while reducing ability to change perspective (cf. Broverman, Klaiber, Kobayashi, & Vogel, 1968).

Children dislike the drugs. McGuiness (1989) cited a report by Eichlseder (1985) on 872 children diagnosed ADD who received stimulants. All complained about how they felt on the drug regimen.

Among the well-documented short-term side effects of stimulants are insomnia, loss of appetite, elevated basal heart rate, and lowered skin temperature. The drugs are often started on children as young as 3 and continued into adulthood, so possible long-term effects must be considered. Little information is available other than that growth may be suppressed (Safer, Allen, & Barr, 1972), probably temporarily (Roche, Lipman, Overall, & Hung, 1979). McGuiness suggested that long-term use of amphetamines might affect production or action of no-repinephrine and dopamine.

▒ Insight-Promoting Drugs

During the period from 1950 to the mid-1960s, psychiatrists administered LSD and other psychedelic drugs to more than 40,000 patients. Their goal was to promote insights into such problems as alcoholism, sexual difficulties, obsessional neuroses, and sociopathy. The psychedelic drug experience may allow direct confrontation of guilt, as in the following example taken from the report of a man who had been seriously neglecting his family (Pahnke & Richards, 1969):

> I opened my eyes and there was a picture over the mantle. . . . There seemed to be in front of the picture many veils hanging and I pushed each veil aside one by one, knowing that as I got the last veil aside I would finally see God. . . . Finally the last veil was to be removed. I knew it was the last veil and tried to prepare myself for the great experience of seeing God. I raised my hand over my head and then leaned backwards to make myself more receptive in order to feel the full force of God. And finally the last veil was pulled aside and there were my three children crying for their father. . . . Before me was going all the selfish feelings—all the selfish attitudes that I had had throughout my entire married life.

Most psychiatrists who tried LSD therapy described the results glowingly. Their patients undoubtedly provided more entertainment than run-of-the-mill sibling rivalries, Oedipal complexes, and so forth; and heightened therapist interest leads to more favorable outcomes. The religious and mystical aspects may have invested patients' lives with new meanings—LSD is more likely than maintenance chlorpromazine to promote spiritual awakening. But well-controlled experimental support for long-range improvement was minimal. Few researchers used control groups, random assignment, double-blinds, objective measures, or post-session follow-ups. Unger (1967) stated that, "not a single, methodologically acceptable controlled study of psychedelic drug-assisted psychotherapy has yet been performed." A few well-designed studies were eventually conducted, but most yielded negative results. For example, Johnson (1969) randomly assigned alcoholics to one of four treatment groups:

1. LSD was given and a nurse was present throughout.
2. LSD was given in the presence of both a nurse and therapist.
3. A combination of amobarbital and methamphetamine was given in the presence of both a nurse and therapist.
4. Patients received routine clinical care.

The patients who received drugs got split doses, the second being adjusted according to the therapist's assessment. This ensured that everybody received an optimal dose. The LSD recipients improved substantially on several measures such as degree of abstinence and response to alcohol, and the changes persisted for at least a year. However, patients in every group improved, and *there were no significant differences among the groups on any measure.* LSD treatment was no better than routine care or the alteration in consciousness induced by the amobarbital-methamphetamine combination. Score another for placebos.

Grinspoon and Bakalar (1986) agreed that the optimism about LSD was excessive, but they criticized laws that ban psychiatrists from conducting studies on new psychedelic drugs. They wrote,

> A generation of physicians and scientists has grown up without the opportunity to pursue human research with these drugs, and the financial and administrative obstacles remain serious. These drugs should not be regarded either as a panacea or as entirely worthless and extraordinarily dangerous. If the therapeutic results have been inconsistent, that is partly because of the complexity of psychedelic drug effects. For the same reason we may not yet have had enough time to sort out the best uses of these drugs.

Grinspoon and Bakalar (1986) noted that psychedelics are used in many preindustrial cultures to enhance psychotherapeutic healing. The drugs facilitate diagnosis, strengthen the therapeutic alliance, and help patients generate memories, fantasies, and insights. Similar objectives motivated several psychiatrists in the United States and Europe, since the early 1970s, to use MDMA (3,4-methylenedioxymethamphetamine). MDMA, structurally similar to amphetamine, is not hallucinogenic. If, as advocates claim, it increases capacity for introspection and intimacy while providing temporary freedom from anxiety and depression, it might serve as a catalyst for psychotherapy. Greer and Tolbert (1990) reported many favorable outcomes following single (nonblind) MDMA sessions in a clinical setting. Gallagher (1986) wrote that MDMA helps "grease the emotional and cognitive gears that produce insight." Gallagher quoted psychiatrist Richard Ingrasci, "You've been seeing this patient for six months, and you think you know him pretty well. Then you give him some MDMA, and suddenly you're hearing all kinds of stuff you haven't heard before. That's when the therapy really takes off."

Grinspoon and Bakalar (1986), concerned about the dwindling opportunities for research on other drugs with possible psychotherapeutic usefulness, concluded their article by writing, "To ignore the possibility of reviving the centuries-old but now neglected tradition of drug-enhanced psychotherapeutic healing would mean unnecessarily limiting the potential of psychotherapy itself to help people gain insight into their problems and bring more perspective to their lives."

Greer and Tolbert (1986) noted that MDMA was patented in 1914 and is no longer patentable; so pharmaceutical manufacturers were uninterested in sponsoring an Investigational New Drug application or in supporting research. In 1985, MDMA was classified as a Schedule I drug of the Controlled Substances Act. Drugs are classified as Schedule I if the administrator of the Drug Enforcement Administration determines that the drug has a high potential for abuse, no currently accepted medical use in treatment, and a lack of accepted safety for use under medical supervision.

Summary

The leading hypothesis about the cause of schizophrenia is that it stems from excess activity of a subtype of dopamine receptors. Most antipsychotic drugs block DA receptors, with clozapine an exception. The most frequently prescribed antipsychotics are thioridazine, haloperidol, chlorpromazine, trifluoperazine, thiothixene, and fluphenazine.

Antipsychotics help relieve patients' fears and anxieties during acute schizophrenic episodes. Therapists disagree about their value as maintenance treatment. The drugs produce many side effects, including movement disorders, impaired memory, weight gain, and sexual problems.

The three main classes of antidepressants are monoamine oxidase inhibitors, tricyclics, and serotonin reuptake blockers. Their effectiveness is established but varies with different subsets of patients. Several factors have been identified that predict patient responsiveness.

Lithium is the drug of choice for treating and preventing the recurrence of bipolar disorder. Carbamazepine is an alternative.

Anxiety conditions are treated with benzodiazepines, which are terribly mis- and overprescribed. The drugs impair behaviors associated with punishment and nonreward. They enhance functioning of GABA.

Panic disorders are best treated with alprazolam or antidepressants. The tricyclic clomipramine and other serotonergic antidepressants effectively treat obsessive-compulsive disorder. Beta-blockers such as propranolol reduce sympathetic activity, so help performers plagued with stage fright.

Attention-deficit disorder is treated with methylphenidate and other stimulants. The drugs reduce hyperactivity, but critics argue that they are neither liked by nor helpful to the recipients.

LSD and similar drugs were once widely used by psychiatrists for helping patients gain insights into their conditions. Many positive outcomes were reported, few based on double-blind studies. The use of such drugs is now forbidden by law.

Mini-Quiz: Psychopharmacotherapy

What is the effect of phenothiazines upon dopamine receptors?

they block DA receptors

T/F: Most psychiatrists claim that antipsychotic drugs act against the specific symptoms of schizophrenia.

true

Movement disorders are a common side effect of _____ drugs.

antipsychotic

Tardive dyskinesia is a _____ that is a frequent side effect of _____ drugs.

movement disorder; antipsychotic

Which are the two key brain sites where phenothiazines block dopamine receptors?

limbic system; extrapyramidal system

T/F: The text presented evidence that side effects of antipsychotic drugs are overreported.

false

About 2% of schizophrenics treated with _____ develop a potentially fatal blood abnormality.

clozapine

Name the main classes of antidepressants.

TCAs, SSRIs, and MAOIs

Most known antidepressants enhance functioning of which NT?

serotonin

A unique antidepressant that inhibits DA uptake is _____.

bupropion

Which antidepressant has as its primary therapeutic use the treatment of bipolar disorder?

lithium

T/F: Patients who don't respond well to one antidepressant generally don't respond well to any other.

false

Most people who respond to antidepressants respond within 4 (hours/days/weeks/months).

weeks

In what ways do the new MAOIs differ from the older ones?

    a. The new ones are selective MAO-A inhibitors.
    b. The new ones inhibit MAO reversibly.
    c. The new ones are much safer.

Evidence was presented that effective _____ reduce REM sleep by more than 50% of pretreatment level.

antidepressants

The drug of choice for treating mania is _____ and an alternative is _____.

lithium; carbamazepine

Match the drug with a serious drawback to its use.

1. lithium	a. tardive dyskinesia
2. phenelzine	b. a potentially fatal blood disorder
3. chlorpromazine	c. rebound anxiety
4. alprazolam	d. small therapeutic window
5. clozapine	e. interaction may cause hypertensive crisis

1d; 2e; 3a; 4c; 5b

Which drug from the previous question has the greatest abuse potential?

alprazolam

Which NT do most antianxiety drugs act on?

GABA

T/F: Generalized anxiety disorder is best treated with an antianxiety drug.

false

The drug of choice for obsessive-compulsive disorder is _____.

clomipramine

Because they diminish sympathetic influence, _____ drugs have been used to treat stage fright.

beta-blocking

The most widely used drug for attention-deficit disorder is _____.

methylphenidate

T/F: The use of LSD and related drugs to treat a variety of psychiatric conditions is supported by dozens of double-blind studies.

false

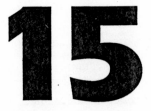

By the time you finish reading this chapter, you should be able to answer the following questions:

According to the information processing model, how many types of memory are there?

What is the process by which short-term memories are converted to long-term ones?

Chronic alcoholism contributes to which three medical conditions that have severe memory problems as a significant component?

What is alcoholic blackout?

What are the effects of glucose on memory?

What are nootropics? What is the effect of stimulant drugs on memory?

What is significant about the observation that stimulants produce the greatest improvements when given right after training?

Which neurotransmitter has been most strongly implicated in the memory impairment of Alzheimer's disease?

With respect to memory, what is significant about the fact that antipsychotic drugs have anticholinergic properties?

T/F: Some drug effects on memory are species-specific.

T/F: Some drug effects on memory are task-specific.

T/F: Material learned while under the influence of a drug will be recalled best while under the influence of the drug.

Memory

Contents

The question, "What is the effect of drug X on memory?" rarely has a simple answer. It depends on a great many factors.

❋ Encoding

Encoding is the process by which information is placed into memory. According to the most influential modern view, the information processing model, there are three stages of encoding. Sensory memory stores sensory information for less than one second. Short-term memory, not quite so impermanent, holds small amounts of information for periods of usually less than 30 seconds. We can remember new telephone numbers long enough to dial them. But an operator who cuts in to ask, "What number are you calling?" is likely to hear an embarrassed silence.

The third stage of encoding is long-term memory. Some short-term memories are converted to long-term ones by a hypothetical process called memory consolidation. Recently consolidated memories are fragile and easily disrupted. For example, Russell and Nathan (1946) reported that more than 70% of people who suffered serious head injury were amnesic for events that occurred within ½ hour of the injury. Long-term memory can store enormous amounts of information indefinitely and can pass it back to short-term memory.

Long-term memories are not always available as needed. When once-established memories such as the names of grade school classmates are not recalled, the explanation may be that stored memories have deteriorated. Alternatively, the memories may be intact but inaccessible to consciousness. The access function is called memory retrieval.

⊞ Types of Information

Several distinct types of information are stored in memory. Procedural memory refers to information about how to do things, such as riding a bicycle. Declarative memory is the ability to remember information. It is subdivided into semantic and episodic memory. Semantic memory involves general knowledge, such as the capital of New Zealand or the name of this book. Episodic memory refers to specific personal experiences, such as the circumstances of your first kiss.

Memory may be classified along other dimensions, such as visual, auditory, and olfactory. Sustained effort is required for processing some but not all memories. Squire (1992) integrated laboratory and clinical work to document the existence of anatomically distinct systems for acquiring and storing fundamentally different kinds of information. The distinctions are important. For example, L-dopa facilitates effortful, episodic but not semantic memories (Newman, Weingartner, Smallberg, & Calne, 1984). Also, the elderly and victims of Korsakoff's syndrome, the dementia of Parkinson's disease, and Alzheimer's disease have selective memory deficits (Kopelman, 1987).

▓ **Methodology**

DRUGS HAVE MANY ACTIONS

Drug-induced changes in performance on memory tasks may result from effects on memory processes. But they may also be secondary to changes in vigilance, pain sensitivity, appetite, judgment, locomotor or sensory abilities, and mood. For example, amphetamine potentiates the functioning of norepinephrine and dopamine, so researchers use it to assess the role of catecholamine neurotransmitters in memory. But amphetamine has many actions. Among other things, it reduces appetite and increases arousal, activity, and ACTH secretion. All may affect performance on a memory task.

DRUG ACTIONS ARE
AFFECTED BY CIRCUMSTANCES

Statements of the type, "adrenergic drugs facilitate learning" overgeneralize on several accounts. First, drug effects may be species-specific. Carbachol placed in the lateral hypothalamus induces drinking in rats (Grossman, 1960), sleeping in cats (Hernandez-Peon, 1965), and foot-thumping in gerbils (Block et al., 1974). Second, drug actions sometimes depend on site of administration. Scopolamine either facilitates or impairs learning in rats, depending on whether it is placed into the ventral or dorsal caudate nucleus (Neill & Grossman, 1970).

Third, learning abilities are task-specific. Rats given yeast RNA learned faster than controls to climb a pole to avoid shock or run a maze for food. But yeast RNA had no effect on discrimination learning or shock avoidance when the appropriate response was something other than pole climbing (Cook & Davidson, 1968; Cook et al., 1963). Or consider goldfish. Bottom-feeding scavengers that normally flee when exposed to an intense stimulus, goldfish rapidly learn to cross a hurdle to avoid electric shock. Siamese fighting fish are much more aggressive fish. Although slower to avoid shock by swimming away, they learn approach responses faster. Fear-reducing drugs might impair or facilitate memory performance by shifting an animal along the goldfish-fighting fish dimension. In fact, antianxiety drugs weaken avoidance behavior (Aron et al., 1971) but enhance maze-learning for food reward (Fox, Abendschein, & Lahcen, 1977).

Fourth, Martinez et al. (1991) noted that a drug may (a) enhance memory at a particular dose and impair it at both higher and lower doses; and (b) enhance memory of weakly learned and impair memory of well-learned tasks. The effects of stimuli such as electric shock also depend on their intensity and the level of learning. Martinez et al. pointed out that drugs and other stimuli can substitute for each other, probably because they act on a common mechanism.

▓ State Dependent Learning

A friend once used amphetamine to help him study through the night for a morning examination, and by test time he knew the material perfectly. Unfortunately, when the exam was distributed his mind became a blank, and that's what he got for a grade. His predicament had been anticipated by Lashley (1917), who reported that rats given strychnine or caffeine learned a maze more rapidly than controls but performed worse when tested while drug-free. Many subsequent researchers have found that responses learned under certain circumstances do not transfer well when the conditions are changed. Drug states constitute an important set of stimuli. The phenomenon, called state-dependent learning (SDL), has been demonstrated in humans following administration of amphetamine and barbiturate (Bustamente et al., 1970), marijuana (Darley, Tinklenberg, Roth, & Atkinson, 1974), alcohol (Lowe, 1981), and nicotine (Peters & McGee, 1982). Lowe (1988) found greater SDL effects when alcohol and nicotine or alcohol and caffeine were combined than when any of the drugs were taken alone.

SDL has important implications for studies on learning and memory. Subjects trained while drugged and then tested in the drug-free state may perform worse than controls who have received placebos during both sessions. An investigator might conclude that the drug interfered with the original training, but SDL might be responsible. See Overton (1974) for suggestions on how to improve experimental designs.

Many psychotherapists believe that therapy helps patients learn new behaviors to replace maladaptive ones. But both antianxiety drugs and phenothiazines produce SDL (cf. Hunt, 1956). So, upon withdrawal from the drugs, the newly learned behaviors may not be remembered. This may partly explain the high relapse rate when patients are withdrawn from the drugs.

▓ Neurochemical Foundations of Memory

Katz and Halstead (1950) speculated that neuronal stimulation causes random configurations of protein molecules to become ordered. Their idea sparked a still-continuing search for molecules that store memories. Over the years, DNA, RNA, proteins, and lipids have all been candidates for long-term memory storage, with proteins probably the most promising. The field is too vast and complex to be given justice here. See Goelet, Castellucci, Schacher, and Kandel (1986) and Davis and Squire (1984) for reviews.

A second area to be discussed only briefly is long-term potentiation (LTP). Stimulation of some neurons causes long-lasting synaptic changes, called LTP (Teyler & Discenna, 1987). Some forms of LTP require activation of N-methyl-D-aspartate (NMDA) receptors and can be blocked by NMDA receptor antagonists. The antagonists also block acquisition of new memories (Morris, Anderson, Lynch, & Baudry, 1986; Walker & Gold, 1991). Some investigators, for example, Brown, Chapman, Kairiss, and Keenan (1988), inferred that the memory-blocking effects are caused by antagonism of NMDA receptors. Others criticized the inference. See Keith and Rudy (1990) and the rejoinders immediately following their paper.

▓ Memory Effects of Common Drugs

ALCOHOL

Alcohol intoxication produces temporary attention and memory deficits (Jones & Vega, 1971), chronic alcoholism longer-lasting ones (Parsons, 1987). Chronic alcoholism also contributes in varying degree to three medical conditions that have severe memory problems as a significant component: Korsakoff's syndrome, Wernicke's disease, and dementia. Schuckit (1979) estimated that alcohol has played a major causal role in 15% to 30% of nursing home patients with organic brain syndrome.

Goodwin (1971) interviewed hospitalized alcoholics and reported that about two-thirds of them had experienced at least one "blackout," a term used to designate severe memory loss. He described an extreme case:

A 30-year old salesman awoke in a strange hotel room. He had a mild hangover but otherwise felt normal. His clothes were hanging in the closet; he was clean-shaven. He dressed and went down to the lobby. He learned from the clerk that he was in Las Vegas and that he had checked in two days previously. It had been obvious that he had been drinking, the clerk said, but he hadn't seemed very drunk. The date was Saturday the 14th. His last recollection was of sitting in a St. Louis bar on Monday the 9th. He had been drinking all day and was drunk, but could remember everything perfectly until about 3 P.M. when "like a curtain dropping," his memory went blank. It remained blank for approximately 5 days. It was still blank 3 years later. He was so frightened by the experience that he abstained from alcohol for 2 years.

The deterioration of cognitive skills is similar in chronic alcoholics and normal elderly people. Oscar-Berman (1990) considered two possibilities: (a) Alcohol accelerates the aging process. (b) Older brains are more vulnerable than younger ones to the harmful effects of alcohol abuse. So at age 40-50, when memory and other deficits due to aging normally begin to appear, alcoholics become more impaired than their peers. Oscar-Berman analyzed patterns of deficits and concluded that the second hypothesis is best supported.

Tarter, Moss, Arria, and Van Thiel (1990) observed that alcoholics perform similarly to nonalcoholics with liver dysfunction on most neuropsychological tests. Moreover, specific liver dysfunctions are associated with specific neuropsychological deficits. They cited evidence showing that effective treatment of the liver problems reduces the deficits. Tarter et al. also noted that 52% of alcoholics meet the criteria for a vitamin E deficiency and perform similarly to vitamin E-deficient nonalcoholics on neuropsychological tests.

ANTIDEPRESSANTS

Antidepressants impair memory (cf. Allen, Curran, & Lader, 1993; Curran, Sakulsriprong, & Lader, 1988; Hoff et al., 1990; Thompson, 1991). TCAs (probably because of their anticholinergic properties—see below) and sedating antidepressants produce the biggest decrements. Thompson noted that much of the evidence comes from short-term studies with healthy volunteers, and he argued that the effects are less serious than they seem. First, the effects weaken over time. Second, volunteers start with intact memory functioning whereas depressed people typically have impaired functioning. (On the other hand, Hoff et al. reported significant decreases in memory scores of clinically depressed people following 4 weeks of nortriptyline treatment.)

BENZODIAZEPINES

Derivatives of benzodiazepine are widely used for treating anxiety and sleep disorders. The benzodiazepines and other drugs that potentiate GABA activity impair memory (Wolkowitz, Tinklenberg, & Weingartner, 1985). Triazolam may be particularly disruptive, especially of episodic memory (Bixler et al., 1991; Weingartner et al., 1992). Other benzodiazepines have potentially clinically relevant consequences (Anthenelli et al., 1991; Taylor & Tinklenberg, 1987). Anxiety sometimes interferes with learning, and in those cases benzodiazepines may facilitate performance (Dimascio, 1963).

CAFFEINE

Caffeine facilitated the performance of college students on tasks that required mental speed, but students with a history of high-dose caffeine consumption did worse on a verbal reasoning task (Mitchell & Redman, 1992). In another study, caffeine improved memory of sleep-deprived women (Rogers, Spencer, Stone, & Nicholson, 1989).

Arnold et al. (1987), working with college students, found different memory effects of caffeine on men and women. Men given a 2 mg/kg dose and asked to learn lists of words did worse than when given either a placebo or a 4 mg/kg dose. Women, who were tested only during the menstrual phase of their cycle, did better with both caffeine doses.

COCAINE

Cocaine abusers who stop using experience a variety of cognitive impairments including short-term memory deficit. Herning et al. (1990) found no improvements during a 3- to 4-week period of abstinence.

MARIJUANA

People intoxicated on marijuana suffer clear memory impairment (cf. Miller & Branconnier, 1983), but chronic effects are less well established. Schwartz (1991) compared adolescent marijuana abusers with controls on tests of visual and auditory memory. The abusers did worse. After 6 weeks of monitored abstinence, they were retested and showed significant improvement. But some impairment remained.

Block et al. (1990) administered standardized tests (Iowa Tests of Educational Development) to 12th-grade students. They also retrieved the students' scores on versions of the same tests taken in the fourth grade, prior to onset of marijuana use. The 4th-grade scores of 12th-grade heavy users (at least five times weekly marijuana use for the past 2 years or more), light users (at least once weekly use for the past 2 years or more), and nonusers (had not used more than twice in their lives) were similar on most of the tests; nonusers had done better on a test of language skills. In the 12th grade, heavy users did worse than the others on a test of verbal expression (closely related to the 4th-grade language skills test) and one of mathematical skills. The three groups were otherwise similar.

NICOTINE

Ney, Gale, and Morris (1989) reviewed research on the effects of nicotine on memory. The most clear-cut conclusion was that variations in experimental conditions—type of memory task; whether subjects were light, moderate, or heavy smokers; and whether they were allowed to smoke before or during the learning and memory phases—matter greatly. A second conclusion was that, "for some subjects, in some learning tasks and with some nicotine concentrations, smoking just prior to learning (and following a period of deprivation) has modest and delayed positive effects on verbal rote learning."

SOLVENTS

Organic solvents such as glues, cements, paint thinners, spray paints, cleaning fluids, typewriter correction fluid, and gasoline are a class of abused compounds (Crider & Rouse, 1988). Most contain toluene, which is also abused in its pure form and may be the key ingredient in all of them. (Nonhuman primates self-administer toluene [Wood, 1978]). Chronic toluene abusers frequently experience short-term memory loss and cognitive impairment (Pryor, 1990).

▓ Facilitation of Memory Consolidation

GLUCOSE

As people age, ability to regulate glucose becomes less efficient and probably results in inadequate brain uptake of glucose from blood (Manning, Hall, & Gold, 1990). Because glucose is the major fuel of the brain, impaired uptake might partly explain why certain functions deteriorate with age.

Gold and Stone (1988) administered glucose to aged rats and mice; they did better than controls on a memory test. Manning et al. (1990) had elderly people drink either glucose- or saccharin-flavored beverages. The glucose group did better on two long-term declarative memory tests on which older people are particularly deficient. The authors noted that the subjects with relatively poor glucose regulation had the poorest memories. In a follow-up study, the optimal dose was determined. It varied but for most people was about 25 grams (Parsons & Gold, 1992).[1]

Drugs administered before training may enhance performance by affecting attention, arousal, or sensory-motor functions rather than memory. So Manning, Parsons, and Gold (1992) administered glucose shortly after presenting material to be learned, then tested subjects 24 hours later when blood glucose levels had returned to baseline. Memory was enhanced.

NOOTROPICS

Giurgea (1973) coined the term *nootropic* to describe a class of drug that facilitates learning and memory while protecting the brain against injury due to disease or external agents. Nootropics promote transfer of information between brain hemispheres and increase synaptic excitability (Okuyama & Aihara, 1988). Piracetam, structurally similar to the neurotransmitter GABA, was the first described. By 1980, hundreds of studies had been run with piracetam and related nootropics. The frequency of research has increased in recent years, and recent reviews indicate that nootropics are effective cognitive enhancers (cf. Coleston & Hindmarch, 1991; Nicholson, 1990).

Nootropic-induced facilitation of learning and memory is well documented in rodents (cf. Giurgea, 1982; Ennaceur, Cavoy, Costa, & Delacour,

1989; Mondadori, Ducret, & Borkowski, 1991; Mondadori & Etienne, 1990; Sansone, Castellano, Battaglia, & Ammassari-Teule, 1990; Sansone & Oliverio, 1989) and monkeys (Fitten, Perryman, Hanna, & Menon, 1990). Several clinical trials with human samples are also quite promising (cf. Abuzzahab, Merwin, Zimmermann, & Sherman, 1977; Chouinard, Annable, Ross-Chouinard, & Oliver, 1983; Dimond & Brouwers, 1976; Itil, Menon, Bozak, & Songar, 1982; Moglia et al., 1986). Wilsher (1986) cited 12 double-blind studies in which piracetam improved performance in dyslexic children. Wilsher et al. (1987) conducted a multicenter double-blind study on dyslexics and reported improvements that lasted for at least 36 weeks.

Piracetam is obtained from *Ginkgo biloba*, the maidenhair tree. Ginkgo, sold over the counter in health food stores in the United States, is used in several other countries for a variety of medical purposes. Recent studies indicate that ginkgo extract may benefit memory. Rai, Shovlin, and Wesnes (1991) worked with middle-aged patients suffering mild to moderate memory impairment. Over a 6-month period, those who received ginkgo outscored a placebo group on several measures of memory. Funfgeld (1989) reported favorable effects of ginkgo on brain wave patterns of patients suffering from Parkinson's disease. Studies with rats and mice (cf. Chopin & Briley, 1992; Winter, 1991) offer additional positive evidence.

STIMULANTS

McGaugh (1973) and his colleagues trained animals, then administered various drugs shortly afterwards. Many stimulants, including amphetamine, caffeine, strychnine, and nicotine, facilitated later performance. Drugs given right after training produced the greatest improvements, showing that activity at the time of retesting is not the key factor. The drugs do help when given just prior to retesting, so they must affect memory retrieval as well as consolidation (cf. Stone, Rudd, & Gold, 1990). Epinephrine may play a key role. The amphetamine effect is greatly weakened if the adrenal medulla, which releases epinephrine, is removed (Martinez et al., 1980). (Epinephrine does not cross the blood-brain barrier, but it does enhance memory when administered shortly after training. So Gold [1991] concluded that its peripheral actions account for the effect. One peripheral action of epinephrine is to cause the liver to release glucose.)

▩ The Role of Acetylcholine

Cognitive processes, like probably all complex behaviors, are controlled by multiple interacting neurotransmitters. Decker and McGaugh (1991) reviewed learning and memory research showing extensive interactions between NTs. Acetylcholine, norepinephrine, dopamine, serotonin, GABA, and several neuropeptides are involved. Acetylcholine, however, may have an especially strong role.

Both memory capacity and cholinergic functioning decline in elderly nonhuman and human animals, and some (disputed) evidence exists that nootropics act through a cholinergic mechanism (cf. Gainotti, Nocentini, & Sena, 1989; Pepeu & Spignoli, 1989). The severe memory impairment of Alzheimer's disease is associated with cholinergic dysfunction (Bartus, Dean, Beer, & Lipa, 1982; Coyle, Price, & DeLong, 1983), and normal adults given the anticholinergic drug scopolamine demonstrate similar deficits (Wesnes & Simpson, 1988).

Leathwood (1989) noted that senile mental decline has many causes, cholinergic dysfunctions occur in many ways, and drugs act by many mechanisms. So it is overly optimistic to assume that a particular cholinergic drug will necessarily correct an existing dysfunction; furthermore, patients likely to benefit from treatment cannot be identified in advance. Nevertheless, cholinergic drugs have positive although short-lasting effects on Alzheimer's patients (Davis et al., 1983; Drachman & Sahakian, 1979).

The severe memory deficits experienced by many schizophrenics are caused at least partly by drugs rather than disease. Walkup (1991) pointed out that antipsychotic drugs have anticholinergic properties—as do the anti-Parkinsonian drugs used to treat movement disorders induced by the antipsychotics. Fayen, Goldman, Moulthrop, and Luchins (1988) compared anticholinergic and dopaminergic drug treatments for the movement disorders and reported fewer memory problems with the latter.

Deutsch (1971) hypothesized that the effects of drugs that modify cholinergic functioning depend on efficiency of ACh synapses at the time the drugs are administered. He trained rats to run a maze, then injected them with DFP, which retards the metabolism of ACh and so enhances cholinergic functioning. He tested DFP-treated and control rats 24 hours later, at which time they were drug-free. His results were most provocative.

Injected shortly before training, DFP did not affect learning. But when injected 30 minutes after rats had made 10 consecutive correct responses, DFP impaired subsequent retest performance. When injected 1 to 3 days after training, it had little effect; yet at 5 or 14 days, it produced near total amnesia; and injected 28 days after training, when control rats have forgotten almost completely, DFP restored the memories. Deutsch injected other rats with the anticholinergic drug scopolamine and reported that the effects mirrored those with DFP. Deutsch (1983) summarized the results of his research program but included no references to work done after 1972. In a personal communication (July 1992), he wrote that further work would have provided only minor increase in information at major effort and cost.

The ACh precursor phosphatidylcholine (lecithin, much more effective than the more frequently used choline) improved learning of elderly mice and retarded the development of age-related neural and behavioral deficits in middle-age mice (Leathwood, 1989). Dozens of other animal studies involving several species and a wide variety of tasks have clearly established an important role for ACh in formation and maintenance of memories (Decker & McGaugh, 1991).

Summary

There are many types of memory, and drug effects vary with memory task, species, brain region, dose, and time of administration.

Responses learned in the presence of some stimulus complexes do not transfer well when the stimulus complexes are changed. The phenomenon, called state dependent learning, has both practical and methodological implications.

Temporary memory impairment, a prominent feature of acute alcohol intoxication, can become long-lasting in alcoholics. Many alcoholics experience occasional blackouts—severe memory loss for events or entire time periods. Older people are more vulnerable than younger ones to the harmful effects of alcohol.

Benzodiazepines generally impair memory but may help people whose learning is impaired by anxiety. Marijuana produces clear-cut short-term memory impairment; effects on long-term users are inconclusive. Nicotine improves performance on some learning and memory tasks. Organic solvents impair memory.

Many stimulant drugs facilitate memory consolidation and retrieval. So does glucose. The stimulants may act at least in part by promoting the release of glucose.

A large body of literature supports the view that certain other drugs and drug classes enhance memory. The nootropics have been studied most.

Cholinergic functioning declines in elderly humans and other animals and is associated with memory declines. Drugs that increase ACh levels have beneficial effects on memory in some elderly individuals.

▧ Note

1. One consequence of writing this book is that my candy and dental bills both increased dramatically.

Mini-Quiz: Memory

A person who learns something while intoxicated with alcohol may not remember if tested when sober. The phenomenon is called _____.

state dependent learning

Chronic alcoholism contributes to three diseases whose victims have severe memory deficits. They are _____, _____, & _____.

Korsakoff's syndrome, Wernicke's disease, and dementia

Many chronic abusers of _____ experience occasional severe memory losses called blackouts.

alcohol

T/F: Older brains are more vulnerable than younger ones to alcohol abuse.

true

T/F: Memory deficits due to acute use of marijuana are well established, but deficits due to chronic use are not.

true

What substance that can be bought inexpensively in supermarkets improves memory in aged rats and people?

glucose

Piracetam and other _____ facilitate memory in rats and people and protect the aging brain against disease.

nootropics

Stimulant drugs facilitate memory most when given (before/during/right after/long after) training.

right after

Dysfunction of which NT is most closely associated with Alzheimer's disease?

   ACh

Which conclusion best summarizes the data? Cognitive processes are under control of:
a. ACh   b. NE   c. serotonin   d. interactions between several NTs

   d

By the time you finish reading this chapter, you should be able to answer the following questions:

How do psychologists measure creativity, and what implication can be drawn from the availability of so many tests?

How did alcohol help (hinder) the creativity of various 20th-century writers?

What types of creative people have been helped by the drug propranolol?

Why is it generally inadvisable to use stimulants such as amphetamine during attempts to be creative?

What is the relationship between psychedelic drugs, imagery, and creativity?

What is brainstorming?

Almost all studies on drugs and creativity have lacked a ___.

How did the subjects of popular music change during the late 1960s, when psychedelic drug use intensified.

What evidence exists for the claim that psychedelic drugs enhance esthetic sensibilities?

Creativity

Contents

The creativity chapter of *Drugs and Behavior* (1982) had the sentence, "Governments have virtually abolished the use of drugs like LSD and mescaline in studies of creativity." In 1994, the word *virtually* can be deleted. I chose to write a chapter anyway, because reports on drug-induced creativity are alluring and laws can be changed. If some drugs enhance creativity safely, people should know about them. Even if the drugs prove dangerous, they might offer clues to designing safer ones and to nonpharmacological creativity-enhancing techniques. If the drugs don't work, we should know that too.

Creativity researchers face a major and perhaps insurmountable difficulty—meanings of terms. Psychologists do not agree on criteria for evaluating creative efforts, a fact underscored by the variety of measurement devices. For example:

327

Remote Associations Test. Subjects are given sets of three words and for each set asked to find a word that links the other three. An appropriate link to "rat," "blue," and "cottage" is "cheese."

Ingenuity Test. Subjects read short paragraphs that have a missing word or phrase at the end. Then they must pick from five words or phrases with some of the letters missing.

> In the process of writing a report, several hundred reference books were used. It was decided that a list of the authors and the titles of the books would be included at the end of the report for bibliographic references. In order to speed up the alphabetizing process for this bibliography, it was decided that each reference would be listed on a small ___.
> a. n—s. b. t—r. c. r—d. d. c—d. e. s—e.
> The correct answer is d (card).

Story-Writing Test. Testees are shown a series of pictures and asked to make up imaginative stories about each one.

Unusual Uses Test. Subjects are asked to list various uses to which each of several common objects, such as bricks and toothpicks, could be put. Both quantity and quality of responses are scored.

Productive Thinking. Hypothetical conditions, such as the synthesis of a new gas with unusual properties, are described and subjects are asked to discuss possible consequences.

Mosaic Design Test. Subjects are given a box of mosaic tiles and asked to create designs; evaluations are made on the basis of originality, organization, and esthetic appeal.

On the first two tests, only one answer is scored correct. Demanding one right answer is, in a fundamental way, the antithesis of creativity. The next four listed tests beg the question: To score for quality of responses or esthetic appeal presupposes agreement on the meaning of those terms. The proliferation of tests and low correlations among them (Hattie, 1980) are evidence that agreement has not been reached.

Neither philosophers of esthetics nor painting, drama, literature, or music critics fare any better when it comes to judging works of art. Many presently acclaimed artists, among them van Gogh, Picasso, Cezanne, Kokoschka, Racine, Beethoven, Stravinsky, and Mozart, received hostile receptions by the critics of their day. Can anyone today be confident how future generations will judge the Beatles, Woody Allen, and Bob Dylan?

Creativity in the narrow sense connotes art galleries, concert halls, and Nobel Prizes. Viewed more broadly, it applies to many forms of problem solving. Some people are highly skilled at finding creative solutions to life's daily problems. Creative problem solving is a valuable skill.

▓ Methodology

Neither the drugs and creativity literature, nor the drugs and sex literature reviewed in the next chapter, are paragons of methodological sophistication. Many of the studies lack experimental rigor, and their inclusion in a book stressing methodology may seem hypocritical. In defense, I offer two points. First, facilitation of creativity and sexual functioning are goals worth pursuing. Second, although scientists should demand the greatest rigor possible, they should not ignore potentially useful information obtained from other than laboratory experiments. Controlled experimentation is a luxury often denied astronomers, paleontologists, geologists, medical researchers, and many others. Those fields progressed because researchers did the best they could with the methods available to them. Most modern philosophers of science recognize that research designs must be adapted to circumstances. Even anecdotal evidence can be useful. Still, research lacking proper controls rarely permits unambiguous conclusions. It must be evaluated judiciously.

The opinions of "experts" about the effects of drugs on creativity range from "pure bunk" to "very beneficial" (cf. Cohen, 1968; Finlater, quoted in "The Drug Revolution," 1970; Leary, 1968; Louria, 1968; Watts, quoted in "The Drug Revolution," 1970; Yolles, 1968). The opinions have little to do with strength of supporting evidence.

▓ Alcohol

Rothenberg (1990) remarked that many highly creative writers, including five of the eight U.S. Nobel prize winners, were alcohol abusers. He listed major writers who almost certainly had severe problems with alcohol: James Agee, Charles Baudelaire, Louise Bogan, James Boswell, Truman Capote, John Cheever, Stephen Crane, Theodore Dreiser, William Faulkner, F. Scott Fitzgerald, Lillian Hellman, Ernest Hemingway, Victor Hugo, Samuel Johnson, Ring Lardner, Sinclair Lewis, Jack London, Robert Lowell, Malcolm Lowry, John O'Hara, Eugene O'Neill, Edgar Allan Poe, William Porter (O. Henry), Edwin Arlington Robinson, John Steinbeck, Dylan Thomas, Tennessee Williams, and Thomas Wolfe. He also mentioned several major painters: Mark Rothko, Arshile Gorky, Jackson Pollock, and Willem de Kooning. Rothenberg analyzed biographical material of all the writers listed and reported that few wrote or even thought about writing while intoxicated. Hemingway, Fitzgerald, and O. Henry were exceptions, if their claims are believed. The potential for bias in biographical studies is substantial, as they depend on anecdotal material derived from secondary sources and selectively chosen and presented by the investigator. Nevertheless, they offer a rich source of data unavailable from laboratory research.

Rothenberg considered the possibility that genes that predispose to alcoholism and creativity are linked. No evidence is available on that point. He also hypothesized that (a) the men became "tough-guy drinkers" to counter the cultural stereotype creative men are effeminate or homosexual; and (b) many were Irish, a cultural group with a high incidence of alcoholism. This hypothesis requires evidence showing that Irish writers are no more likely to be alcoholic than Irish in other occupations.

From extensive interviews with John Cheever, Rothenberg developed a third possible explanation for the writing/drinking connection. Plausible and compatible with the others, it too lacks supporting evidence. He wrote that creativity involves a gradual unearthing of unconscious processes; creative people embark on activities leading to discovering and knowing themselves in fundamental ways. Inevitably, a host of negative emotions are generated including anxiety, guilt, antagonism, jealousy, and hostility. At times, they threaten to overwhelm, and alcohol brings sedation and relief. So, "The muse may not be in the bottle itself, but the alcohol may be the acceptable way to deal with her glory and threat" (Rothenburg, 1990).

Ludwig (1990) analyzed biographical data of 20th-century eminent creative artists who had had reputations as heavy drinkers. His sample consisted of 28 writers, 2 artists, and 4 composer/performers (31 men and 3 women). He documented both positive and negative effects of alcohol on creative performance but expressed reservations about some of the former. He cited the cases of John Cheever, who claimed that drinking inspired him but wrote his most acclaimed novel, *Falconer*, after becoming abstinent; Eugene O'Neill and John O'Hara, who were very productive after they stopped drinking; and Jackson Pollock, who once thought that drinking made his paintings possible but painted four of his masterworks during an extended sober period.

Ludwig's findings are summarized below, with examples and quotes taken from his article. (The percentages add up to more than 100%, because most of the people displayed more than one alcohol/creativity relationship during the course of their lives.) The most prominent finding is that alcohol impaired creative performance in 76.5% of his sample.

1. Alcohol increased creative output directly in 8.8% by somehow facilitating the creative process.

A. E. Housman: Having drunk a pint of beer at luncheon, I would go out for a walk. As I went along ... there would flow into my mind, with sudden and unaccountable emotion, sometimes a line or two of verse, sometimes a whole stanza.

2. Alcohol increased creative output indirectly (by relieving pain or inhibition, increasing motivation, etc.) in 50%.

E. B. White: Before I start to write, I always treat myself to a nice dry martini. Just one, to give me the courage to get started. After that, I am on my own.

3. Alcohol decreased creative output directly in 76.5%.

Eugene O'Neill: I will never, nor never have written anything good when I am drinking or even when the miasma of drink is left.

4. Alcohol decreased creative output indirectly (by impairing general health, mood, motivation, etc.) in 17.6%.

Carson McCullers: Her drinking affected her health, which affected her writing.

5. Alcohol had no effect on creative output in 44.1%.

Frederic Remington: He was a heavy, steady drinker and productive artist.

Ernest Hemingway: He wrote 500 words every morning even when he'd drunk heavily the night before.

6. Alcohol intake increased directly in 5.8%. They used it to cope with the intense brain activity generated by creative output.

Truman Capote said that once he began writing in earnest, his mind "zoomed all night every night, and I don't think I really slept for several years. Not until I discovered that whiskey could relax me."

7. Alcohol intake increased indirectly in 32.4% as a result of creative activities (which caused depression or anxiety, use of other drugs, or the need to conform to the cultural expectation that creative people drink heavily).

John Cheever usually became depressed after completing a novel; he used alcohol to relieve his distress.

8. Creative output directly decreased alcohol intake in 11.8%, either because the two were mutually incompatible or because the creative activity satisfied whatever drive is responsible for alcohol intake.

Dashiell Hammett deliberately remained abstinent during the writing of his fifth novel.

9. Creative output indirectly decreased alcohol intake in 2.9% by improving self-confidence, providing proof that a writing block was over, or relieving an underlying psychopathology.

William Faulkner drank heavily during frequent bouts of depression. Writing relieved his depression.

10. Factors such as motivational state, personality, and presence or absence of various conditions independently affected creative activity and alcohol intake in 38.2%.

When manic, Delmore Schwartz sometimes wrote, sometimes drank, sometimes did both.

▩ Antianxiety Drugs and Lithium

Striving for perfection before large and often critical audiences may induce disabling sympathetic nervous system symptoms such as racing heart, hand tremor, and palpitations. To prevent these from occurring while they perform on stage, many actors and musicians take propranolol and related drugs. Of 2,122 members of the International Conference of Symphony and Opera Musicians, 27% admitted using propranolol and 19% of those said they use it daily (Lockwood, 1989). Conventional antianxiety drugs may not be effective. Working with 15 professional musicians who suffered from stage fright, Clark and Agras (1991) found that cognitive behavior therapy reduced anxiety and improved the quality of performance; but buspirone was ineffective.

Schou (1979) presented 24 case reports of manic-depressive artists who took lithium to prevent recurrences of their illness. He wrote that artistic productivity increased in 12, was unaltered in 6, and decreased in 6. He attributed the productivity increases to the ability of lithium to bring debilitating depression under control. He speculated that the decreases were due to lack of inspiration, reduced motivation, or elimination of prolonged periods of pain that could be used creatively. Schou strongly advocates lithium treatment, so possible bias is a concern.

▩ Stimulants

Stimulants such as amphetamine and caffeine might occasionally sustain somebody during an outpouring of creative effort, where failure to remain alert would result in loss of motivation or valuable ideas. But routine reliance on stimulants to improve creativity is unwise. An extensive literature shows that high doses of amphetamine produce stereotyped behaviors. Rats, guinea pigs, and cats repeat the same movements for hours at a time (Randrup & Munkvad, 1967). In humans, amphetamine psychosis inevitably appears during chronic high-dose use and is characterized by elements of compulsivity such as repetition of single words or phrases (Connell, 1958). Amphetamine improves ability to attend to dull, well-learned tasks such as naming colors, but it reduces effectiveness when solutions require new perspectives (discussed in Broverman et al., 1968). So amphetamine and related stimulants are unlikely candidates for creativity enhancers.

▧ Opiates

Hayter (1968) wrote that opium had significant effects on the works of Coleridge, DeQuincey, and Poe. One of the most beautiful and famous poems in the English language is Coleridge's "Kubla Khan." Its genesis is well known. Coleridge had been ill and received a drug, probably opium, from which he fell into a profound sleep in the midst of reading a passage about the emperor Kubla Khan. He had unusually vivid dreams that he fully recollected upon awakening. He began writing them down but was interrupted by a visitor. When he returned to writing, he was able to reconstruct only the fragment that still survives.

▧ Nitrous Oxide

William James experimented with nitrous oxide and experienced mystic revelations. But for a long time, he was unable to record the moments of illumination or remember them upon awakening. He finally succeeded and wrote down his monumental thoughts just before losing consciousness. Upon arising, he rushed to his paper and found written:

> Hogamous, Higamous
> Man is polygamous,
> Higamous, Hogamous
> Woman is monogamous.

The anecdote, reported in Gibbons and Connelly (1970), illustrates the blunting effect that drugs often have on self-criticism. As a result, first-person accounts are unreliable. Still, it's worth noting that many highly creative people besides James experimented with nitrous oxide: poet Robert Southey, Coleridge, Roget (of thesaurus fame), Watt the steamboat man, and Wedgewood the potter.

Hansen et al. (1984-1985) assigned dental patient volunteers to groups that received oxygen alone or oxygen plus nitrous oxide. They then asked the subjects to solve a series of water jar problems (see Table 16.2). The main finding was that the nitrous oxide subjects were much more sensitive to the set breaking problem and switched problem-solving strategies more quickly and with fewer errors. Hansen et al. noted that cognitive blocks are powerful barriers to psychotherapeutic change as well as to artistic creativity.

Table 16.1 Altered States of Consciousness and Creativity

Person	Achievement	Altered State
Robert Louis Stevenson	Dreamed and remembered complete stories, e.g., *Dr. Jekyll and Mr. Hyde*	Dreaming
Wagner	Rheingold theme	Dreaming
Tartini	Heard sonata, which gave inspiration for "Devil's Thrill"	Dreaming
Mozart, Schumann, and Saint-Saëns	All first heard some of their music during dreams	Dreaming
Niels Bohr	Conceptual model of atom	Dreaming
Otto Loewi	Concept of chemical transmission in nervous system	Dreaming
Kekule	Discovery of structure of benzene ring	Dreaming
Mendeleev	Periodic Table of the Elements	Dreaming
Elias Howe	Sewing machine	Dreaming
A. R. Wallace	Formulation of theory of evolution by natural selection	Malarial fever
Tissot	Painting: *The Ruins*	Daydream
Rachmaninoff	Concerto No. 2 in C Minor for Piano and Orchestra	Hypnosis

▒ Psychedelics

REASONS FOR BELIEVING THAT PSYCHEDELIC DRUGS MIGHT STIMULATE CREATIVITY

Many historic ideas and inventions have been preceded by and attributed to an altered state of consciousness (see Table 16.1). Fischer and Scheib (1971) reported that the poet Saint-Paul-Roux hung a sign on his door before going to sleep: "Poet at work." Harman et al. (1966) suggested specific ways in which consciousness-altering drugs such as marijuana, LSD, peyote, and mescaline might improve creative output. These, some of which are discussed further below, include increased access to unconscious data; increased ability to play spontaneously with hypotheses, metaphors, paradoxes, and so forth; heightened ability for visual imagery and fantasy; relaxation and openness; heightened empathy; and reduced tendency to censor creations by premature negative judgment. Harman et al. also noted that some effects, such as reduced capacity for logical thought, might hinder creativity.

Imagery

Researchers have noted strong connections between imagery and creativity. For example, Khatena (1977) wrote:

> Much of brain activity relative to the creative imagination has to do with imagery or the re-experiencing of images. My recent research on the creative imagination has led me to define the functions of the imagination as the chemistry of mental processing where interactive intellectual and emotional forces participate in stimulating, energizing and propagating the creative act.

Psychedelic drugs elicit pulsating visual images followed by childhood memories of scenes rich with emotionality (Siegel, 1977). Aldous Huxley (1963) gave a vivid description of imagery following LSD or mescaline:

> First and most important is the experience of light. . . . All colors are intensified to a pitch far beyond anything seen in the normal state, and at the same time the mind's capacity for recognizing fine distinctions of tone and hue is notably heightened.
>
> The typical mescaline or lysergic-acid experience begins with perceptions of colored, moving, living geometrical forms. In time, pure geometry becomes concrete, and the visionary perceives, not patterns, but patterned things, such as carpets, carvings, mosaics. . . . Fabulous animals move across the scene. Everything is novel and amazing.

Play of Ideas

Brainstorming is a technique widely assumed to enhance creativity (cf. Parnes & Meadow, 1959), although claims should be evaluated in the context of the definitional problems discussed above. Once a problem is raised for consideration, brainstorming participants are instructed to behave according to three rules: (a) generate as many ideas as possible; (b) seek remote, bizarre, and wild ideas; (c) do not criticize. The rationale for brainstorming is epitomized in a Chinese proverb: The best way to catch fish is to have many lines.

Subsequent evaluation is crucial and invariably reveals many ideas to be unworkable; still, brainstorming and its variants justify their popularity if they foster discovery of good ideas that might not have been produced otherwise. Similarly, ingestion of various drugs may impair critical judgment and lead to the creation of many inferior artworks. But some superior works may owe their existence to temporary drug-induced suspension of judgment.

New Perspectives

A major barrier to creativity is the tendency to perceive things in a set way. Shekerjian (1990), who interviewed 40 winners of the prestigious Macarthur Award, concluded:

> Overfamiliarization with something—an idea, say, or a method, or an object—is a trap. Where creativity is concerned, that is the irony of skill: the more adept you are at something, the less likely you are to appreciate a varying interpretation; the greater your mastery of the skills and routines associated with a particular discipline, the less likely you will be tempted to generate new approaches.

Adams (1986) noted that creativity techniques "are intended to result in the production of concepts that deviate from the usual." He added that the techniques all result in effort being focused in new directions, and they modify the usual habitual process of problem solving.

Beveridge (1980) summarized the results of a symposium in which 24 eminent scientists including 4 Nobel prize winners discussed the creative process in science and medicine:

> It has long been known that breaking out from conventional thinking is a major factor in creative thinking, and this was reaffirmed at the Kronberg symposium. Many scientists, philosophers, and psychologists have emphasized that the mental act of invention, of intuition, is a non-rational activity. The advocates of wild thinking believe it can best be sought by deliberately invoking a chaotic, irrational mood in which bizarre analogies that are normally censored by the subconscious are brought into the conscious mind.

Consider three examples. (a) In the classic nine-dot problem (see Figure 16.1), subjects are asked to connect all nine dots with just four straight lines and without taking their pen from the paper. (b) The problem shown in Figure 16.2 (adapted from Kohler, 1969) is difficult. But changing how it is represented simplifies considerably (see Figure 16.3). (c) The third task is to use water jars with the capacities shown in columns A-C to obtain the amounts shown in column D (from Luchins, 1946) (see Table 16.2). The most efficient way to solve the first three

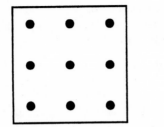 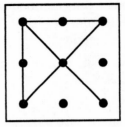

Figure 16.1. Connect the nine dots by drawing four straight lines without lifting your pencil

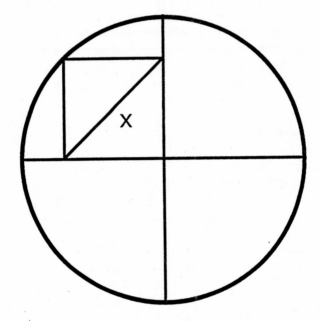

Figure 16.2. The diameter of this circle is 10 inches. How long is line X?

does not work for the fourth. There is an easy solution to the fourth problem, but people often overlook it.

In ancient Persia, people confronted with a difficult decision weighed the evidence and made a choice. The next day, they got drunk and chose again. The choice was implemented only if it was the same on both occasions. Otherwise, believing that problems viewed from both sober and drunk perspectives are understood better than from either alone, they

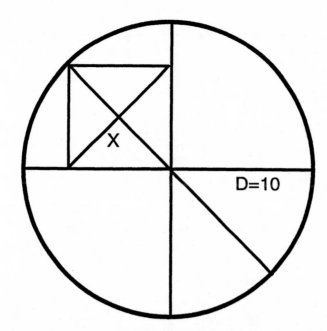

Figure 16.3. The diameter of this circle is 10 inches. How long is line X?

NOTE: Line X is the same length in both cases. Figure 16.3 emphasizes that it is a diagonal of the rectangle, so it is equal to the rectangle's other diagonal. That diagonal is a radius of the circle, so it and line X are both 5 inches long.

Table 16.2 Given water jars of the sizes listed in columns A, B, and C, obtain the exact amounts in column D.

A	B	C	D
37	4	9	15
59	11	6	36
83	16	2	63
41	93	11	30

NOTE: Answers to problems in Table 16.2
The solutions to the first three problems follow a simple pattern: Fill jar A, then pour enough water from A to fill jar C twice, then pour enough from A to fill jar B once. Jar A then has the desired amount. People who discern a pattern often try to apply it where it doesn't work, as in the fifth problem. There is an easy answer to the fourth: Fill jar A and pour enough water from it to fill jar B. Jar A then has the desired amount.

alternated between states until agreement was reached. I believe that many creative people would go further; given the chance, they would gladly change gender for a day or briefly become a cat or fish or tree. Impossible, but psychedelic drugs might offer a close substitute.

New Experiences

Psychedelics supply unique, rich, and emotionally intense experiences that artists can build on. Nietzsche wrote, "Poets act shamelessly toward their experiences: they exploit them."

I'm not particularly creative but would like to share an experience. Several years ago, a psychiatrist friend evaluated the powerful drug ibogaine for his practice. One of his volunteer subjects reported that ibogaine provoked one of the worst ordeals of his life. For a period of about 3 hours, he felt like "the last molecule in an otherwise utterly desolate universe." Upon hearing his description, and under no illusion that my experience would be less painful, I asked to take ibogaine. I arranged for friends to check up on me throughout the day. One, a powerfully built African-American former all-pro football player, came at the height of the trip and joked around at a time when simple talk would have served me better. After he left, I endured an extended period during which vivid scenes flashed through my mind of violent wars between ancient tribes of blacks and whites. Having thought myself totally free of racial prejudice, the images disturbed profoundly. They provoked constant introspection and discussion with friends of different races during the following few weeks. The result was a deeper understanding and creative synthesis of important issues.

Brain Laterality

Popular accounts of functional differences between the left and right brain hemispheres often oversimplify, but differences exist and some are relevant to creativity research. Falcone and Loder (1984) found that people who spent more time gazing leftward while taking a test of creativity were more likely to earn high scores; gazing leftward is a sign of right hemisphere activity. Similarly, Martindale, Hines, Mitchell, and Covell (1984) reported greater EEG activity in the right than left hemisphere when creative people performed creative tasks.

Serafetinides (1965) administered LSD to patients who had had a temporal lobe removed to alleviate epilepsy. Psychedelic responses to LSD occurred after left but not right temporal lobe removal, suggesting that LSD acts primarily on the right hemisphere. Other drugs have unequal effects on the two hemispheres (Nelson, Phillips, & Goldstein, 1977; several cited in Geschwind & Galaburda, 1987).

The data on drug-enhanced creativity are, unfortunately, less impressive than the rationale.

EXPERIMENTS WITH
OBJECTIVE DEPENDENT VARIABLES

The few studies with objective tests have been flawed methodologically. Aldrich (1944) gave a synthetic marijuana-like compound to 12 jazz musicians who had used it previously. They did not get better at discriminating between the pitch, intensity, and timbre of musical notes but, significantly, 8 of the 12 believed they had improved. The study was not double or even single blind, and the test measured discriminatory ability rather than creativity.

Zegans, Pollard, and Brown (1967) and McGlothlin, Cohen, and McGlothlin (1969) both studied the effects of LSD on male volunteers, and both reported essentially negative effects on tests of creativity. Both suffered from shortcomings:

- Negative studies are always somewhat inconclusive, because failure to find an effect can be caused by insensitive tests or inadequate control over relevant variables. In the Zegans et al. study, men who scored well on a predrug personality test improved after receiving LSD. But only eight such men participated, so only a very powerful effect would have been statistically significant.

- Both sets of authors relied on timed tests. Whether or not the tests are generally valid, claims of enhanced creativity from LSD do not have increased speed of response as one of the bases; and creativity is not fostered by the filling in of forms.

- The laboratory setting is hardly ideal for inspiring creative outflow. Consider the comment of Dutch poet Simon Vinkenoog, who participated in an LSD experiment (Krippner, 1968): "In 1959, LSD was inflicted on me by a team of unqualified doctors-to-be who messed up some of my most beautiful experiences ever by having me fill in silly forms, by hooking me up to an electroencephalograph going momomomomomomomomo, etc."

- LSD induces profound perceptual, motor, and cognitive changes, so much so that subjects like Simon Vinkenoog resent having to attend fully to paper and pencil tests. First-time users especially might be unable or unwilling to ignore the effects. They might experience anxiety, which can interfere with performance. First-time marijuana users often perform poorly whereas chronic users do not (Weil, Zinberg, & Nelson, 1968). All the subjects in the McGlothlin et al. study were first-time users.

- In both studies, subjects were given a battery of tests prior to and again after taking LSD. Changes in performance furnished the basis of comparison between drug and placebo subjects. This paradigm biases the results, because LSD subjects probably benefited least from their first exposure to the tests. People who learn things under the influence of a drug frequently have impaired recall when tested undrugged (see p. 314).

The one positive study is also flawed. Harman et al. (1966) gave three creativity tests to several professional people who had been stymied in their work by problems requiring creative solutions. A few days later, the subjects received mescaline in a comfortable home, then relaxed and listened to quiet music while waiting for it to take effect. They then retook the tests and improved on all of them. But the improvement may have resulted from their prior exposure. In addition, the study lacked a control group—people given placebo and instructed to relax and listen to music in comfortable surroundings.

EXPERIMENTS WITH
SUBJECTIVE DEPENDENT VARIABLES

In the Harman et al. study, the 27 subjects worked on their professional problems for 4 hours while under the influence of mescaline. The results, as indicated by responses to a questionnaire 6 to 8 weeks later, sound impressive. Of 44 problems attempted, there were 20 new avenues for investigation opened; 2 working models completed; 1 developmental model to test solution authorized; 6 solutions accepted for construction or production; and 10 partial solutions obtained, being developed further, or being applied.

The subjects also listed benefits such as increased ability to communicate and respond to pressure. Four architects claimed that LSD aided them in visualizing three-dimensional space and heightened their perceptivity. But the lack of control group and clear drug bias make the results questionable. The same problems compromise both favorable and unfavorable conclusions from several other studies:

- Barron (1964) administered psilocybin to a ballet dancer, then filmed her during the next 5 hours. Later, her troupe members viewed the film and said she had performed unusual and worthwhile movements.

- Berlin et al. (1955) gave LSD or mescaline to four well-known graphic artists. Other artists judged their works to have greater esthetic value than what they had done previously.
- Hartmann (reported in *Time*, 1969) observed that nearly all of 34 artists he tested declined in skill after receiving LSD, and most overestimated the worth of their drug-induced productions.
- Tonini and Montanari (1955) reported that neither LSD nor mescaline improved the works of a painter.

Over a 7-year period, Janiger and De Rios (1989) administered LSD to professional artists, provided them with a comfortable setting in which to work, and collected 250 paintings and drawings. Participants generally expressed enthusiasm about the results, exemplified by one man's quote, "This is four years of art school!" Many judged their LSD works more interesting and esthetically superior to their usual mode of expression. Janiger and De Rios submitted 81 of the works, including 56 before-and-after samples, to a professor of art history (who knew the drug state under which each work was produced). He noted several stylistic changes, the most frequent being from representational or abstract to expressionistic or nonobjective.

CREATIVE PRODUCTS

Reports from outside the laboratory should not be ignored but must be scrutinized carefully. As noted several times above, the capacity for self-criticism is often blunted by drugs. So, first-person accounts are unreliable. Moreover, an artist's productivity after taking a drug is not proof that the drug was the cause. Many of the artists had been previously successful. For example, much has been made of the fact that Aldous Huxley wrote parts of three books, *Heaven and Hell*, *The Doors of Perception*, and *Island* while under the influence of mescaline. To credit the drug is to ignore his prior standing as one of the most important and prolific writers of the 20th century. *Brave New World* and several other of Huxley's novels have received greater critical acclaim than any of the three books associated with his mescaline use. At least, the three books show that drug use is not incompatible with creativity.

The writing of a novel, the composition of a symphony, or the execution of a major painting occupies a much greater time span than the duration of a single drug trip. Yet accounts of drug-induced creativity are rarely explicit about what is and is not due to drugs. Did the drug inspire the conception of the masterpiece? Was the drug active during part or all of the physical labor? Did the artist remain intoxicated while editing or retouching the work?

Many writers have used psychedelics. Poets Robert Graves, Michael McClure, and Henri Michaux wrote under the influence of the *Psilocybe* mushroom, peyote, and marijuana, respectively. Ken Kesey took peyote and LSD just prior to writing several passages of *One Flew Over the Cuckoo's Nest*. LSD was also the muse of Allan Ginsberg (*Kaddish and Other Poems*) and Alan Watts (*The Joyous Cosmology*), who also wrote under the influence of mescaline and psilocybin. William Burroughs attributed much of his *Naked Lunch* to marijuana, and a variety of psychedelics fueled science fiction writer Phillip Dick's stories.

Timothy Leary (1968) wrote that more than 70% of nonacademic artists have used psychedelics. Allen Ginsberg (1966) claimed that most of the major poets, painters, musicians, cineastes, sculptors, singers, and publishers in America and England are long-time marijuana users. Krippner (1968) quoted a "well-known pop recording artist" as saying that most of the top rock-n-roll groups use marijuana regularly and have tried LSD at least once. This echoes Rosevear's (1967) claim that marijuana was and is extremely popular among musicians. Richard Alpert ("The Drug Revolution," 1970) asserted that 90% of the rock industry is linked to LSD.

The accuracy of such claims is uncertain and, even if true, of problematic significance. They do not demonstrate that drug use improves creativity. A plausible alternative is that artists, being an unconventional lot, eagerly try new experiences. In addition, many artists have evolved elaborate rituals to accompany attempts at creative work. Vornoff (1941) gave some examples:

- To diminish the circulation of blood to his feet and increase it to his head, Schiller kept his feet in ice while writing. Composer Andre Crety did the same.
- Bossuet stood in a cold room and covered his head with fur.
- Descartes, Leibniz, Milton, and Rossini meditated under piles of blankets.
- Balzac and Poincare needed coffee.
- Tycho Brahe required total silence.
- The naturalist Buffon donned ceremonial apparel.
- Poet Gerard de Nerval wrote only while dressed in pearl-gray clothing.

The rituals surely did not enhance creativity directly, but they probably helped people who believed in them. Rituals are comforting and reassuring. Psychedelic drugs, because they induce such distinctive states, might be particularly effective as rituals.

Nevertheless, psychedelic drugs have left a powerful imprint on our culture. Lomberg (1983) contrasted the lyrics of Western popular music during periods of strong and weak interest in psychedelics. (He did not say which music he thought better, noting only that drugs inspired a special type.) Before the mid-1960s, most pop music was about courtship and love, dating and heartbreak. As drug use intensified in the late 1960s, musicians turned to interior experiences and the meaning of reality. They experimented with instruments (sitar, electronics, synthesizer), arrangements, and studio productions. Popular songs from that era include "Magical Mystery Tour" (Beatles), "Legend of a Mind" (Moody Blues), "Eight Miles High" (Byrds), "Cosmic Wheels" (Donovan), "Schizoforest Love Suite" (Jefferson Airplane), and "A Very Cellular Song" (Incredible String Band). In the 1970s, as interest in psychedelics diminished, the focus of popular music once again turned to love and sex.

In the visual arts, Lomberg pointed to drug-stimulated emphases on surrealistic, visionary, Far Eastern, and Native American art. He noted similarities between special effects in film and LSD visions, suggesting that one originated from the other.

▓ Psychedelic Artists

Masters and Houston (1968) published a book, *Psychedelic Art*, featuring the works of artists who believed that their works had been helped by psychedelic experiences, primarily psychedelic drugs. Several of the artists have since become prominent, and four of their paintings are reproduced as Figures 16.4-16.7. But nothing conclusive can be said about the role of drugs on their careers. There were, of course, no control groups.

Krippner (summarized in Krippner, 1985) surveyed 180 unnamed but, in his estimation, prominent artists. All but 18 had taken a psychedelic drug at least once, with LSD and marijuana the most popular. Many worked while intoxicated. Several fields of creative activity were represented: painting, light shows, mixed media, films, prose, photography, instrumental music, poetry, collage, sculpture, theater, and happenings.

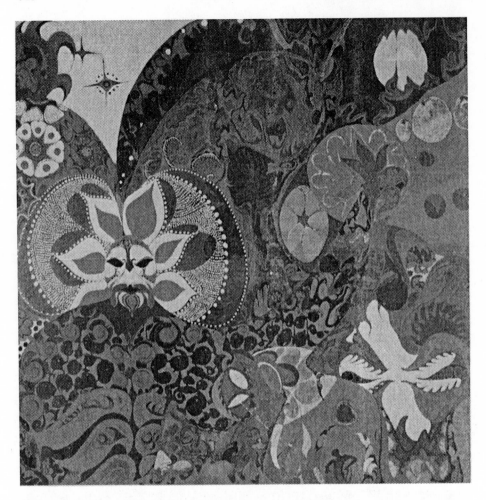

Figure 16.4. Isaac Abrams. *All Things are Part of One Thing*. Oil on canvas. 50 × 50".
1966. Collection Reed Erickson, Baton Rouge, Louisiana.

None of the artists believed their work had suffered, although several admitted that others did not share their view. More than two-thirds said their techniques, particularly use of colors, had improved noticeably. Many, such as painter Arlene Sklar-Weinstein, said their approach to art had changed. Her single LSD session "opened thousands of doors for me and dramatically changed the content, intent, and style of my work." Writer Ronny van den Eerenbeemt (quoted in Krippner, 1985) said:

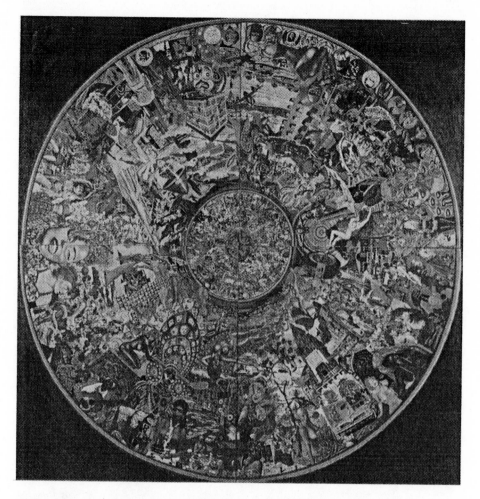

Figure 16.5. Mati Klarwein. *A grain of Sand.* Oil on composition board. 72 × 72". 1965.

When very young, I started writing stories and poems. The older I got, the more I had a feeling of not being able to find something really worthwhile to write about. My psychedelic experiences taught me that what I used to do was no more than scratch the surface of life. After having seen and felt the center of life, through the psychedelics, I now think I do have something worthwhile to write about.

Unfortunately, the vast potential for bias in Krippner's surveys makes them less than fully convincing. He advocates the use of psychedelic drugs for enhancing creativity, and he selected the artists. Those he

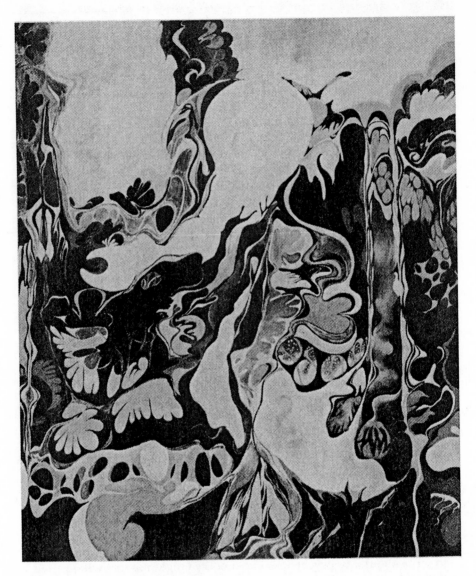

Figure 16.6. Isaac Abrams. *Spring Painting*. Oil on canvas. 50 × 60". 1967. Collection Arthur Eaton, New York.

knew directly or through friends probably shared many of his attitudes. The artists might have felt a need to justify their use of drugs. What better way than to say that their creativity had been enhanced.

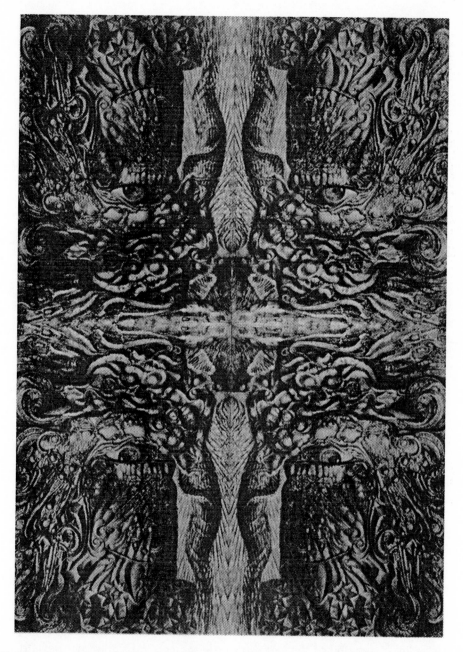

Figure 16.7. Ernst Fuchs. *Cherub (like a rhinoceros).* Pencil. 8 ½ × 10". 1962. Collection Aoki Gallery, Tokyo.

AWAKENING OF
ESTHETIC SENSIBILITIES

A good spectator also creates.
—Swiss proverb

Boszormenyi (1960) reported an awakened interest in art and writing in subjects who had taken diethyltryptamine. Two started to paint seriously and a third said, "I felt an enormous drive to write, to put down the marvelous feelings."

Drug-heightened appreciation for music and color is common and sometimes lasts well beyond the acute intoxication. Izumi (1970) claimed that LSD helped him appreciate certain qualities in the paintings of El Greco and Utrillo for the first time, and that ballet music became more emotionally moving for him. Burroughs (1966) affirmed that mescaline gave him a permanent ability to see a painting fully. Korngold (1963) said that patients given LSD frequently felt intense beauty and creative originality. Barron (1965) abstracted from various subjective reports of mescaline, LSD, and psilocybin users:

Colors become more vivid and glowing; the play of light on objects is enchanting; surface details become sharply defined; sensual harmonies, of sound, light, color, become marked. There are beautiful synesthesias, in which patterns of association usually confined to a single sense modality may cross over to others: music is "heard" as colored light, for example.

In some cases, ugliness will become intensified. A garish light may seem horrible, an unmusical sound unbearable; a false tone in a human may seem like a shriek; a false expression on a face may make it into a grotesque mask.

Both beauty and ugliness in objects are thus more than usually important and the esthetic qualities of the perceived world take on much greater value.

Psychologist Frances Vaughan (1983) wrote:

My aesthetic sensibilities were profoundly enhanced (by LSD), not only during the few hours of the session, but afterwards as well. This effect has lasted over a period of 15 years. My appreciation of music, art, nature, and human beings has continued to grow since that time. I remember being particularly struck by the joy of hearing music as I had never heard it before. I could laugh at my old self-image, which included "not being musical."

Allen Ginsberg (1966) wrote:

> Marijuana is a useful catalyst for specific optical and aural aesthetic percep-
> tions. I apprehended the structure of certain pieces of jazz and classical
> music in a new manner under the influence of marijuana, and these appre-
> hensions have remained valid in years of normal consciousness. I first
> discovered how to see Klee's *Magic Squares* as the painter intended them
> (as optically three-dimensional space structures) while high on mari-
> juana. I perceived ("dug") for the first time Cezanne's "petit sensation" of
> space achieved on a two-dimensional canvas (by means of advancing and
> receding colors, organization of triangles, cubes, etc., as the painter describes
> in his letters) while looking at *The Bathers* high on marijuana. And I saw
> anew many of nature's panoramas and landscapes that I'd stared at
> blindly without even noticing before; thru the use of marijuana, awe and
> detail were made conscious. These perceptions are permanent—and deep
> aesthetic experience leaves a trace, and an idea of what to look for that
> can be checked back later. I developed a taste for Crivelli's symmetry; and
> saw Rembrandt's *Polish Rider* as a sublime Youth on a Deathly horse for
> the first time—saw myself in the rider's face, one might say—while
> walking around the Frick Museum high on pot. These are not "hallucina-
> tions"; these are deepened perceptions that one might have catalyzed not
> by pot but by some *other* natural event (as natural as pot) that changes the
> mind, such as an intense love, a death in the family, a sudden clear dusk
> after rain, or the sight of the neon spectral reality of Times Square one
> sometimes has after leaving a strange movie. So it's all *natural*.

Hunter Thompson (cited in Byrne, 1982) offered a more vivid account:
"A cap of good acid (LSD) costs five dollars and for that you can hear
the Universal Symphony with God singing solo and the Holy Ghost on
drums." (Byrne added a rejoinder by William Buckley: "Though one
should be prepared to vomit rather frequently and disport with pink
elephants and assorted grotesqueries while trying, often unsuccess-
fully, to make one's way to the toilet.")

The reports of three different questionnaire studies with LSD participants (Ditman, Hayman, & Whittlesey, 1962; McGlothlin et al., 1969;
Savage et al., 1963) appear to bolster the preceding claims. To the question,
"Was the LSD experience a thing of great beauty?" 66% in one study
(Ditman et al., 1962) and 81% in another (Savage et al., 1963) answered
"quite a bit" or "very much." Ditman et al.'s (1962) subjects reported
increased interests in nature (38%), art (34%), and music (33%).
McGlothlin's subjects, questioned 6 months afterwards, reported a
greater appreciation for music (62%) and art (46%). In addition, they

spent more time than previously—and more time than controls who had not taken LSD—in museums, attending musical events, and buying records. The results are impressive, but there always seems to be a worm in the apple: in this case, in the form of a second study by Ditman et al. (1972). To the statement, "I felt the beauty and meaning of music as never before," most LSD subjects responded positively; but just as many positive responses were given by subjects who thought they might be getting LSD but actually received chlordiazepoxide.

Summary

A major problem with research on drug effects on creativity is defining terms. Experts disagree about the nature of creativity and how to measure it.

A high proportion of eminent 20th-century writers and many artists were alcoholic. Biographical studies suggest that alcohol facilitated creativity in some, impaired it in some, and had little effect on some.

Many actors and musicians take antianxiety drugs to overcome sympathetic symptoms caused by stage fright; the symptoms might otherwise interfere with their performances.

Stimulants provide energy to sustain long bursts of creative activity, but they also lead to stereotyped thinking.

If consciousness-altering drugs like LSD and marijuana improve creativity, several plausible mechanisms can be cited: The drugs increase imagery, promote play of ideas, offer new perspectives and experiences, and change the balance of activity between the brain hemispheres.

In a controlled experiment, nitrous oxide helped people break sets that impeded problem solutions.

Experiments with psychedelic drugs have all been seriously flawed.

Many substantial literary, musical, artistic, and other works have been created by people under the influence of psychedelics. But it does not necessarily follow that the drugs were responsible.

People have claimed that their esthetic sensibilities were awakened by psychedelics; the issue remains in doubt.

Mini-Quiz: Creativity

A concern about the Remote Associations Test and Ingenuity Test as measures of creativity is that _____.

> **only one answer is accepted as correct**

A concern about the Unusual Uses and Productive Thinking tests as measures of creativity is that _____.

> **they assume that the scorer knows how to measure creativity**

T/F: Scores on the various tests of creativity generally correspond quite well.

> **false**

T/F: Many highly creative writers have abused alcohol, and in most cases alcohol has improved their writing.

> **true to the first part, but the evidence suggests that alcohol impaired the writing of most of them**

The data that Rothenberg and Ludwig used to assess the effects of alcohol on creativity came from _____.

> **biographies**

How can the work of Ludwig be summarized as to the effects of alcohol on creativity?

> **The effects varied tremendously between individuals and on the same individual at different times.**

Why do many actors use propranolol?

> **to prevent sympathetic nervous system symptoms from occurring while they perform**

T/F: Most artists who took lithium to control depression found their creativity impaired.

> **false**

High doses of stimulant drugs produce _____ behaviors.

stereotyped

What drug is associated with the poem "Kubla Khan"?

opium

What are the three rules of brainstorming?

1. **Generate as many ideas as possible.**
2. **Seek remote, bizarre, and wild ideas.**
3. **Do not criticize.**

T/F: Studies have shown that some drugs act differently on the two cerebral hemispheres.

true

T/F: Studies with objective dependent variables on the effects of psychedelic drugs demonstrate that the drugs enhance creativity.

false; the results have been largely negative and all the studies have been methodologically flawed

What methodological flaws have compromised studies with subjective dependent variables?

not double-blind; no control group; strong pro-drug bias

T/F: People who use psychedelic drugs often report a heightened appreciation for music and color.

true

The text cites three questionnaire studies in which esthetic sensibilities were apparently enhanced by LSD. What additional information calls the first conclusion into question?

People who thought they might have gotten LSD but actually received chlordiazepoxide claimed similar enhancements.

By the time you finish reading this chapter, you should be able to answer the following questions:

Which prescription drugs are most likely to cause sexual problems?

Under what circumstances are hormones effective for treating sexual problems?

Which drugs of abuse do users rate as having generally unfavorable effects on sexuality?

Why is it important to distinguish between physiological and psychological effects of drugs on sexuality?

Are there any effective aphrodisiacs?

Which neurotransmitters are most clearly involved in sexual behavior?

Sexual Behavior

Contents

The alchemists' quest to transmute lead to gold was never more diligent than the search of men everywhere for a reliable aphrodisiac. Results have been comparable. Freedman (1976) claimed that almost every well-known drug was at one time used as an aphrodisiac. Some common and exotic substances with reputed aphrodisiac qualities are celery, parsley, asparagus, strychnine, wild oats, irises, mandrake root, honeyed wine, oysters, cloves, nutmeg, and peppermint. *Parade Magazine* (1980) reported that Sweden shipped 250 live reindeer to Japan at a cost of $660 each plus $100,000 for air-freight. Purchasers believe that the ground horns "make impotent men potent and drive frigid women into passionate embraces."

Dog testes, the magic substance in 1889, successfully renewed the sexual vigor of a 72-year-old man and thereby stimulated interest in the embryonic science of endocrinology (Turner, 1966). But the renewed vigor, although genuine, was due to faith rather than pharmacology. Any substance or ritual believed to enhance sexual desire, pleasure, or performance is likely to do so. Not surprisingly, however, neither the dog testes report nor most others on aphrodisiacs have included placebo controls.

▩ Methodology

Sexual desire and performance do not always correspond, as in the case of the old man who tried to violate a young woman and was charged with assault with a dead weapon. Pleasure is a third key aspect of sexuality, and writers have not always made clear which aspects drugs modify. Much of the information comes from animal experiments. The desire and performance of laboratory rats can be easily measured and evaluated, but quantifying their pleasure is another matter.

Spanish philosopher Ortega y Gasset wrote, "Nine-tenths of that which is attributed to sexuality is the work of our magnificent ability to imagine." Drug administration may affect sexuality by modifying ability to imagine rather than through pharmacology. Other possible indirect mechanisms include lessened inhibitions or guilt, reduced depression, improved state of health, perceptual changes, and increased ability to focus. Some examples follow:

- The Indian Hemp Drugs Commission (1893-1894/1969) reported that marijuana was used by religious ascetics in the 19th century to exorcise sexual desire; and, during the same time period, in brothels as a sexual stimulant.
- Wilson and Lawson (1976) had college men drink either alcohol mixed with tonic water or tonic water alone. Half of the men in each group were told they were drinking alcohol and half were told they were drinking tonic water. Then they were shown erotic videotapes. Alcohol had little effect, but those who believed they had drunk alcohol had stronger erections.
- Shortly after discovering that L-dopa is an effective treatment for Parkinson's disease, several clinicians reported that their patients showed improved sexual functioning. Some concluded that the drug is an aphrodisiac. More probably, the effects on sexuality were secondary to general improvements in health and mood (cf. Hyyppa, Falck, & Rinne, 1975).
- Langevin et al. (1985) found that men who drank moderate or high doses of alcohol were aroused by sexually deviant stimuli. The disinhibition may partially explain previous observations that a high proportion of sex offenders abuse alcohol (cf. Amir, 1967; Berlin, 1983).

- Gartrell (1986) reported that 6 of 13 women treated with the antidepressant trazodone experienced increased libido.

Surveys in which drug users are asked about their sexuality are correlational and may mislead on several grounds. First, as is true of all correlational studies, they do not demonstrate causality. Users and abstainers differ in many ways, such as eagerness to try new experiences, even before they ever use (see Chapter 10). The preexisting differences, rather than drug use, may account for Goode's (1972b) finding that number of types of drugs used by college students correlated with their number of sex partners. A second problem is that many survey respondents have been polydrug users. Third, some people try and then stop using drugs because of negative effects on sexuality, so generalizations should not be made from continuing users to the population as a whole. Fourth, because of possible political ramifications of surveys, continuing users are likely to slant their answers to emphasize positive drug effects.

▨ Effects of Prescribed Drugs on Human Sexuality

Depression, anxiety, and other deviations from well-being are frequently accompanied by sexual dysfunctions. Loss of sexual desire is a symptom of depression, and impotence is often caused or exacerbated by performance anxiety. In such cases, drugs that relieve the emotional problem may restore sexual vigor and enjoyment. On the other hand, many prescribed drugs impair sexuality, and patients may stop taking them rather than tell their physicians. Slag et al. (1983) estimated that 25% of cases of impotence in a medical outpatient clinic were caused by drugs. Of the 401 men who acknowledged erectile difficulties in response to specific questions, only 6 had previously volunteered the information. Similarly, Kotin et al. (1976) reported that 60% of their male patients treated with thioridazine developed sexual problems. Few had complained until actively questioned.

Buffum (1986), Segraves (1989), and Bissada and Finkbeiner (1988) listed a variety of prescription drugs that have depressed male libido in at least some patients. Among them are antihypertensives (the drugs most frequently reported as causing sexual side effects), antihistamines, CNS depressants, antipsychotics, antianxiety drugs, antidepressants, and amphetamines. Drugs that have caused erectile impotence include anticholinergics, antihistamines, antihypertensives, anti-Parkinsonian drugs, CNS depressants, antipsychotics, antianxiety drugs, antidepressants, and amphetamines. The evidence comes from spontaneous accounts rather than double-blind experiments, by patients with illnesses that sometimes affect sexuality. Most probably, the patients underreport sexual side effects.

The literature on drug-induced sexual dysfunction is far less extensive for women than men. Drugs that decrease libido in men may do so in women, but women appear less vulnerable (Mann et al., 1982). Drugs that inhibit erection in men can decrease lubrication in women (Mann et al., 1982). Drugs may promote bacterial or yeast infections, resulting in painful intercourse. Segraves (1985, 1988c) and Shen and Sata (1990) reported that female orgasm is frequently delayed or inhibited by antidepressants, benzodiazepines, and antipsychotics. Discontinuing the drug or reducing the dose usually restores orgasmic capacity. Lesko, Stotland, and Segraves (1982) suggested that sexual side effects are probably grossly underreported in women because of their reluctance to discuss such matters with male physicians.

▨ Effects of Hormones on Human Sexuality

MEN

The testes of male mammals, stimulated by pituitary hormones, secrete several steroid hormones collectively called androgens. Testosterone is the most important for sexual behavior. Plasma testosterone increases immediately after sexual activity (Fox et al., 1972) or watching erotic films (Pirke, Kockett, & Dittmar, 1974).

Following castration, both androgen levels and sexual responsiveness decline; testosterone replacement therapy restores activity (Sturup, 1979). But though a threshold level of testosterone is necessary for normal expression of sexual behavior (not always—some castrated men remain sexually active—cf. Bremer, 1959), additional amounts have little effect. For example, Grunt and Young (1952) ranked male guinea pigs for sexual activity, then castrated the animals and injected each with the same doses of testosterone; the sexual rankings did not change. Similarly, testosterone treatment benefits some hypogonadal men but does not enhance libido in men with normal levels (Davidson, Camargo, & Smith, 1979; Segraves, 1988b). In men without overt pathology, no relationship was found between plasma testosterone levels and reported sexual activity (Monti, Brown, & Corriveau, 1977).

Some men who are impotent or complain of diminished libido have excessive blood levels of the pituitary hormone prolactin (Carter et al., 1978; Franks, Jacobs, Martin, & Nabarro, 1978). The drug bromocriptine may help in such cases (cf. Segraves [1988a] for discussion).

WOMEN

Segraves (1988b) reviewed the evidence on sexual responsiveness throughout the menstrual cycle. The reliable cyclic variations in levels of estrogens and progesterone are not paralleled by reliable behavioral changes. But testosterone, which is produced in small amounts by the adrenal glands, is highest during midcycle and tends to coincide with peak sexual activity (Bancroft, Sanders, Davidson, & Warner, 1983). Testosterone may be helpful in treating sexually unresponsive women or women whose libido declines during menopause (Crenshaw, 1986; Speroff, 1988).

As the ovaries run out of eggs during menopause, estrogen production and vaginal lubrication gradually decline (McCoy & Davidson, 1985; McCoy, Cutler, & Davidson, 1985). So does sexual interest, but only partly because of the physiological changes. Expectations play a big role. Koster and Garde (1993) interviewed 474 women three times each, at ages 40, 45, and 51. Most reported no change in sexual desire during the study period, and changes that did occur were unrelated to menopausal status. The women's health, previous sexual activity, and anticipations of declines were all relevant. Beard and Curtis (1989) reported that estrogen therapy helps most women experiencing decreased libido secondary to declining estrogen levels.

In 1982, about 5% of the world's women of reproductive age used oral contraceptives—drugs for birth control, containing varying amounts of estrogens and progestogens ("Oral Contraceptives in the '80s," 1982). About 25% discontinue use within a year (Trussell & Kost, 1987), especially women with a tendency to premenstrual symptoms (Sanders, Warner, Backstrom, & Bancroft, 1983) or history of postnatal depression (Kutner & Brown, 1972). Bancroft and Sartorius (1990) reviewed the effects of oral contraceptives on mood and sexuality. They concluded that some women react adversely, which contributes to the high discontinuation rates, but most experience few adverse effects and may even benefit.

▨ Effects of Recreational Drugs on Human Sexuality

OVERVIEW

Gay and Sheppard (1973) and Gay et al. (1975) questioned people seeking help at a free medical clinic about their drug-sex practices. They asked about drug effects on sexual desire, sexual pleasure, chance of achieving orgasm, and so forth. Many respondents indicated that they used drugs to make sex better. Cocaine ranked highest for that purpose, followed in order by mescaline, marijuana, LSD, amphetamine, alcohol, and amyl nitrite.

Barbiturates, heroin, and methaqualone were the only drugs of abuse rated as having generally unfavorable effects on sexual pleasures. That may relate to Ungerer, Harford, Brown, and Kleber's (1975) finding that polydrug users who scored highest on a test measuring sex guilt preferred heroin and barbiturates; the lowest sex guilt scorers preferred cocaine and amphetamines.

Alcohol

Crowe and George (1989), in reviewing the effects of alcohol on human sexuality, considered physiological and psychological effects separately. Shakespeare anticipated the distinction: he had the gatekeeper in *Macbeth* say that alcohol "provokes the desire, but it takes away the performance." Crowe and George also distinguished between acute and chronic effects, pharmacological and expectational effects, and effects on men and women. Their main conclusions follow:

In men, small amounts of alcohol increase physiological sexual responsiveness but larger amounts impair it. In women, even small amounts reduce vaginal blood flow. Low doses reduce inhibitions in both men and women, which is interpreted as increased feelings of sexual arousal. Thus, alcohol and other CNS depressants may be useful for treating mild sexual disorders marked by anxieties and inhibitions (Brady, 1967). Alcohol-induced disinhibition is partly pharmacological and partly due to expectations—in several studies, people became sexually aroused after drinking a placebo they thought was alcohol.

In men, chronic alcohol consumption impairs testosterone production and metabolism. As a result, their breasts may enlarge and testicles atrophy. Erectile dysfunction and ejaculatory difficulties occur sufficiently often that Masters and Johnson (1970) called alcohol abuse the second leading cause of impotence among men who came to them for treatment. Alcoholic women menstruate abnormally and show reduced sexual arousal, interest, and orgasm. (Crowe & George [1989] noted that the alcoholics in these studies came primarily from treatment and recovery programs, so may not be representative of alcoholics in general; many were using disulfiram, which in high doses impairs gonadal functioning and sexuality.)

Amphetamine

Amphetamine users reported that the drug increases both sexual drive and sexual aggressiveness (Gay & Sheppard, 1973; Gay et al., 1975). Amphetamine promotes confidence while reducing inhibitions, leading some to experiment with bisexuality and group sex. Rylander (1969) asserted that intravenous use of amphetamine or other central stimulants is associated with intense sexual pleasure—"the shot goes straight from the head to the scrotum."

Amyl Nitrite

The vasodilator amyl nitrite, inhaled shortly before orgasm, prolongs and intensifies it. Amyl nitrite has few serious side effects, although contradindicated in people with cardiovascular problems. Some users experience a large fall in blood pressure or complain of headaches (Everett, 1975). Gay and Sheppard (1973) gave some representative comments:

It's an exotic addition to the [sex] act.

I blew my mind at the intensity and sheer abandonment.

I felt like a car with brand new super-chargers and barrels added.

Cocaine

Some South American Indian tribes represent the goddess of love with coca leaves in her hand. The confidence-promoting and disinhibiting effects of cocaine are similar to those of amphetamine. Wesson and Smith (1985) reported that low doses of cocaine enhance sexual desire, but higher doses impair erection and ejaculation in men and orgasm in women. Siegel (1982) reported several cases of impotence and frigidity in chronic cocaine users.

Psychedelics

Timothy Leary (1968) wrote: "Compared with sex under LSD, the way you've been making love—no matter how ecstatic the pleasure you think you get from it—is like making love to a department store window-dummy." Several psychiatrists claimed that LSD is extremely effective for treating frigidity and impotence (Stafford & Golightly, 1967). Unfortunately, no mention was made of nasty little details like placebo controls, double-blinds, or statistical analyses. Gay and Sheppard (1973) gave some representative quotes:

When I come [on LSD] my whole soul and body seem to fuse [with my partner].

I can "fantasize that I've found the perfect lover, and I would dig the cat for days after the trip."

To make love on LSD is to make perfect love and gain protoplasmic unity.

I can't get it together enough on LSD to sexually perform.

Marijuana

Although some respondents dissented, most agreed that marijuana increases both sexual desires and pleasures (Goode, 1970, 1972a; Halikas, Weller, & Morse, 1982; Kolodny, Master, Johnson, & Biggs, 1979; Koff, 1974; Tart, 1971). Gay and Sheppard (1973) included some representative comments:

An orgasm lasts forever.

My sensations are heightened—such as the savor of lips, nipples, skin texture, and the sunlight reflecting off pubic hair.

It's like being tickled all over. I'm really loose.

MDMA

Buffum and Moser (1986) distributed questionnaires on MDMA and sexuality to people in the San Francisco Bay Area. Although many respondents indicated that MDMA increases emotional closeness, enhances the sensual aspects of sex, and would be chosen as a sexual enhancer, only 28% of women and 23% of men reported an increased interest in initiating sexual activity while on MDMA.

Opioids

Heroin addiction lowers sexual drive and potency (Chein & Wilner, 1964; Mathis, 1970; Parr, 1976). Both heroin addicts and methadone users, male and female, are less likely to have intercourse, masturbate, or achieve orgasm (De Leon & Wexler, 1973; Wieland & Yunger, 1970). Nevertheless, heroin addict couples often develop a close, warm, physical relationship (Gay & Sheppard, 1973).

In male rats, the narcotic antagonist naloxone increases sexual activity (Gessa, Paglietti, & Pellegrini-Quarantotti, 1979; McIntosh, Vallano, & Barfield, 1980). In men, powerful rebound effects occur during withdrawal from opioids: Ejaculations may occur during sleep or in response to minimal genital stimulation (Gebhard, 1965). Gay and Sheppard (1973) quoted an addict: "Sex is best when the junk wears off, just before getting sick."

▓ Drugs Used to Treat Impotence

Yohimbine has a reputation as an aphrodisiac. It works in male rats, increasing sexual arousal in sexually experienced males and inducing sexual activity in previously inactive ones (Clark, Smith, & Davidson, 1984). It may work in people, too. Morales, Surridge, Marshall, and Fenemore (1982) and MacFarlane, Reynolds, and Rosencrantz (1983) reported improved erections in some organically impotent men given yohimbine; and Reid et al. (1987) reported positive effects in psychogenic impotence. The mechanism of action is unknown but probably within the central nervous system to improve libido rather than at the penile level (Lue, 1988).

Virag (1982) pioneered a technique involving drug injections directly into the corpora cavernosa of the penis of impotent men. Summarizing results with 533 men who received regular treatments over an 8-year period, Virag, Shoukry, Nollet, and Greco (1991) reported a restoration of sexual activity in 91% with few side effects or other complications. Only 11% dropped out, which is lower than the rate reported by most investigators and was attributed to experience and continued improvement of technique. The smooth muscle relaxant papaverine was the first drug tried. Others include prostaglandin E1, a vasodilator and smooth muscle relaxant (Earle et al., 1990), papaverine plus the alpha-adrenergic blocker phentolamine (Zorgniotti & Lefleur, 1985), and all three drugs in combination (Bennett, Carpenter, & Barada, 1991). Virag et al. (1991) reported that results were best with a drug mixture, ceretine. Ceretine contains papaverine plus five substances that affect blood vessels.

In a double-blind study, men treated with small doses of the antidepressant drug clomipramine reported prompt relief from premature ejaculation. Similar results were reported with the antidepressant sertraline. Both studies were described at a meeting of the American Urological Association (Althof; Swartz; May 17, 1994).

▩ Neurotransmitters

Segraves (1989) reviewed the effects of different classes of drugs on sexual behavior and speculated that several neurotransmitter systems are involved. The key evidence follows (see Segraves [1989] for references).

ACETYLCHOLINE

Studies with both men and women have failed to demonstrate a direct cholinergic effect on human sexual responsiveness. But when sexual dysfunctions occur because of an abnormality in another neurotransmitter system, cholinergic drugs may be helpful.

DOPAMINE

In animals, drugs that amplify dopamine (DA) activity increase male sexual behavior. Prior administration of various DA blockers prevents the behavioral changes; but domperidone, a DA blocker that does not cross the blood-brain barrier, does not. This suggests that the DA effects occur within the central nervous system.

Some cases of impotence, associated with excessive blood levels of the pituitary hormone prolactin, have responded to the drug bromocriptine. Bromocriptine lowers prolactin levels—but is also a DA agonist. Recently another DA agonist, apomorphine, elicited penile erections in 11 of 12 psychogenically impotent men (Segraves, Bari, Segraves, & Spirnak, 1991). L-dopa increases both central DA activity and sexual responsiveness in men. Drugs that deplete or block DA, including reserpine, methyldopa, and many antipsychotics, frequently cause erectile dysfunction or diminished libido.

EPINEPHRINE AND NOREPINEPHRINE

Two distinct types of receptors respond to epinephrine and norepinephrine. Drugs that block alpha receptors (alpha-adrenergic blockers) promote erections in man. The alpha-adrenergic blockers phenoxybenzamine, phentolamine, trazodone, and yohimbine all improve erectile capacity. Two others, idazoxan and imiloxan, induced erections and increased sexual arousal in rats (Smith, Lee, Schnur, & Davidson, 1987a, 1987b). As noted above, drugs used to treat hypertension are the most common pharmacological cause of erectile dysfunction. Most are either alpha-adrenergic agonists or beta-blockers.

SEROTONIN

In male laboratory animals, drugs that lower brain serotonin levels increase sexual activity; and destruction of serotonergic pathways within the medial forebrain bundle facilitates ejaculation. There is little methodologically adequate data on humans. Some evidence suggests that increased serotonin activity (a consequence of most antidepressant drugs) is associated with impaired orgasm in both men and women.

Summary

Claims have been made about many substances that they increase sexual desire, pleasure, or performance. The substances may do so, in almost all cases because users believe in them rather than as a result of their pharmacological properties. Yohimbine may be a genuine aphrodisiac.

Impotence secondary to depression may improve following treatment with an antidepressant. But many psychiatric drugs, probably to a much greater extent than what is reported in the literature, impair sexual functioning. Among the worst offenders are antihypertensives, antihistamines, CNS depressants, antipsychotics, antianxiety drugs, antidepressants, and amphetamines.

Antipsychotics and antidepressants frequently delay or inhibit female orgasm.

A threshold level of testosterone is needed for normal expression of sexual behavior in men, but additional amounts have little effect. In women, testosterone levels are highest during midcycle, when sexual activity tends to peak.

Some impotent men and men with diminished libido have excessive blood levels of prolactin.

Estrogen therapy helps most women experiencing decreased libido secondary to declining estrogen levels.

Among recreational drugs, users rated cocaine highest for enhancing sexual pleasures. The only drugs rated negatively were barbiturates, heroin, and methaqualone.

Alcohol reduces physiological sexual responsiveness, and chronic alcoholism leads to dysfunction, but people anxious about their sexuality may benefit from small amounts of alcohol.

Psychedelics such as LSD were once widely used by psychiatrists to treat a broad spectrum of sexual problems. There are no good placebo-controlled studies demonstrating effectiveness.

Most marijuana users report that it enhances sexual pleasure.

Some drugs, especially smooth muscle relaxants, are beneficial in treating impotence. They are injected directly into the corpora cavernosa of the penis of impotent men.

Drugs that increase brain dopamine activity improve erectile capacity. So do alpha-adrenergic blockers and drugs that reduce serotonergic activity.

Mini-Quiz: Sexual Behavior

Which antidepressant increased libido in several women?

trazodone

The drugs most frequently reported as causing sexual side effects are _____.

antihypertensives

T/F: Evidence suggests that sexual side effects of drugs are overreported.

false—they are probably underreported

T/F: Women are less vulnerable than men to libido-reducing side effects of drugs.

true

Male hormones are collectively called _____.

androgens

The most important androgen for sexual behavior is _____.

testosterone

Some impotent men have excessive blood levels of the hormone _____.

prolactin

Impotent men who have excessive blood levels of prolactin may be helped by the drug _____.

bromocriptine

Peak sexual activity in women tends to occur when levels of the hormone _____ are highest.

testosterone

As a woman's production of _____ declines, so do vaginal lubrication and sexual interest.

estrogen

Among drugs used to make sex better, people ranked _____ highest.

cocaine

A drug rated as having unfavorable effects on sexuality was _____.

barbiturates/heroin/methaqualone

Low doses of _____ may help people who have severe sexual anxiety, but large doses cause dysfunction.

alcohol

Some people inhale the vasodilator _____ shortly before orgasm, to intensify the effects.

amyl nitrite

Psychiatrists used _____ to treat impotence and frigidity, but they rarely evaluated results with properly controlled experiments.

LSD

T/F: Heroin addiction lowers sexual drive.

true

The narcotic antagonist _____ increases sexual activity in rats.

naloxone

Both rat and human data support the view that _____ is an aphrodisiac.

yohimbine

Drug injections into the _____ of the penis have helped impotent men.

corpora cavernosa

A drug that, injected into the corpora cavernosa of the penis, helps impotent men, is _____.

papaverine/prostaglandin/phentolamine

Which neurotransmitters have been most clearly implicated in male sexuality?

dopamine, norepinephrine

By the time you finish reading this chapter, you should be able to answer the following questions:

By what three independent mechanisms might a drug increase violence?

Which drug(s) affect aggression by a direct, pharmacological mechanism?

What are the effects of anabolic steroids on aggression?

What is the significance of cholesterol-lowering diets on aggression?

T/F: Most violent incidents between gangs are drug related.

T/F: People's beliefs about what they have drunk greatly influence the alcohol/violence connection.

Aggression and Violence

Contents

▩ Drug-Related Violence

Although concerns about drug-related violence are of paramount importance to many U.S. citizens, the nature of the relationship is more complex than most realize. Consider alcohol, the drug most clearly associated with violence. Many anxious, irritable, aggression-prone people take alcohol to calm themselves, but not always successfully. For some, alcohol provides an excuse for the aggression. Violent alcoholics may be more likely than violent nonalcoholics to get caught (Roizen & Schneberk, 1977), partly because police may heavily patrol establishments that serve liquor (Myers, 1986). If caught, violent alcoholics may be more likely to get convicted (Greenberg, 1981).

Goldstein (1985) introduced a model that specified three independent mechanisms—psychopharmacological, economic compulsive, and systemic—by which a drug might increase violence.

- Psychopharmacological model: Use of certain drugs (a) promotes excitable, irrational, and violent behavior; or (b) marks the user as an easy victim for violent predators; or (c) promotes violence by causing anxiety and irritability during withdrawal.
- Economic compulsive model: Drug users commit violent crimes for money to support their habits.
- Systemic model: Violence occurs because drug users buy, sell, and distribute illegal substances involving large sums of money. Dealers assault users to collect debts and fight over territories and quality of drugs. Buyers and sellers are robbed. Disputes occur over paraphernalia.

At least four other factors strengthen the drugs-violence connection. First, the drug business attracts violence-prone people (cf. Fagan & Chin, 1990). Second, antisocial personality disorder is a risk factor for drug abuse, and drug abusers with antisocial personality disorder are particularly prone to violence (Abram & Teplin, 1990). Third, drug abusers often live with people whose behavior precipitates violence (cf. Miller, 1990). Fourth, because drug selling is illegal, nonviolent methods for settling disputes are unavailable.

In-depth confidential interviews with drug users and sellers have led most researchers to conclude that psychopharmacological violence (except for that caused by alcohol) is relatively uncommon. Fagan and Chin (1990) emphasized systemic factors, especially for the rapidly expanding and unstable crack cocaine market.

> The potential for high profits from selling crack attracted young initiates into drug dealing in social areas in which legitimate economic activity had decreased. For many young inner-city residents in this decade, the informal economy offered the most lucrative income opportunities (Sassen-Koob, 1989). Involvement in the high-profit informal crack market offered economic opportunities to replace formal opportunities lost as capital flowed out of inner-city neighborhoods in the decades preceding its emergence.

Along the same lines, Haller (1989) argued that the huge profits and heavy penalties from drug trafficking created a multilayered distribution system. This requires many transactions, often involving large sums of money and people who don't know each other well. Under similar conditions, even florists might become violent. Collins (1990) wrote that drug traffickers come disproportionately from among the economically disadvantaged, and selling drugs is an attractive option for them despite the risks. He criticized politicians and the media for their sensationalist approach to the drug problem. For example, he cited a 1989 report to the President on the involvement of gangs:

> California is home to one of the most dangerous and menacing developments in drug trafficking, the large scale organized street gang. . . . The Los Angeles gangs are radiating out from the areas where they originated—up the West Coast as far as Seattle and Vancouver, into the heartland as far as Denver, Kansas City, and Chicago, and even to cities on the East Coast. . . . One of the most frightening aspects of California street gangs is their willingness to direct their violence at each other, at the police, at members of the public—at anyone who stands in the way of their operations.

Collins discounted the statement, claiming that it was not based on evidence. He cited Moore (1990) and Fagan (1989), both of whom studied gangs. Moore concluded that organized gang involvement in drug distribution is not the norm. Fagan wrote that most violent incidents between gangs are not drug related.

Inciardi (1990) interviewed 611 multiple drug-using Miami teenagers who were heavily involved in the criminal justice system. During the previous year, 5.4% had been violent due to psychopharmacological causes and 4.6% had been victims of such violence; 59.1% had robbed at least one person and collectively they had robbed 6,669, mostly for drug money; 9.0% had been victims of and 8.3% had perpetrated systemic violence.

After reviewing police records, Spunt, Goldstein, Belluci, and Miller (1990b) estimated that psychopharmacological, systemic, and economic compulsive drug-related causes accounted for 19%, 10%, and 4%, respectively, of all homicides committed in New York State in 1984. Most of the psychopharmacological homicides (62 of 75) involved alcohol. In two further studies, Spunt and colleagues (Spunt, Goldstein, Belluci, & Miller, 1990a; Spunt, Tarshish et al., 1990) asked drug abusers to report their involvement in violent incidents over an 8-week period. Of the drug-related episodes, psychopharmacological causes again predominated and most involved alcohol.

▩ Drugs That May Increase Aggressive Tendencies

ALCOHOL

The National Commission on the Causes and Prevention of Violence (1970) implicated alcohol in 65% of murders. Lindqvist (1991) analyzed 52 homicides committed in Sweden by alcohol abusers. Not one offender had been sober during commission of the crime, and at least three had acted on alcohol-induced illusions or hallucinations. Forty-three of the victims had been drinking with them.

Several studies using diverse methods indicate a strong relationship between alcohol and domestic violence (cf. Miller, 1990). Women alcoholics are much more likely than other women to experience spousal abuse (Miller, 1990) and to report having physically abused their children (Bland & Orn, 1986).

Alcohol increases aggression in the laboratory. Zeichner and Phil (1979) gave volunteers either alcohol or placebo drinks, then exposed them to aversive stimuli. They thought the stimuli had been administered by another subject. When given the opportunity to retaliate, intoxicated subjects gave nearly three times as much shock as sober ones.

Alcohol's effects may depend more on expectations than pharmacology. In one of a series of studies reviewed by Marlatt and Rohsenow (1981), heavy social drinking men were randomly assigned to one of four conditions: Groups 1 and 2 were told they would be drinking vodka mixed in tonic, Groups 3 and 4 that they would be drinking straight tonic water. But actually, Groups 1 and 3 received vodka and tonic, Groups 2 and 4, tonic alone. Then half the subjects in each group were deliberately provoked by a confederate of the experimenter posing as another subject. Next, the confederate was given a learning task and the subject told to shock him whenever he made a mistake. (The confederate pretended to be hurt but did not actually receive shocks.) Regardless of what they had actually drunk, both provoked and unprovoked men gave longer and more intense shocks when they thought they had drunk alcohol.

AMPHETAMINE

Lemere (1966), Siomopoulos (1981), and others have documented many cases of aggressive and violent behavior following high-dose, intravenous, chronic amphetamine use. On the other hand, several authors (Allen, Safer, & Covi, 1975; Beezley, Gantner, Bailey, & Taylor, 1987; Griffiths et al., 1977; Laties, 1961) found that low doses promote friendliness and cooperation.

In a recent literature review, Miczek and Tidey (1989) concluded that nonhuman animals become timid when given amphetamine. Threatened by another, amphetamine-injected animals either try to escape or assume a defensive posture. But if confronted repeatedly, they become more likely than controls to attack.

ANABOLIC STEROIDS

Males of most mammalian species are more combative than females, at least partly because males have higher testosterone levels. Anabolic steroids are drugs with testosterone-like actions. Their possible value in treating certain medical conditions has been overshadowed in recent years by their abuse potential. People, including more than 6% of male high school seniors (Buckley et al., 1988), take anabolic steroids to build muscle mass and improve athletic performance. The gains are achieved at considerable cost to physical and mental health, including increased aggression. In an uncontrolled study, Pope and Katz (1988) interviewed steroid-using athletes. Many had demonstrated manic symptoms and committed violent acts while on steroids. Several cases currently being litigated involve defendants who committed crimes while taking anabolic steroids. Elofson and Elofson (1990) wrote about their son who, preceding his senior year in high school, began taking steroids. He gained 30 pounds in a short period of time but became uncharacteristically aggressive. The following year, he committed suicide.

COCAINE

Several authors linked the swelling of the national homicide rate in the late 1980s to increased cocaine abuse (cf. Harruff et al., 1988). Roehrich and Gold (1988) reported that 27% of adolescent callers to the national cocaine hot line had become violent while using. Interpretation is complicated by the fact that a sizeable majority also frequently used alcohol, which is rapidly metabolized and undetectable after several hours. Brody (1990) analyzed records of 252 patients who visited a medical emergency unit in Atlanta, GA, over a 2-year period with acute cocaine intoxication; 37 (6.8%) were violent, aggressive, or agitated during their visit, and in most cases their behaviors had impelled others to bring them to the hospital. (Most of the patients had also used alcohol or other drugs.)

LSD

An exchange in the *Journal of the American Medical Association* illustrates the need for caution before attributing violent behavior to LSD or any other drug. An LSD-intoxicated man killed his girlfriend, and Klepfisz and Racy (1973) blamed the drug. But Klamt (1973) pointed out that the man had previously taken LSD more than 100 times without becoming assaultive, that he was not questioned about the use of other drugs, and that examiners, because they had focused on LSD, may have overlooked a serious underlying thought disorder.

MARIJUANA

Long-time Federal Narcotic Bureau Commissioner Harry Anslinger played a key role in shaping U.S. attitudes toward marijuana. His article, "Marijuana: Assassin of Youth" (Anslinger & Cooper, 1937), gave several vivid accounts such as the following:

> An entire family was murdered by a youthful (marijuana) addict in Florida. When officers arrived at the home they found the youth staggering about in a human slaughterhouse. With an ax he had killed his father, mother, two brothers, and a sister. He seemed to be in a daze. . . . He had no recollection of having committed the multiple crime. The officers knew him ordinarily as a sane, rather quiet young man; now he was pitifully crazed. They sought the reason. The boy said he had been in the habit of smoking something which youthful friends called "muggles," a childish name for marijuana.

With an estimated 10 million current U.S. marijuana users and 68 million who ever used, it would appear that the chance of any of us lasting out the week are pretty slim. But all may not be lost: Chopra and Chopra (1939) and Charen and Perelman (1946) argued that marijuana deters crimes of violence, perhaps because users become preoccupied with their own thoughts (Babor, Mendelson, Uhly, & Kuehnle, 1978). In the laboratory, marijuana reduces aggression (Tinkleberg, 1974).

PHENCYCLIDINE (PCP)

PCP is inexpensive, so PCP-related violence is probably due more to psychopharmacological than economic factors. Violence does occur, partly because violence-prone people are attracted to PCP (Fram & Stone, 1986), partly because it engenders feelings of power and invulnerability (Gorelick, Wilkins, & Wong, 1986). Siegel (1978b) described the PCP state:

> The PCP-intoxicated user's orientation toward the immediate present and disregard for long range consequences of his/her behavior would make it difficult for him/her to premeditate criminal acts. But the tendency to react strongly to sensory stimuli in the immediate environment, the inclination to refer everything to oneself that often develops into paranoia, and the need to do something due to intense psychomotor stimulation can all produce an aggression-prone individual.

McCarron et al. (1981) wrote that 35% of acutely intoxicated PCP abusers examined on prison wards became violent; Simonds and Kashani (1980) wrote that they commit more violent crimes than abusers of any other drug; and Lerner and Burns (1986) identified more than 400 court cases in which PCP abusers had committed violent crimes. A common defense strategy, evolving from reports that PCP renders people unaware of the consequences of their conduct and unable to control it, was to blame the crime on the drug. Wish (1986), however, has contrary data. From urinalyses of 4,847 male arrestees in New York City, he found that 56% tested positive for at least one drug: 12% for PCP, 42% for cocaine, 21% for opiates, and 23% (including 49% of the PCP users) for two or more drugs. Relatively few (11%) of the PCP arrestees had been violent, with robbery their most frequent offense. Wish speculated that the behavior of emotionally stable users is not substantially altered by low doses.

▨ Drugs Used to Treat Aggressive Disorders

Eichelman (1986) distinguished between acute and chronic treatment of aggression. He suggested that acute episodes, which generally occur in a medical setting, be treated with sodium amobarbital, benzodiazepines such as diazepam and lorazepam, or a high potency antipsychotic drug such as haloperidol. Garza-Trevino et al. (1989) reported

Table 18.1 Preferred Drugs for Treating Aggression Due to Various Underlying Disorders

Underlying Disorder	Drug or Drug Class
Delirium tremens	benzodiazepines
Anxiety associated with agitation	benzodiazepines
Acute schizophrenia with paranoid delusions	antipsychotic drugs
Manic states	antipsychotic drugs
Attention-deficit disorder	methylphenidate or amphetamine
Organic brain injury	propranolol
Hyperthyroidism	direct medical attention to primary illness

that lorazepam combined with haloperidol produced more rapid and effective sedation than either drug alone.

Eichelman made the important point that chronic treatment should be directed at the underlying disorder if known or suspected. Table 18.1 lists preferred drugs for aggression associated with various conditions.

Clinicians use a variety of antipsychotic drugs to suppress aggression in schizophrenic, manic, demented, retarded, and personality-disordered individuals. None is clearly superior, so Eichelman suggested they be chosen on the basis of ease of administration and side effects. Because chronic use of antipsychotics increases the risk of tardive dyskinesia, he cautioned clinicians to try alternatives with non-psychotic patients.

Veterinarians frequently use benzodiazepines to calm aggressive animals, and aggressive people respond also. Eichelman wrote that benzodiazepines are effective with violent patients of many diagnostic classes, but a small percentage of people respond with even greater rage.

Lithium tames aggressive animals and people and may do so even at nonclinical levels. Dawson, Moore, and McGanity (1972) and Schrauzer and Shrestha (1990) reported a significant inverse correlation between lithium concentrations in regional drinking water supplies and homicide rates in 27 Texas counties. In a separate study (Cromwell, Abadie, Stephens, & Kyle, 1989), hair lithium levels were lower in violent compared with nonviolent criminals.

Brain electrical dysfunction and seizures sometimes cause aggression; in such cases, anticonvulsants such as phenytoin, primidone, and carbamazepine may suppress it. Eichelman (1986) reviewed several positive reports but noted the existence of negative ones. Several studies show that propranolol reduces episodic violent behavior, particularly in patients with organic brain syndromes.

Fava, Anderson, and Rosenbaum (1990) worked with four people who suffered from anger attacks—brief outbursts of anger associated with rapid heart beat, sweating, flushing, and a feeling of being out of control. Speculating that anger attacks are variants of panic disorder, Fava et al. treated the patients (non-blind and uncontrolled) with tricyclic antidepressants and reported dramatic improvements.

As indicated above, testosterone increases aggression. In many species, removal of the testes abolishes fighting and testosterone injections restore it (Davis, 1964). The drugs medroxyprogesterone and cyproterone block the actions of testosterone, producing functional castration. When administered to violent people, especially sexual offenders, they reduce aggression (Kelly & Cavanaugh, 1982; Money, 1970). Whether done surgically or pharmacologically, castration raises serious ethical questions. Also, it is not fail-safe: Bremer (1959) reported 9 deaths caused by aggressive interactions among 16 men who had been castrated to reduce their aggressiveness.

⊠ Neurotransmitters

Eichelman (1986, 1987) noted that there are many types of aggression, and neurotransmitter changes may decrease the frequency of one type while increasing that of another. For example, tricyclic antidepressants suppress predatory aggression in rats but enhance shock-induced fighting. As the human and nonhuman animal literatures are consistent (cf. Eichelman, 1990), the following discussion focuses on humans.

Evidence for cholinergic involvement in human aggression is sparse. In animals, increased brain levels of ACh facilitate aggression. The antiaggressive effects of antipsychotic drugs are probably due to antagonism of dopamine; and those of benzodiazepines are due to enhancement of GABA activity.

Beta-adrenergic antagonists such as propranolol, and lithium, which decreases the availability of NE, inhibit some aggressive behaviors. Aggressive people have higher levels than others of both a major NE metabolite (3-methoxy-4-hydroxyphenylglycol) and phenylethylamine, an endogenous amphetamine-like compound.

Neurophysiological preparations that reduce levels of brain serotonin (lesions of the raphe nucleus, administration of serotonin neurotoxins, tryptophan-deficient diets) enhance aggression in animals. Raising serotonin levels reduces aggression. In people, both levels of serotonin in brain and blood and serotonin metabolites are inversely correlated with aggressive behaviors. Reduced activity of postsynaptic serotonin receptors correlates with impulsive aggressiveness (Coccaro, 1989). Roy, Virkkunen, and Linnoila (1987) suggested that the aggressiveness of some alcoholics is caused by a defect in their brain serotonin system. Administration of serotonin precursors reduces some forms of human aggression. From measures of serotonin turnover, Virkkunen et al. (1989) were able to predict with 84% accuracy which of a group of released prisoners were most likely to commit violent crimes. The lower the turnover, the higher the likelihood of committing a violent crime—possibly because serotonin inhibits impulsive behavior (Charney, Woods, Krystal, & Heninger, 1990).

Cholesterol is needed for serotonin synthesis. Muldoon, Manuck, and Matthews (1990) reviewed all well-controlled studies in which men were treated to lower cholesterol levels. Not surprisingly, mortality from coronary heart disease was less in the cholesterol lowering than control groups. But total mortality was virtually identical, because the cholesterol-lowering groups suffered more deaths from suicides, homicides, accidents, and trauma. In a more recent review that included both men and women, Newman, Browner, and Hulley (1992) reported similar findings.

Kaplan, Manuck, and Shively (1991) found that monkeys fed a low-fat diet are more aggressive than those receiving cholesterol-rich diets; and Muldoon, Kaplan, Manuck, and Mann (1992) reported that brain serotonergic activity is significantly lower in monkeys fed low-fat diets.

Virkkunen (1987) suggested a relationship between levels of cholesterol, blood sugar, and serotonin, alcohol intoxication, and violence. Habitually violent compared with nonviolent criminal offenders have low cholesterol levels and, in response to a glucose tolerance test, relatively strong, long-lasting reactive hypoglycemia and enhanced insulin secretion. Alcohol increases insulin secretion and serotonin inhibits it.

Summary

According to an influential model, drugs may increase violence by any of three independent mechanisms:

1. psychopharmacological—drug use (a) promotes excitable, irrational, and violent behavior; or (b) marks the user as an easy victim for violent predators; or (c) promotes violence by causing anxiety and irritability during withdrawal.
2. economic compulsive—drug users commit violent crimes to support their habits.
3. systemic—violence occurs because drug users buy, sell, and distribute illegal substances involving large sums of money.

The psychopharmacological is the least common reason for violence, the systemic the most. Psychopharmacological factors are most strongly documented for alcohol. Anabolic steroids, cocaine, and phencyclidine increase tendency toward violence in some users.

Many drugs are used to treat violence-prone people, and different ones are effective with different subpopulations. So chronic treatment should be directed at the underlying disorder.

Reduced levels of brain DA and NE are associated with reduced aggression. So too are increased levels of GABA and serotonin.

Mini-Quiz: Aggression and Violence

List and define the three independent mechanisms by which a drug might increase violence (as suggested by Goldstein).

psychopharmacological—drugs may promote violent behavior; mark users as easy victims; or promote violence during withdrawal

economic compulsive—users may commit violent crimes to support their habits

systemic—drug transactions involve illegal activities and large sums of money; these promote violence

Most researchers agree that psychopharmacological violence is relatively _____ except for _____.

rare; that caused by alcohol

The drug involved in most homicides is _____.

alcohol

Which of Goldstein's three mechanisms best explains violence due to anabolic steroids?

psychopharmacological

Which family of drugs is used by veterinarians to calm aggressive animals?

benzodiazepines

A study was mentioned in which an inverse correlation was found between concentration of _____ in drinking water and homicide rate.

lithium

Cyproterone blocks the actions of _____, so causes functional castration.

testosterone

If levels of brain serotonin are reduced, level of aggression _____.

increases

By the time you finish reading this chapter, you should be able to answer the following questions:

What important limitation restricts conclusions from laboratory studies on effects of drugs on human sleep?

What is the equipment called that measures sleep patterns in the laboratory?

What special benefit does the multiple sleep latency test confer for interpreting effects of drugs on human sleep?

What should be the first step in treating insomnia?

What is the most widely used class of drugs for treating insomnia?

Are there effective naturally occurring sleep-inducers?

How effective are over-the-counter sleeping preparations?

What is narcolepsy?

Does tolerance develop to the alerting effects of caffeine?

Why should people who snore heavily not use hypnotic drugs?

Which neurotransmitters are most clearly implicated in sleep and dreaming? What are hypnotoxins?

T/F: Physicians tend to underprescribe drugs for their patients with insomnia.

T/F: The sleep produced by hypnotic drugs is indistinguishable from normal.

Sleep

Contents

Research on drug-induced modifications of sleep has been motivated by four largely independent aims: (a) to develop drugs that facilitate sound, restful sleep; (b) to develop drugs that fend off sleep; (c) to describe effects on sleep patterns of widely used prescription and recreational drugs; and (d) to clarify the physiological underpinnings of the sleep-dream cycle.

✖ Normal Sleep

Laboratory researchers use a device called a polysomnograph to record sleep patterns. They place electrodes on various parts of the body to carry small bioelectric signals into a bank of amplifiers—the polysomnograph.

The amplified signals, recorded on chart paper or a special tape recorder, change during the various stages of sleep. Polysomnograph recordings show that brain waves vary in frequency from about 3 to 40 cycles per second (cps) according to state of arousal.

When a person rests quietly with eyes closed, the dominant wave form is called alpha. Alpha waves have high amplitudes and low frequencies (about 10 cps). As the level of arousal increases, the waves shift to lower amplitudes and faster frequencies. They shift in the reverse direction as an individual drifts off to sleep. The deepest sleep stage, characterized by high amplitude and low frequency (1-2 cps) delta waves, is called slow wave sleep. It is also called stage 3 and 4 sleep. Brain waves during dreaming resemble those during arousal.

Waking, sleeping, and dreaming are cyclic processes. Normal human adults dream about every 90 minutes, four or five times during the night, for a total dream time of about 90 minutes. Dreaming is a period of intense activity. Respiratory and heart rate increase and males have penile erections. There are rapid, jerky eye movements—REMs—from which the name REM sleep comes. Browman, Gordon, Tepas, and Walsh (1977) surveyed working adults and reported that they slept an average of 7.1 hours per night. The range was 4.0 to 10.0 hours, with nearly 70% saying they slept between 7 and 8 hours. Kripke, Simons, Garfinkel, and Hammond (1979) reported greater mortality among people who averaged less than 4 or more than 9, compared with 7 or 8, hours per night. Both duration and pattern of sleeping and dreaming change with age. Newborn babies spend about 16 hours of each day sleeping, and about one-half of that time is spent dreaming. Ninety-year-olds sleep about 5 hours per day and dream for only about an hour (Roffwarg, Muzio, & Demont, 1966).

▨ Methodology

Leading sleep researcher William W. Dement (1972), in entitling a book *Some Must Watch While Some Must Sleep,* called attention to the fact that laboratory subjects in sleep studies must be monitored throughout entire nights. Because observing is both expensive and tedious, most studies have been conducted with only a few subjects and rarely for periods longer than 5 weeks. The typical subjects are chronic insomniacs in sleep disorder clinics or recruited through advertisements. The data they provide may have little relevance for treating transient insomnias, which are the most common.

However recruited, subjects do not adjust rapidly to a sleep regimen in which wires are attached to their heads and strange people watch over them and take recordings. Because the first night's sleep is abnormal, researchers typically allow one or two adaptation nights during which data are not evaluated. But patterns of REM sleep sometimes don't stabilize for months and may be influenced by several nonpharmacological factors (Hartmann & Cravens, 1973). Moreover, tolerance develops to the sleep-altering effects of many drugs, so results from short-term studies may not apply to chronic insomnias that last for months or even years.

Polysomnograph stages have been defined for normal, nondrugged sleep, but some drugs produce new patterns. Also, discrepancies arise between polysomnograph records and subjective estimates of sleep. In one study, drugs reduced amounts of deep sleep according to brain wave activity, but subjects reported that they had spent more time in deep sleep (Itil, 1976).

Measurement should not end when the alarm clock rings. Some drugs are metabolized or excreted slowly, affecting next-day performance. Others are eliminated rapidly and induce withdrawal effects. Carskadon and Dement (1982) argued that proper evaluation of sleeping pills requires assessment of functioning throughout the entire 24-hour day. One method is the multiple sleep latency test (MSLT). Five or six times at 2-hour intervals throughout the day, subjects are asked to try to fall asleep while lying in bed in a quiet, darkened room. Latencies to sleep onset reflect daytime sleepiness; they change with amount of sleep the previous night.

Sleep is powerfully influenced by suggestion. Hartmann and Cravens (1973) reported that placebos influence sleep parameters; and that placebo discontinuation is followed by an increase in REM sleep. Mark Twain told a story that further underscores the power of placebos. Twain was convinced that he could sleep only in well-ventilated rooms. Finding himself in a small hotel room with a window that was stuck shut, he tried in vain to fall asleep. Finally, unable to bear it any longer, he reached under his bed, picked up a shoe, and heaved it at the window. The ensuing crash relieved him and he quickly fell asleep. He awoke refreshed, only to find that he had missed the window and shattered a mirror instead.

▨ Drugs for Initiating and Maintaining Sleep

OVERVIEW

About a third of the population has sleep problems. As a result, hypnotics (sleeping pills) are among the most frequently prescribed of all drugs (Smith, 1979). Mellinger, Balter, and Uhlenhuth (1985) estimated that 4.3% of U.S. adults use a prescribed drug to improve their sleep, and another 3.1% use over-the-counter sleeping pills. Such reliance on sleeping pills is probably unwise. Scientists are uncertain about the function of sleep but know that it is essential to health. Sleep that differs from normal may not be as valuable as natural sleep. As discussed below, hypnotic-induced sleep is abnormal. In a correlational study (Kripke et al., 1979), almost 1 million adults were asked if they used sleeping pills. Mortality rates 5 to 10 years later were 1.5 times greater for people who had answered "yes."

Dement (1983) stressed that hypnotics provide only symptomatic relief of insomnia. They have no specific therapeutic effects and are contraindicated in several conditions. They should not be given to people with sleep apnea (repeated stoppage of breathing for periods of more than 10 seconds during sleep), who use alcohol excessively, who are subject to being aroused and required to perform in the middle of the night, or to pregnant women. Rational treatment of insomnia varies with the cause and specific symptoms, so proper diagnosis should be the first step.

The two major causes of transient insomnia are (a) a disturbing influence such as grief, anxiety, noise, or stimulation; and (b) a change in schedule in which a person shifts sleep hours or travels rapidly to another time zone. The causes of chronic insomnia are more diverse: The Diagnostic Classification Steering Committee (1990) listed 88 types of sleep disorders, 33 related to insomnia. Of 1,214 patients at 11 sleep disorder centers whose primary problem was initiating or maintaining sleep, psychiatric disorders were diagnosed in 35% (Coleman et al., 1982). Psychophysiological insomnias (of unknown origin but possibly due to transient insomnias that become persistent when patients start trying to fall asleep) occurred in 15%. Drug dependence was the primary cause of insomnia in 12%, nocturnal myoclonus (periodic repetitive leg movements) in 12%, and sleep apnea in 6%. The polysomnograph failed to reveal any sleep pathology in 9% of patients with complaints of insomnia.

Everitt, Avorn, and Baker (1990) presented 501 primary care physicians and 298 office-based nurse practitioners with a hypothetical case of a man (either 37 or 77 years old) complaining of sleeping difficulties. Respondents were encouraged to ask for additional information and list therapeutic recommendations. The interviewers were instructed to say, if asked, that the patient typically goes to bed at 9:00 p.m., then wakes at 4:00 a.m. and is unable to get back to sleep. If asked about medical problems, they were to respond that he has severe arthritis. They were to say that he takes Tylenol for the arthritis, that he has two cups of coffee with dinner, that his spouse was recently diagnosed as having lung cancer, and that his exercise consists of getting in and out of a car several times a day.

The patient had many reasons for sleep problems, such as under-treated chronic pain, evening caffeine consumption, psychological stress, and lack of exercise. Yet most respondents never found out, because they asked zero to two questions (nurse practitioners asked more than physicians). Fewer than half the physicians asked about the patient's sleep pattern, one-third about other drugs, and fewer than one-quarter about diet (so they did not learn about the coffee with dinner). Almost two-thirds of physicians and 17% of nurse practitioners recommended a hypnotic; 46% of physicians said a hypnotic would be the most effective therapy for the older patient. Yet the problem may not even have been real, as the patient was getting 7 hours of sleep per night.

Only 29% of physicians suggested changes in level of exercise or pattern of sleep, and only 17% recommended reduction of evening caffeine consumption. For those presented with the older patient, only 15% recommended changes in caffeine, exercise, or sleep pattern as the single most effective therapy.

NONPHARMACOLOGIC INTERVENTIONS

Nonpharmacologic interventions for insomnia include the following:

- Exercise regularly, but not right before bedtime.
- Do something quiet and relaxing during the last hour before bedtime.
- Avoid caffeine-containing beverages for several hours before bedtime.
- Don't eat heavily at night.

- Go to sleep at the same time each day.
- Don't use the bedroom for eating, watching television, serious reading, or other stimulating activities besides sex.
- Don't nap any time other than about 8 hours after awakening and for no more than 10 to 15 minutes; naps 10 to 12 hours after awakening are especially likely to interfere with the next major sleep period (Zarcone, 1989).

HYPNOTIC DRUGS

Benzodiazepines

Barbiturates, once the most widely used hypnotics, have been supplanted by benzodiazepines. Benzodiazepines have a much wider margin of safety and produce comparatively few adverse effects. However, benzodiazepine-induced sleep is abnormal. Total sleep-time and percentage of bed-time spent sleeping increase, but deepest sleep and dream-time decrease (Itil, 1976; Tsoi, 1991). Nicholson (1989) claimed that benzodiazepines are best for treating insomnia of recent origin and should not be used nightly for more than 2 weeks. He related the pharmacokinetics of different benzodiazepines to their clinical actions:

- Sleep onset difficulties should be treated with a rapidly absorbed drug.[1]
- Sleep onset difficulties respond also well to rapidly eliminated hypnotics.[2] But, to ensure that sleep is sustained, physicians often prescribe higher doses than needed for sleep initiation. These may cause respiratory depression and residual effects such as amnesia and rebound insomnia when the drug is discontinued.
- If the main problem is frequent nightly awakenings, the drug should have a reasonable duration of action. Flurazepam and nitrazepam, though commonly prescribed, are eliminated slowly; so repeated ingestion leads to residual effects and accumulation. Rapidly eliminated drugs are preferable.[3]
- When severe anxiety accompanies insomnia, drugs that are slowly eliminated or have slowly eliminated metabolites are best.[4]

Bliwise et al. (1983; 1984) compared both nighttime and daytime effects of flurazepam, triazolam, and oxazepam. The drugs had similar effects on nighttime sleep of insomniacs; flurazepam, however, increased daytime sleepiness. Other studies corroborate flurazepam-induced deficits in daytime performance (Church & Johnson, 1979; Linnoila, Erwin, & Logue, 1980). Brookhuis, Volkerts, and O'Hanlon (1990) tested driving performance at several times after administration of flurazepam.

Driving was impaired, more so in women than men and in the morning than afternoon. Tolerance did not develop even after a week of continuous use. The principal metabolite of flurazepam has a much longer half-life than do triazolam, oxazepam, or any of their metabolites.

Transient insomnia often follows rapid travel across time zones (jet lag) or sudden changes in sleep schedule. Seidel et al. (1984) induced transient insomnia in normal sleepers by requiring them to postpone sleep for 12 hours. Their sleep and alertness were impaired for at least 3 days and not helped by placebo. Flurazepam improved sleep but not next-day alertness or performance. Triazolam subjects slept and performed normally. An alternative to benzodiazepines for minimizing jet lag is the pineal hormone melatonin. Volunteers on transcontinental flights who received melatonin outperformed placebo subjects on both objective and subjective measures over a period of several days (Petrie, Conaglen, Thompson, & Chamberlain, 1989).

Benzodiazepine-discontinuation sometimes causes rebound insomnia, although rarely after low dose, limited use. Anxiety, sometimes exceeding baseline levels, is another occasional rebound effect; the most frequent culprits are the rapidly absorbed and eliminated benzodiazepines (Kales et al., 1991). Hypnotics have considerable abuse potential and, in one study, nearly a third of abusers had received their first prescription for insomnia (Ladewig, 1983). Benzodiazepines increase heart rate during sleep (Muzet, Johnson, & Spinweber, 1982) and may impair breathing in patients with sleep apnea (Robinson & Zwillich, 1989). Because triazolam causes both serious memory deficits and depression in some users (Scharf, Fletcher, & Graham, 1988), it was banned in Britain in October 1991. Other benzodiazepines may produce the same effects, though to a smaller extent (Greenblatt, Harmatz, Engelhardt, & Shader, 1989).

Morgan (1990) constructed a table, reproduced as Table 19.1, showing comparative elimination half-lives of hypnotic drugs in young and elderly subjects. Half-lives are considerably longer in the elderly, increasing the likelihood that they will experience impaired daytime performance, rebound insomnia, and several other harmful effects.

Trazodone

Depression often distorts sleep patterns (Ford & Kamerow, 1989), and many antidepressants add to the distortion (Kupfer et al., 1978; Ware et al., 1989). But trazodone, the antidepressant with the shortest half-life,

Table 19.1 Comparative Elimination Half-Lives of Hypnotic Drugs in Young and Elderly Subjects (data taken from Brigs et al., 1980; Cook, 1986; Gaillot et al., 1983; Houghton et al., 1985; Parker & Roberts, 1983)

| | Elimination Half-Life (hours) [range][a] | |
Drug	Young Patients	Elderly Patients
Flurazepam[b]	83 (37-144)	140 (71-289)
Nitrazepam	26 (19-31)	38 (26-64)
Loprazolam	11 (7-21)	20 (11-45)
Temazepam	13 (6-25)	16 (8-38)
Lormetazepam	10 (6-15)	13 (5-24)
Zopiclone	4-7	8-9[c]
Chlormethiazole	3 (2-5)	4 (2-6)
Triazolam	3 (2-10)	4 (4-12)
Midazolam	3 (2-5)	4 (3-12)

SOURCE: "Hypnotics in the Elderly: What Cause for Concern," by K. Morgan, 1990, *Drugs, 40*, pp. 688-696.
NOTES: a. All values rounded.
b. Values shown are for the metabolite N-dealkylflurazepam.
c. Higher values include older patients with chronic liver disease.

improves the quality of sleep. Scharf and Sachais (1990) administered trazodone to six depressed patients, and Ware and Pittard (1990) gave it to six healthy volunteers. Both groups reported an increase in deep sleep with no reduction in REM (dream) sleep.

Zopiclone

Zopiclone is one of a new class of hypnotics, the cyclopyrrolones. Allain et al. (1991) questioned 20,513 insomniac outpatients who received zopiclone over a 21-day period. Of the 93.8% who responded, more than 80% of both patients and their physicians judged the efficacy of the treatment as "excellent" or "good." Adverse effects, none serious, were reported by 9.2% of patients.

OVER-THE-COUNTER DRUGS AND OTHER REMEDIES

Prescription hypnotics compete for sales with over-the-counter sleeping preparations. Despite advertising claims, the latter are all quite similar. They contain one or a combination of scopolamine, diphenhydramine or other antihistamine, and a salicylate. They are much less effective than benzodiazepines and elicit many unpleasant side effects (Allen, Greenblatt, & Noel, 1979; Kales, Tan, Swearington, & Kales, 1971).

L-Tryptophan

Several studies demonstrate that the essential amino acid L-tryptophan reduces sleep latency in both normal sleepers and insomniacs (Hartmann & Greenwald, 1984). (Gaillard, Nicholson, & Pascoe [1989] claimed that many negative results with tryptophan were never published.) Tryptophan, which does not cause physical dependence or withdrawal symptoms, was promoted as a natural sleep aid and until recently sold without prescription in health food stores.

But after a 1989 announcement of severe and even fatal reactions in more than 300 users ("Update," 1989), sales were discontinued. The reactions may have been caused by an impurity in the preparation rather than by the L-tryptophan itself (Eidson et al., 1990; Kamb et al., 1992). But because L-tryptophan is a natural substance unprotected by patent laws, pharmaceutical firms have no incentive to do research on it or dispel rumors.

Vitamin B_{12}

Several case reports suggest that vitamin B_{12} may be useful for treating sleep disorders (Ohta et al., 1991; Okawa et al., 1990; Okawa, Mishima, Hishikawa, & Takahashi, 1991). No double-blind studies have been done. Interestingly, vitamin B_{12} is widely promoted as a psychic energizer.

Glucose

Several studies show that sleep is (a) sensitive to the effects of circulating glucose levels and (b) impaired in old age. So Stone, Wenk, Stone, and Gold (1992) examined whether glucose would improve sleep in aged rats. The results were positive. Compared with sleep values after saline injections, aged rats given glucose improved on several measures, especially REM sleep.

SOMNAMBULISM
AND NIGHT TERRORS

Both somnambulism (sleepwalking) and night terrors usually arise out of slow wave (deep) sleep. Somnambulism occurs in 1% to 6% of the population, more in boys than girls and children than adults (Kleitman, 1963). Somnambulists arise from a sleeping position and walk clumsily, occasionally injuring themselves or others. Sometimes they mumble incomprehensibly or scream. They are not easily awakened and exhibit complete amnesia for the episode.

Although night terrors are similar to intense nightmares, they differ in several ways (see Table 19.2). Fisher, Kahn, Edwards, and Davis (1973) wrote:

> In its fully developed and most severe form, the stage 4 night terror is a combination of extreme panic, fight-flight reactions in the form of motility and somnambulism, and sleep utterances in the form of gasps, moans, groans, cursing, and blood-curdling piercing screams. . . . The subject may be hallucinating, delusional, and out of contact with the environment while he acts out the night terror which is accompanied by extreme autonomic discharge with the heart rate attaining levels up to 160 to 170/minute within 15 to 30 seconds, a rate of acceleration greater than in any other human response, including severe exercise or orgasm.

Several drugs may induce somnambulism or night terrors. They include a number of antipsychotics, antidepressants, and hypnotics. Benzodiazepines and imipramine help reduce or eliminate episodes (Nino-Murcia & Dement, 1987).

▨ Drugs for Promoting Alertness

Two sleep disorders are characterized by excessive sleeping. Hypersomniacs sleep adequately at night but awaken in a confused state and require additional daytime sleep. The more than 125,000 narcoleptics in the United States (Richardson, Fredrickson, & Lin, 1990) experience frequent irresistible urges to sleep, often at inappropriate times such as while running or driving. They often react to emotional stimuli with brief episodes of muscle paralysis without loss of consciousness, called cataplexy. Normal sleepers invariably progress from waking to light to

Table 19.2 Differences Between Night Terrors and Nightmares

Night Terrors	Nightmares
1. Also known as *pavor nocturnus*	Anxiety dreams
2. Occurs during state 3 or 4 sleep	Occurs during REM sleep
3. Evident during 1st third of the night	Often present during the last third of the night
4. Could be accompanied by sleepwalking/enuresis	No major motoric activity
5. Severe anxiety and vocalization (screaming)	Although present, less anxiety/vocalization
6. Severe autonomic discharge	Less autonomic discharge
7. Complete amnesia for the episode or only fragmentary recall	Vivid and detailed dream recall
8. Confusion if awakened	Good intellectual function at awakening
9. 75% actual or potential injury	Minimal injury potential
10. Violent behavior in 55% of the patients	No violent behavior

SOURCE: Reprinted from "Psychophysiological and Pharmacological Aspects of Somnambulism and Night Terrors in Children," by G. Nino-Murcia & W. Dement (1987), *Psychopharmacology: The Third Generation of Progress*, edited by H. Meltzer. New York: Raven Press. Copyright © Raven Press. Used with permission.

deep to REM sleep, but narcoleptics often shift directly from waking to REM sleep.

Stimulants such as dextroamphetamine and methylphenidate help most narcoleptics and some hypersomniacs, although no drug brings narcoleptics to normal levels of sleepiness (Mitler & Hajdukovic, 1991). Tolerance develops, so drug holidays are encouraged. But sudden withdrawal may induce depression (Dement, Carskadon, Guilleminault, & Zarcone, 1976). Cataplexy is treated with antidepressants (Aldrich, 1992).

Although stimulants taken before bedtime disturb sleep, they are necessities of life in the morning. Caffeine in low doses reduces sleepiness, improves mental clarity, and counteracts the impaired functioning caused by night shift work hours or sleep deprivation (Kornetsky, Mirsky, Kessler, & Dorff, 1959; Rosenthal et al., 1991; Walsh et al., 1990).

Considerable tolerance develops to the alerting effects of caffeine. But its effectiveness may be maintained because of conditioning. Subjects who received caffeine for 2 days and placebo on the 3rd were more alert on day 3 than those who received 3 straight days of placebo

(Zwyghuizen-Doorenbos, Roehrs, Lipschutz et al., 1990). Caffeine has a short half-life, so the difference was probably not due to accumulation in the body. Zwyghuizen-Doorenbos, Roehrs, Lipschutz et al. speculated that stimuli accompanying the caffeine administration elicited a conditioned alerting response.

Weiss and Laties (1962) asked about the costs of the performance enhancement of caffeine and another stimulant, amphetamine. The answer:

> is mostly negative. Both from the standpoint of physiological and psychological cost, amphetamines and caffeine are rather benign agents. Except for reports of insomnia, the subjective effects of the amphetamines in normal doses are usually favorable.... Caffeine seems somewhat less benign.... Caffeine also produces a significant increase in tremor. At dose levels that clearly enhance performance, the amphetamines seem not only more effective than caffeine, but less costly in terms of side effects.

Unfortunately, users develop tolerance to amphetamine and are tempted to increase dosage, so abuse potential is severe. The morning cup of coffee shall be with us for a while.

Lyons and French (1991) reviewed the literature on modafinil, a centrally active alpha-adrenergic agonist. They noted that most of the information comes from sources that did not face editorial scrutiny. In three double-blind studies, however, modafinil reduced subjective sleepiness and improved concentration and performance. In another, it decreased the number of sleep attacks of narcoleptics. Modafinil appears to have low abuse potential (laboratory animals do not self-administer it). Tolerance does not develop, and it produces no serious side effects nor interferes with normal sleep. Pharmaceutical houses do little research on stimulants, because the market is restricted by legal issues and drug abuse liability. As a result, no reliable long-term information on modafinil is available.

▓ Effects of Commonly Used Drugs on Sleep Patterns

Nicholson, Bradley, and Pascoe (1989) reviewed the effects of several drugs and drug classes on sleep.

ALCOHOL

Small doses of alcohol, in both alcoholics and nondrinkers, reduce latency to sleep and amount of REM sleep. They increase total sleep time. But moderate drinking before bedtime (defined as 6 ounces of vodka, 12 ounces of port, 20 ounces of wine, or 48 ounces of beer) is typically followed by strong sympathetic nervous system activity that interrupts sleep; some people awaken from intense dreaming with sweating and headache (Zarcone, 1989).

Chronic alcoholism causes sleep abnormalities that often last for months after sobriety is achieved.

Alcohol's sedative effect is enhanced in sleepy people (Zwyghuizen-Doorenbos, Roehrs, Timms, & Roth, 1990). One factor that determines sleepiness is circadian rhythm. Even well-rested people typically get sleepy between 11:00 p.m. and 8:00 a.m. (Walsh, Sugarman, Muehlbach, & Schweitzer, 1988); and moderate alcohol doses increase early morning sleepiness. At those times, even low blood alcohol levels may seriously impair driving competence (Walsh et al., 1991).

Victims of sleep apnea snore heavily, and alcohol impairs their breathing. So Zarcone (1989) advised heavy snorers to forgo alcohol or any other sedative hypnotic before bedtime.

OPIOIDS

Morphine derives its name from Morpheus, the god of dreams. Heroin addicts talk of "being on the nod," to describe the acute effects of that drug. But single doses of heroin, morphine, and methadone are stimulating and decrease REM activity (Kay, 1975a, 1975b, 1979).

APPETITE SUPPRESSANTS (DIET PILLS)

Almost all appetite suppressants are stimulants, and for most drugs the two actions are inseparable. They cause insomnia as a frequent side effect.

ANTIDEPRESSANTS

Abnormal sleep patterns—difficulty falling asleep, waking frequently during the night, and experiencing less deep sleep than normal—

are indicators of depression. Antidepressants have inconsistent effects on most sleep parameters (Mendels, 1974; Oswald, 1968), but they all suppress REM sleep. The extent of suppression may predict patients' clinical responses (Kupfer & Spiker, 1981).

ANTIANXIETY DRUGS

All the benzodiazepines used to treat anxiety are hypnotics at slightly higher doses. Seidel, Cohen, Wilson, and Dement (1985) compared the benzodiazepines alprazolam (short half-life) and diazepam (long half-life) on normal volunteers. Both drugs had similar effects on nighttime sleep and caused daytime sleepiness. By day 7, tolerance developed to the daytime effects of alprazolam but not diazepam. Sedation may account for the increased likelihood of automobile accidents among users of antianxiety drugs (Honkanen et al., 1980), so tolerance to the effect is desirable. In a later study (Dement et al., 1991), both alprazolam and diazepam-treated subjects had significantly slowed reaction times even on day 7. Buspirone, however, an antianxiety drug unrelated to benzodiazepines, produced little impairment.

ANTIHYPERTENSIVES

Many antihypertensives (drugs taken to lower blood pressure) disturb sleep. Some increase wakefulness, some reduce the duration of REM sleep (Monti, 1987).

ANTIPSYCHOTICS

Most antipsychotic drugs reduce wakefulness and increase slow wave sleep. Clozapine and chlorpromazine are more sedating, haloperidol, spiroperidol, trifluoperazine, and fluphenazine less so.

MARIJUANA

The first night of marijuana use is accompanied by an increase in deep sleep and reduction in REM sleep. With chronic use, levels return to normal (Zarcone, 1973).

NICOTINE

Nicotine relaxes in low doses and arouses in higher ones. Zarcone (1989) noted that many people smoke a lot while drinking alcohol before bedtime. They fall asleep easily, but the alcohol is metabolized more rapidly than the nicotine and then they awaken.

▩ Neurotransmitter Systems

The next sections rely heavily on chapters by Gaillard et al. (1989) and Gaillard (1989b), but omit many of the important complexities they discussed. References are given below only to material not cited in their work. The Gaillard et al. chapter begins with a statement on the importance of drug studies for understanding sleep mechanisms.

ACETYLCHOLINE (ACh)

Throughout the central core of the brain stem, extending from the medulla to the thalamus, is a complex network of neurons called the reticular formation (RF). The RF controls state of arousal. ACh is heavily concentrated in the RF and plays a major role in regulating sleep and waking. ACh changes cyclically throughout NREM sleep, REM sleep, and wakefulness. Administration of drugs that affect ACh synthesis, release, and metabolism changes sleep patterns.

NOREPINEPHRINE (NE)

Many stimulant drugs facilitate transmission of NE and other catecholamines. The drugs most effective in treating narcolepsy stimulate the central release of both NE and dopamine (Mitler & Hajdukovic, 1991). Monoamine oxidase inhibitors and tricyclic antidepressants increase NE levels and cause a prolonged and profound decrease in REM sleep.

5-HYDROXYTRYPTAMINE (SEROTONIN)

The raphe system is a group of serotonin-rich neurons near the midline of the brain. In cats, lesions of the raphe nuclei produce profound insomnia. So do drugs that inhibit serotonin synthesis, whereas the serotonin precursor tryptophan increases drowsiness. But the matter is complicated. Some drugs increase both levels of brain serotonin and wakefulness.

DOPAMINE

High doses of the dopamine agonist apomorphine are arousing. Methylphenidate and pemoline also increase DA activity and are the most effective drugs for treating narcolepsy (Mitler & Hajdukovic, 1991). Amphetamine releases DA and stimulates, whereas the DA antagonist pimozide reduces wakefulness.

HISTAMINE

In rodents, histamine levels are highest during periods of maximal spontaneous activity. Inhibition of histamine synthesis leads to increased sleep, and agonists increase waking. Antihistamines produce drowsiness as a common side effect.

ADENOSINE

Adenosine agonists induce sleep. Caffeine and related stimulants antagonize adenosine receptors.

GAMMA-AMINOBUTYRIC ACID (GABA)

The most widely used hypnotics, the benzodiazepines, activate GABA receptors and GABA-ergic transmission. GABA antagonists have an alerting effect.

▓ Hypnotoxins

Many scientists believe that naturally occurring substances accumulate in the blood during waking and promote sleep. These have been named hypnotoxins. Pappenheimer, Miller, and Goodrich (1967) removed cerebrospinal fluid from sleep-deprived goats and injected it into the brains of rats. The rats curled up and slept naturally. Other extracts caused hyperactivity (Pappenheimer et al., 1974). Similarly, cerebrospinal fluid extracts from inactive rats reduced, and from active rats increased, the activity of recipient rats (Sachs, Ungar, Waser, & Borbely, 1976). Fluid collected from the reticular formation of sleeping cats induced sleep in waking cats, and fluid from active cats awoke sleepers (Drucker-Colin & Spanis, 1976).

Monnier et al. (1977) isolated one of the sleep-inducing substances. Called delta sleep-inducing peptide, it induces deep sleep when injected into freely moving rabbits. Pappenheimer (1979) identified a different substance, which he called Factor S. In doses of 1/20 millionth of a gram, it induces deep sleep in rabbits.

Borbely and Tobler (1989) reviewed data on various classes of endogenous compounds implicated in sleep regulation. Many promote physiological sleep, possibly as a secondary effect. (All are involved in functions other than sleep, and none have been rigorously shown to vary reliably during normal sleep and waking.)

Summary

The typical subjects recruited for drug studies on sleep may provide data with little relevance for treating transient insomniacs.

The polysomnograph records and amplifies bioelectric signals. Hooked up to sleeping subjects, it is the primary device for measuring sleep patterns. The multiple sleep latency test evaluates sleepiness throughout the day following administration of hypnotic drugs.

Hypnotics should be used only for symptomatic treatment of insomnia. Physicians should always (but frequently do not) establish the cause of sleeping difficulties before prescribing drugs. Many nonpharmacological interventions relieve insomnia.

Benzodiazepines are the most widely used hypnotic drugs. They have a wide margin of safety and produce few adverse effects. But benzodiazepine-induced and normal sleep differ. Also, benzodiazepines are addictive and may cause rebound insomnia and anxiety.

The natural substance L-tryptophan may be a useful hypnotic. Over-the-counter drugs are much less effective than benzodiazepines.

Several drugs increase the likelihood of experiencing night terrors. Benzodiazepines and imipramine are helpful in reducing their incidence.

Various stimulant drugs temporarily relieve the symptoms of narcolepsy and hypersomnia.

Acetylcholine has an important role in the regulation of wakefulness, sleep, and dreams. The exact nature of its role is not clear.

Most stimulant drugs enhance functioning of norepinephrine, dopamine, or both.

Lesions of serotonin-rich neurons or administration of antiserotonergics produces profound insomnia.

Caffeine and related drugs antagonize adenosine receptors.

The benzodiazepines facilitate GABA-ergic transmission.

Naturally occurring substances, hypnotoxins, may accumulate in the blood during waking and promote sleep.

⊞ Notes

Nicholson made the following recommendations:[1] flunitrazepam, midazolam, and soft gelatin capsules of lormetazepam and temazepam;[2] midazolam, triazolam, and zolpidem;[3] brotizolam and zopiclone;[4] clorazepate and desmethyldiazepam.

Mini-Quiz: Sleep

T/F: Subjects in sleep studies are typically given adaptation nights until their sleep patterns stabilize.

false; they are given adaptation nights, but REM patterns sometimes don't stabilize for months

The device for measuring sleep patterns is called a _____.

polysomnograph

What is the multiple sleep latency test?

Five or six times at 2-hour intervals throughout the day, subjects are asked to try to fall asleep while lying in bed in a quiet, darkened room. Latencies to sleep onset are recorded.

T/F: Hypnotic drugs provide only symptomatic relief of insomnia.

true

Hypnotic drugs should not be given to people who suffer from sleep _____.

apnea

Is transient or chronic insomnia more common? Which type has more diverse causes?

transient; chronic

Which family of drugs are the most commonly prescribed hypnotics?

benzodiazepines

If the main problem is sleep onset, the drug chosen should be absorbed _____.

rapidly

The widely used hypnotic _____ helps people fall asleep quickly; but it has a long half-life, so next day performance is impaired.

flurazepam

The hormone _____ minimized problems with jet-lag.

melatonin

Two types of rebound effects following benzodiazepine discontinuation are _____ and _____.

insomnia; anxiety

T/F: Benzodiazepines have considerable abuse potential.

true

T/F: Over-the-counter drugs are about as effective as benzodiazepines.

false

Many studies indicate that the natural amino acid _____ is an effective hypnotic.

L-tryptophan

An inexpensive, readily available substance that improves many deficits due to aging, including sleep problems, is _____.

glucose

T/F: Somnambulism and night terrors are effectively treated with methaqualone.

false—they are occasionally induced by it

Which sleeping disorders are helped by methylphenidate?

narcolepsy; hypersomnia

T/F: Tolerance develops to the alerting effects of caffeine.

true

The most consistent effect of antidepressants on sleep is _____.

suppression of REM sleep

T/F: Chlorpromazine is more sedating than haloperidol.

true

A complex network of neurons found throughout the central core of the brain stem, that plays a major role in sleep and waking, is the _____.

reticular formation

Which NTs are released by drugs used to treat narcolepsy?

NE and DA

In cats, lesions of the _____ nuclei produce profound insomnia.

raphe

Caffeine antagonizes _____ receptors.

adenosine

On which NT do benzodiazepines exert their primary effect?

GABA

Factor S is a _____.

hypnotoxin

Glossary

Absorption: Absorption refers to the uptake of a drug into the bloodstream.

Abstainer: Someone who refrains from using a drug.

Action Potential: The firing of a neuron when the charge within it becomes more positive than the charge outside the neuronal membrane.

Active Placebo: Something that produces discernible effects, but not on the condition being treated. For example, if a drug's primary effect were to relieve headache, the drug would be an active placebo if used to treat skin rash.

Acute Effects: Acute drug effects occur shortly after the drug is administered.

Adipose Tissue: Tissue packed with fat cells.

Affinity: The strength with which an NT binds to a receptor.

Agonist: A substance that acts on a receptor to produce similar effects to those of the NT that normally acts on the receptor.

Alcohol Dehydrogenase: The enzyme that breaks down alcohol before it enters the bloodstream.

Alpha (Beta) Receptor: Two receptor types respond to NE. Drugs that act on alpha receptors lower blood pressure and sedate. Drugs that act on beta receptors stimulate the heart and increase blood pressure.

Analgesic: A drug that relieves pain. Pain-relieving.

Androgens: A group of hormones that stimulate the development and functioning of male characteristics.

Antagonist: A substance that blocks a receptor from responding to the NT that normally acts upon it.

Antianxiety Drug: A drug used to reduce anxiety and tension without causing a loss of mental alertness. In slightly higher doses, most antianxiety drugs induce sleep.

Antidepressant Drug: A drug that relieves the symptoms of depression. See tricyclic antidepressants, selective serotonin reuptake inhibitors, and monoamine oxidase inhibitors.

Antipsychotic Drug: A drug used to sedate and relieve the symptoms of schizophrenia and other psychotic disorders.

Asymptomatic Drinking: Drinking without showing any of the symptoms of alcoholism.

Attention-Deficit Disorder: A disorder marked by inability to concentrate for long periods of time and often accompanied by hyperactivity.

Autonomic Nervous System: The part of the nervous system that controls the activity of glands, internal organs, and smooth muscles.

Autoreceptor: Distributed over the surface of presynaptic neurons, autoreceptors monitor concentrations of NTs from those neurons.

Axon: A long slender tube that extends from the cell body of the neuron and carries signals to other neurons.

Behavioral Tolerance: Tolerance that occurs despite unchanged pharmacokinetics.

Benzodiazepines: A group of structurally similar compounds used as antianxiety drugs and hypnotics.

Benzodiazepines: A group of structurally similar compounds used as antianxiety drugs and hypnotics.

Beta-Blocking Drugs: Norepinephrine, which is the transmitter at postganglionic sympathetic sites, acts on two types of receptors, alpha and beta. One subtype of beta receptor is found in the heart. By preventing stimulation of beta receptors, beta-blockers slow heart activity.

Blood Alcohol Concentration: The percentage of alcohol in blood plasma. A BAC of about 0.05% (5 parts per 1,000) of alcohol in the blood is generally associated with reduced inhibitions and good feelings. At 0.1% sensory and motor functions are severely impaired.

Blood-Brain Barrier: The capillary wall in most brain areas that prevents most drugs from entering the brain. Lipid soluble drugs pass through the blood-brain barrier most easily.

Bronchodilator: A drug that relaxes bronchial smooth muscle, so helps people breathe who have chronic bronchitis or asthma.

Carcinogen: A substance that induces cancer.

Catecholamines: A family of substances comprised of a catechol nucleus to which an amine group is attached. Three important catecholamines are epinephrine, norepinephrine, and dopamine.

Central Nervous System: The brain and spinal cord.

Chemical Name: A name given to a drug that indicates its chemical structure.

Cholinergic: Nerve fibers that release ACh as a neurotransmitter. Drugs that increase activity of cholinergic fibers are called cholinergic drugs.

Chronopharmacology: The study of drug effects as a function of body time and upon the body's time structure.

Cognitive: Referring to perception, learning, thinking, and reasoning.

Congeners: Related drugs.

Correlational Research: Research in which two or more variables are measured to see if there is a relationship between them. It is inappropriate to draw conclusions about cause from correlational research.

Cross Tolerance: Tolerance developed to one drug may be exhibited toward related drugs.

Dendrites: The branchlike extensions of neurons that receive signals from other neurons.

Dependence Liability: The likelihood that a drug will promote physical or psychological dependence.

Distribution: Movement of a drug throughout the body.

Dose-Response Curve: The graphic display of effects as a function of drug dosage.

Double-Blind Study: An experiment in which neither the researcher nor the subjects know which subjects have received drug and which have received placebo.

Down- (Up-) Regulation: A decrease (increase) in the number or sensitivity of receptors when levels of neuronal stimulation are high (low).

Drug Discrimination: Tests to see if animals can reliably discriminate between different drug states. The animals are required to make one response when they have received drug X and a different response when they have received drug Y.

DSM-IV: A manual published by the American Psychiatric Association for classifying mental disorders.

Dysphoria: A state of anxiety and depression.

Endogenous Depression: Depression that arises from causes within the body rather than from external events.

Endorphins: Substances produced within the body that have pain-relieving properties similar to those of the opiates.

Estrogen: A hormone that stimulates the functioning of female characteristics.

Excretion: The removal of drugs from the body, primarily through the kidneys.

Experiment: A research design in which subjects are randomly assigned to groups. They are treated exactly the same except for variables manipulated by the experimenter. Experimentation is the only research design that permits conclusions of the type that one variable causes changes in another.

Extroverts: People who are talkative and sociable, who flourish around other people.

False Positive: A screening test that leads to the incorrect conclusion that a drug is harmful is said to have given a false positive.

Fetal Alcohol Effects: Like fetal alcohol syndrome, but less severe.

Fetal Alcohol Syndrome: A cluster of symptoms occurring in infants of alcoholic mothers; the leading known cause of mental retardation.

Ganglia: Aggregations of neurons.

Gas Chromatography: A technique for analyzing unknown substances based on comparative adsorption rates of the unknown and a known substance.

Half-Life: The time in which the concentration of a drug in tissues is reduced by one-half.

Hallucinogen: See psychedelic.

Hypersensitivity Reaction: An abnormally large response to a drug.

Hypertension: High blood pressure.

Hypnotic: Hypnotic drugs induce sleep.

Hypotension: Low blood pressure.

Hypothermia: Reduction of body temperature below the normal range.

Idiosyncratic Response: An unusual and unexpected response.

In Vitro: Describing biological phenomena that are observed in test tubes.

Incidence: The frequency with which new users appear in a population. Contrast with prevalence.

Interaction: If the effect of one drug is influenced by the presence of another, the two drugs are said to interact. Many types of interactions occur—see antagonist, synergist.

Intravenous Injection: Injection directly into a vein.

Introverts: People whose thoughts and interests are directed inward.

Ion: An electrically charged particle.

Ion Channel: A passageway on the neuronal membrane through which ions pass, generally one type of ion per channel.

Law of Initial Value: In general, the higher the initial level of a body function, the smaller is the response to function-raising drugs, the greater is the response to function-depressing drugs.

LD50: The dose of a drug that is lethal to 50% of subjects.

Ligand: A substance that binds to a receptor.

Limbic System: A group of structures that form a border around the lower forebrain and are involved in emotional behavior and motivation.

Locus Coeruleus: A group of neurons on each side of the base of the brain in which norepinephrine cell bodies cluster heavily.

Mass Spectrometry: A technique for analyzing unknown substances based on the separation of charged particles in an electromagnetic field.

Metabolism: Various chemical reactions that generally, although not always, make a drug less active. Metabolism facilitates excretion of drugs by converting them from lipid-soluble to water-soluble. Most metabolic reactions take place in the liver.

Monoamine Oxidase Inhibitor: A family of antidepressants that block the metabolism of several neurotransmitters.

Morbidity: The state of being diseased.

Muscarinic Receptors: Receptors for ACh found in organs innervated by postganglionic parasympathetic fibers.

Neuromodulator: A substance that modifies the function or effects of an NT.

Neuromuscular Junction: The meeting point of a nerve fiber and the muscle fiber that it supplies.

Neuron: A nerve cell.

Neurotransmitter: A chemical released by a neuron to transmit a signal to other neurons.

Nicotinic Receptors: Receptors for ACh found at the neuromuscular junction.

Obsessive-Compulsive Disorder: A disorder characterized by persistent and uncontrollable thoughts that compel the victim to perform repetitive, compulsive rituals that interfere with normal functioning.

Obstetric Drugs: Drugs given to mothers during labor and delivery.

Official Name: A name given to a drug by a special committee that identifies the active drug ingredient.

Orphan Drug: A drug used to treat a rare disease.

Panic Disorder: A disorder characterized by the sudden onset of severe anxiety.

Perinatal: The period from about 3 months before birth to 1 month after birth.

Peripheral: The peripheral nervous system comprises all parts of the nervous system except for brain and spinal cord. Peripheral effects refer to effects on the peripheral nervous system.

Pharmacogenetics: The field that studies the relationship between the genetics of organisms and their response to drugs.

Pharmacokinetics: The process of absorption, distribution, metabolism, and excretion of drugs.

Pharmacological Tolerance: Tolerance due to pharmacokinetic changes.

Pharmacotherapy: Treating patients with psychiatric drugs.

Phase I Testing: Before a drug is approved for widespread distribution it must undergo three phases of testing. In Phase I testing, a small number of volunteers are exposed for about a month to a limited number of doses. The goals are to evaluate toxicity and pharmacokinetics.

Phase II Testing: A few hundred sick people are given a drug for a few months while matched controls receive placebo. The goals are to ensure that the drug works without producing serious toxicity and to identify side effects.

Phase III Testing: Thousands of people are tested in settings almost identical to those in which the drug will be used if released for general marketing.

Placebo: Any form of therapy without specific activity for the condition being treated.

Plasma Proteins: Substances within the bloodstream that may bind with drugs; while bound, the drugs cannot diffuse out of the bloodstream.

Polypharmacy: Administration of more than one drug to an individual.

Pre- (Post-)ganglionic: Preganglionic nerve fibers end in a ganglion and synapse with postganglionic fibers. The postganglionic fibers continue to the effector organ, muscle, or gland.

Pre- (Post-)synaptic Neuron: The axon of the presynaptic neuron releases neurotransmitter into the synaptic cleft where it acts upon the postsynaptic neuron.

Precursor: A substance that is metabolized to a neurotransmitter.

Prevalence: The number of users in a population. Contrast with incidence.

Prodrug: An inert substance that is converted within the body into an active drug.

Progesterone: A hormone that prepares the inner lining of the womb for pregnancy.

Prophylactic: Something that prevents the development of a condition.

Protocol: A preliminary description of the procedures to be used in conducting a study.

Psychedelic (Hallucinogen, Psychotomimetic): A drug that distorts cognitions and perceptions while promoting introspection and feelings of profundity.

Psychoactive Drug: A drug that acts on the CNS to change mood, perceptions, thoughts, or behaviors.

Psychomotor Retardation: A slowing of muscular and motor activity.

Psychophysiological Measures: Physiological measures such as heart rate, skin resistance, and pupil size that correlate with behavioral events.

Radioimmunoassay: A technique in which radioactive tracers are used to determine levels of particular substances in the blood.

Raphe Nuclei: A cluster of cells in the upper brain stem containing serotonergic neurons.

Receptor: A site on a neuron at which NTs act.

Residual Effects: Drug effects often persist after discontinuation of use. These are called residual effects.

Reticular Activating System: Part of the brain that plays a vital role in the control of sleep and wakefulness.

Reverse Tolerance: In some cases, responsiveness to a drug increases after repeated administrations. This is called reverse tolerance.

Screening Test: A simple test carried out on animals and used to predict how a drug is likely to affect people.

Second Messenger: Substances whose release is triggered by neurotransmitters that change the likelihood that the postsynaptic cell will fire.

Self-Medication: Using a drug without a doctor's prescription, because it helps relieve symptoms of a psychiatric condition.

Serotonin Selective Reuptake Inhibitors (SSRIs): A family of antidepressants that increase activity of serotonin.

Side Effect: An unwanted effect produced by a drug in addition to its desired therapeutic effect.

Site of Action: The place where a drug acts.

Somatic System: The part of the peripheral nervous system that controls skeletal muscle movement.

Subcutaneous Injection: Injection under the skin.

Synaptic Cleft: The small gap between the axon terminal of the presynaptic neuron and the dendrites of the postsynaptic neuron.

Synaptic Vesicles: Tiny sacs on the axon terminal filled with neurotransmitter.

Synergist: Two drugs given in combination may produce greater effects than the sum of the effects of the two given separately. The phenomenon is called synergy, and the drugs are called synergists.

Synergistic: If the effects of two drugs given in combination are greater than the sum of their individual effects, the drugs are called synergists.

Tachyphylaxis: Development of very rapid tolerance.

Tardive Dyskinesia: A disorder characterized by facial tics and involuntary movements of the mouth and shoulders. Chronic use of antipsychotic drugs causes tardive dyskinesia.

Targeting: Designing a prevention, treatment, or promotional strategy for specific types of people, for example, beer commercials aimed specifically at young, upwardly mobile men.

Teratogen: A substance that increases the likelihood that an offspring will be born malformed.

Testosterone: The principal male sex hormone.

Therapeutic Index: The ratio between the dose of a drug needed to produce a therapeutic effect (usually, in 50% of recipients) and the toxic dose (usually, in 50% of recipients).

Therapeutic Window: The range between the therapeutic and toxic doses of a drug.

Tolerance: Responsiveness to a drug often changes after repeated administrations. When a drug produces a smaller effect than it did initially, the phenomenon is called tolerance.

Tricyclic Antidepressants: A family of structurally similar antidepressants that increase activity of norepinephrine and serotonin.

References

Aach, R., Girard, D., Humphrey, H., et al. (1992). Alcohol and other substance abuse and impairment among physicians in residency training. *Annals of Internal Medicine, 116,* 245-254.

Abel, E. (1984). *Fetal alcohol syndrome and fetal alcohol effects.* New York: Plenum.

Abel, E., Moore, C., Waselewsky, D., et al. (1989). Effects of cocaine hydrochloride on reproductive function and sexual behavior of male rats and on the behavior of their offspring. *Journal of Andrology, 10,* 17-27.

Abraham, H. (1983). L-5-hydroxytryptophan for LSD-induced psychosis. *American Journal of Psychiatry, 140,* 456-458.

Abram, K., & Teplin, L. (1990). Drug disorder, mental illness, and violence. In M. De la Rosa, E. Lambert, & B. Gropper (Eds.), *Drugs and violence: Causes, correlates, and consequences.* NIDA Research Monograph 103.

Abrams, R., Cook, C., Davis, K., et al. (1985). Plasma THC in pregnant sheep and fetus after smoking a marijuana cigarette. *Alcohol and Drug Research, 6,* 361-369.

Abuzzahab, F., Merwin, G., Zimmermann, R., & Sherman, M. (1977). A double-blind investigation of piracetam (nootropil) vs placebo in geriatric memory. *Pharmakopsychiatry, 10,* 49-56.

Ackoff, R., & Emshoff, J. (1975). Advertising research at Anheuser-Busch Inc., (1963-1968). *Sloan Management Review, 16,* 1-15.

Acord, L., & Barker, D. (1973). Hallucinogenic drugs and cerebral deficit. *Journal of Nervous and Mental Disorders, 156,* 281-283.

Adams, J. (1986). *The care and feeding of ideas.* Menlo Park, CA: Addison-Wesley.

Adkins-Regan, E. (1988). Sex hormones and sexual orientation in animals. *Psychobiology, 16,* 335-347.

Albert, A. (1987). *Xenobiosis: Foods, drugs, and poisons in the human body.* New York: Chapman & Hall.

Aldrich, C. (1944). The effect of a synthetic marihuana-like compound on musical talent as measured by the Seashore test. *Public Health Report, 59,* 431-433.

Aldrich, M. (1992). Narcolepsy. *Neurology, 42,* 34-43.

Aleksandrowicz, M. (1973). *Neonatal behavior patterns and their relation to obstetrical medication.* Unpublished doctoral dissertation, University of Kansas.

Aleksandrowicz, M. (1974). The effect of pain relieving drugs administered during labor and delivery on the behavior of the newborn: A review. *Merrill-Palmer Quarterly, 20,* 121-138.

Allain, H., Delahaye, C., Le Coz, F., et al. (1991). Postmarketing surveillance of zopiclone in insomnia: Analysis of 20,513 cases. *Sleep, 14,* 408-413.

Allen, D., Curran, H., & Lader, M. (1993). Effects of lofepramine and dothiepin on memory and psychomotor function in healthy volunteers. *Journal of Psychopharmacology, 7,* 33-38.

Allen, M., Greenblatt, D., & Noel, B. (1979). Self-poisoning with over-the-counter hypnotics. *Clinical Toxicology, 15,* 151-158.

Allen, R., Safer, D., & Covi, L. (1975). Effects of psychostimulants on aggression. *Journal of Nervous and Mental Disorders, 160,* 138-145.

Altman, H., & Evenson, R. (1973). Marijuana use and subsequent psychiatric symptoms: A replication. *Comprehensive Psychiatry, 14,* 415-420.

AMA, pharmaceutical association form "solid front" on gift-giving guidelines. (1991). [Editorial]. *Journal of the American Medical Association, 265,* 2304-2305.

Amaro, H., Fried, L., Cabral, H., & Zuckerman, B. (1990). Violence during pregnancy and substance use. *American Journal of Public Health, 80,* 575-579.

American Pharmaceutical Association. (1986). *Smoking and drug interactions* (1986-181-287:50011). Washington, DC: Government Printing Office.

American Psychiatric Association. (1987). *Diagnostic and statistical manual of mental disorders* (3rd ed., rev.). Washington, DC: Author.

American Psychiatric Association. (1990). Clinical pharmacology of benzodiazepines. In *Benzodiazepine dependence, toxicity, and abuse*. Washington, DC: American Psychiatric Association.

Amir, M. (1967). Alcohol and forcible rape. *British Journal of Addiction, 62*, 219-232.

Anderson, K. (1988). Influences of diet and nutrition on clinical pharmacokinetics. *Clinical Pharmacokinetics, 14*, 325-346.

Andrucci, G., Archer, R., Pancoast, D., & Gordon, R. (1989). The relationship of MMPI and sensation seeking scales to adolescent drug use. *Journal of Personality Assessment, 53*, 253-266.

Anslinger, H., & Cooper, C. (1937). Marijuana: Assassin of youth. *American Magazine, 124*, 18-19.

Anthenelli, R., Monteiro, M., Blunt, B., et al. (1991). Amnestic effects of intravenous diazepam in healthy young men. *American Journal of Drug and Alcohol Abuse, 17*, 129-136.

Anthony, C., & Trinkoff, A. (1989). *United States epidemiologic data on drug use and abuse: How are they relevant to testing abuse liability of drugs?* NIDA Research Monograph 92.

Apsler, R. (1991). Evaluating the cost-effectiveness of drug abuse treatment services. In W. Cartwright & J. Kaple (Eds.), *Economic costs, cost-effectiveness, financing, and community-based drug treatment*. NIDA Research Monograph 113.

Armitage, S. (1952). The effect of barbiturates on the behavior of rat offspring as measured on learning and reasoning situations. *Journal of Comparative and Physiological Psychology, 45*, 146-152.

Arnold, M., Petros, T., Beckwith, B., et al. (1987). The effects of caffeine, impulsivity, and sex on memory for word lists. *Physiology and Behavior, 41*, 25-30.

Aron, C., Simon, P., Larousse, C., et al. (1971). Evaluation of a rapid technique for detecting minor tranquilizers. *Neuropharmacology, 10*, 459-469.

Arora, P. (1990). Morphine-induced immune modulation: Does it predispose to HIV infection? In *Drugs of abuse: Chemistry, pharmacology, immunology, and AIDS*. NIDA Research Monograph 96.

Ashcroft, G., Eccleston, D., & Waddell, J. (1965). Recognition of amphetamine addicts. *British Medical Journal, 1*, 57.

Augusta Chronicle. (1994, April 5).

Avorn, J., Chen, M., & Hartley, R. (1982). Scientific versus commercial sources of influence on the prescribing behavior of physicians. *American Journal of Medicine, 73,* 4-8.

Avorn, J., Dreyer, P., Connelly, K., & Soumerai, S. (1989). Use of psychoactive medication and the quality of care in rest homes: Findings and policy implications of a statewide study. *The New England Journal of Medicine, 320,* 227-332.

Ayd, F. (1974). Single daily doses of antidepressants. *Journal of the American Medical Association, 230,* 263-264.

Babor, T., Mendelson, J., Uhly, B., & Kuehnle, J. (1978). Social effects of marijuana use in a recreational setting. *International Journal of Addiction, 13,* 947-959.

Bachman, J., Wallace, J., O'Malley, P., Johnston, L., Kurth, C., & Neighbors, H. (1991). Racial/ethnic differences in smoking, drinking, and illicit drug use among American high school seniors, 1976-1989. *American Journal of Public Health, 81,* 372-377.

Baer, P., Garmezy, L., McLaughlin, R., et al. (1987). Stress, coping, family conflict, and adolescent alcohol use. *Journal of Behavioral Medicine, 10,* 449-466.

Baker, A., & Thorpe, J. (1957). Placebo response. *American Medical Association Archives of Neurology and Psychiatry, 78,* 57-60.

Balabanova, S., Parsche, F., & Pirsig, W. (1992). First identification of drugs in Egyptian mummies. *Naturwissenschaften, 79,* 358.

Baldessarini, R. (1990a). Drugs and the treatment of psychiatric disorders. In A. Gilman, T. Rall, A. Nies, & P. Taylor (Eds.), *The pharmacological basis of therapeutics.* Elmsford, NY: Pergamon.

Baldessarini, R. (1990b). Update on antidepressants. *The Harvard Medical School Mental Health Letter, 6,* 4-6.

Baldessarini, R., & Cohen, B. (1986). Regulation of psychiatric practice. *American Journal of Psychiatry, 143,* 750-751.

Baldessarini, R., Cohen, B., & Teicher, M. (1988). Significance of neuroleptic dose and plasma level in the pharmacological treatment of psychoses. *Archives of General Psychiatry, 45,* 79-91.

Baldessarini, R., & Frankenburg, F. (1991). Clozapine: A novel antipsychotic agent. *New England Journal of Medicine, 324,* 746-754.

Baldessarini, R., Gelenberg, A., & Lipinski, J. (1976). Letter: Grams of antipsychotics. *New England Journal of Medicine, 294,* 113-114.

Balestrieri, M., Ruggeri, M., & Bellantuono, C. (1989). Drug treatment of panic disorder—A critical review of controlled clinical trials. *Psychiatric Development, 4,* 337-350.

Balster, R. (1987). The behavioral pharmacology of phencyclidine. In H. Meltzer (Ed.), *Psychopharmacology: The third generation of progress.* New York: Raven.

Balster, R., Mansbach, R., Gold, L., & Harris, L. (1992). Preclinical methods for the development of pharmacotherapies for cocaine abuse. In L. Harris (Ed.), *Problems of drug dependence 1991.* NIDA Research Monograph 119.

Balster, R., & Woolverton, W. (1981). Tolerance and dependence to phencyclidine. In E. Domino (Ed.), *PCP (phencyclidine): Historical and current perspectives.* Ann Arbor, MI: NPP Books.

Ban, T. (1990). Clinical pharmacology and Leonhard's classification of endogenous psychoses. *Psychopathology, 23,* 331- 338.

Bancroft, J., Sanders, D., Davidson, D., & Warner, P. (1983). Mood, sexuality, hormones, and the menstrual cycle: III. Sexuality and the role of androgens. *Psychosomatic Medicine, 45,* 509-516.

Bancroft, J., & Sartorius, N. (1990). The effects of oral contraceptives on well-being and sexuality. In S. Milligan (Ed.), *Oxford reviews of reproductive biology.* New York: Oxford University Press.

Bandura, A., Jeffery, R., & Wright, C. (1974). Efficacy of participant modeling as a function of response induction aids. *Journal of Abnormal Psychology, 83,* 56-64.

Banys, P. (1988). The clinical use of disulfiram (Antabuse): A review. *Journal Psychoactive Drugs, 20,* 243-260.

Barnes, J., & Denz, F. (1954). Experimental methods used in determining chronic toxicity. *Pharmacological Review, 6,* 191-242.

Barone, J., & Roberts, H. (1984). Human consumption of caffeine. In P. Dews (Ed.), *Caffeine.* New York: Springer.

Barrett, J. (1981). Differential drug effects as a function of the controlling consequences. *NIDA Research Monograph, 37,* 159-181.

Barron, F. (1964). The relationship of ego diffusion to creative perception. In C. Taylor (Ed.), *Widening horizons in creativity.* New York: John Wiley.

Barron, F. (1965). The psychology of creativity. In T. Newcomb (Ed.), *New directions in psychology II.* New York: Holt, Rinehart & Winston.

Bartels, S. (1989). Organic mental disorder: When to suspect medical illness as a cause of psychiatric symptoms. In J. Ellison (Ed.), *The psychotherapist's guide to pharmacotherapy*. Chicago: Year Book Medical Publishers.

Barton, J., & Sibai, B. (1991). Low-dose aspirin to improve perinatal outcome. *Clinical Obstetrics and Gynecology, 34,* 251-261.

Bartus, R., Dean, R., Beer, B., & Lippa, A. (1982). The cholinergic hypothesis of geriatric memory dysfunction. *Science, 217,* 408-417.

Bateman, N., & Peterson, D. (1971). Variables related to outcome of treatment for hospitalized alcoholics. *International Journal of the Addictions, 6,* 215-224.

Bates, W., Smeltzer, D., & Arnoczky, S. (1986). Appropriate and inappropriate use of psychotherapeutic medications for institutionalized mentally retarded persons. *American Journal of Mental Deficiency, 90,* 363-370.

Baumrind, D. (1985). *Familial antecedents of adolescent drug use: A developmental perspective*. In NIDA Research Monograph 56.

Beard, M., & Curtis, L. (1989). Libido, menopause, and estrogen replacement therapy. *Postgraduate Medicine, 86,* 225-228.

Beecher, H. (1955). The powerful placebo. *Journal of the American Medical Association, 159,* 1602-1606.

Beecher, H. (1961). Surgery as a placebo. *Journal of the American Medical Association, 176,* 1102-1107.

Beers, D. (1991, September 15). [Editorial]. *This World Magazine.*

Beers, M., Ouslander, J., Fingold, S., et al. (1992). Inappropriate medication prescribing in skilled-nursing facilities. *Annals of Internal Medicine, 117,* 684-689.

Beezley, D., Gantner, A., Bailey, D., & Taylor, S. (1987). Amphetamines and human physical aggression. *Journal of Research in Personality, 21,* 52-60.

Bell, C., & Battjes, D. (Eds.). (1985). *Prevention research: Deterring drug abuse among children and adolescents*. NIDA Research Monograph Series 63.

Belsher, G., & Costello, C. (1988). Relapse after recovery from unipolar depression: A critical review. *Psychological Bulletin, 104,* 84-96.

Benfield, P., & Ward, A. (1986). Fluvoxamine: A review of its pharmacodynamic and pharmacokinetic properties, and therapeutic efficacy in depressive illness. *Drugs, 32,* 313-334.

Bennett, A., Carpenter, A., & Barada, J. (1991). An improved vasoactive drug combination for a pharmacological erection program. *Journal of Urology, 146,* 1564-1565.

Benowitz, N. (1990). Clinical pharmacology of inhaled drugs of abuse: Implications in understanding nicotine dependence. *NIDA Research Monograph, 99,* 12-29.

Benowitz, N. (1992). How toxic is cocaine? In *Cocaine: Scientific and social dimensions.* Ciba Foundation Symposium 166. New York: John Wiley.

Benowitz, N., Hall, S., & Modin, G. (1989). Persistent increase in caffeine concentrations in people who stop smoking. *British Medical Journal, 298,* 1075-1076.

Benson, H., & Epstein, M. (1975). The placebo effect: A neglected asset in the care of patients. *Journal of the American Medical Association, 232,* 1225-1227.

Benson, H., & McCallie, D. (1979). Angina pectoris and the placebo effect. *The New England Journal of Medicine, 300,* 1424-1429.

Benton, D., & Cook, R. (1991). The impact of selenium supplementation on mood. *Biological Psychiatry, 29,* 1092-1098.

Beresford, T., & Hall, R. (1990). Clinical concerns in psychopharmacology. *Psychiatric Medicine, 8,* 1-11.

Berger, F. (1960). Classification of psychoactive drugs according to their chemical structures and sites of action. In D. Efron (Ed.), *Psychopharmacology: A review of progress* (USPHS Pub. No. 1836). Washington, DC: Government Printing Office.

Berger, P., Gawin, F., & Kosten, T. (1989). Treatment of cocaine abuse with mazindol. *Lancet, 1,* 283.

Berlin, F. (1983). Sex offenders: A biomedical perspective and a status report on biomedical treatment. In J. Greer & I. Stuart (Eds.), *The sexual aggressor: Current perspectives on treatment.* New York: Van Nostrand Reinhold.

Berlin, L., Guthrie, T., Weider, A., et al. (1955). Studies in human cerebral function: The effects of mescaline and lysergic acid on cerebral process pertinent to creative activity. *Journal of Nervous and Mental Disorders, 122,* 487-491.

Best, J., Thomson, S., Santi, S., et al. (1988). Preventing cigarette smoking among school children. *Annual Review of Public Health, 9,* 161-201.

Beveridge, W. (1980). *Seeds of discovery.* London: Heinemann Educational.

Bibb, J., & Chambless, D. (1986). Alcohol use and abuse among diagnosed agoraphobics. *Behaviour Research and Therapy, 24,* 49-58.

Bielski, R., & Friedel, R. (1979). Depressive subtypes defined by response to pharmacotherapy. *Psychiatric Clinics of North America, 2,* 483-497.

Biron, P. (1973). A hopefully biased pilot survey of physicians' knowledge of the content of drug combinations. *Canadian Medical Association Journal, 109,* 35-39.

Bissada, N., & Finkbeiner, A. (1988). Urologic manifestations of drug therapy. *Urologic Clinics of North America, 15,* 725-736.

Bixler, E., Kales, A., Manfredi, R., et al. (1991). Next-day memory impairment with triazolam use. *Lancet, 337,* 827-831.

Blakey, R., & Baker, R. (1980). An exposure approach to alcohol abuse. *Behaviour Research and Therapy, 18,* 319-323.

Bland, R., & Orn, H. (1986). Psychiatric disorders, spouse abuse and child abuse. *Acta Psychiatrica Belgica, 86,* 444-449.

Bliwise, D., Seidel, W., Greenblatt, D., & Dement, W. (1984). Nighttime and daytime efficacy of flurazepam and oxazepam in chronic insomnia. *American Journal of Psychiatry, 141,* 191-195.

Bliwise, D., Seidel, W., Karacan, I., et al. (1983). Daytime sleepiness as a criterion in hypnotic medication trials: Comparison of triazolam and flurazepam. *Sleep, 6,* 156-163.

Block, J., Block, J., & Keyes, S. (1988). Longitudinally foretelling drug usage in adolescence: Early childhood personality and environmental precursors. *Child Development, 59,* 336-355.

Block, M., Vallier, G., & Glickman, S. (1974). Elicitation of water ingestion in the Mongolian gerbil (Meriones unguiculatis) by intracranial injections of angiotensin II and l-norepinephrine. *Pharmacology, Biochemistry, and Behavior, 2,* 235-242.

Block, R., Farinpour, R., & Schlechte, J. (1991). Effects of chronic marijuana use on testosterone, luteinizing hormone, follicle stimulating hormone, prolactin and cortisol in men and women. *Drug and Alcohol Dependence, 28,* 121-128.

Block, R., Farnham, S., Braverman, K., et al. (1990). Long-term marijuana use and subsequent effects on learning and cognitive functions related to school achievement: Preliminary study. In J. Spencer & J. Boren (Eds.), *Residual effects of abused drugs on behavior.* NIDA Research Monograph 101.

Blum, K. (1984). *Handbook of abusable drugs.* New York: Gardner Press.

Blumenfield, M., et al. (1972). Marijuana use in high school students. *Diseases of the Nervous System, 33,* 603-610.

Borbely, A., & Tobler, I. (1989). Endogenous sleep-promoting substances and sleep regulation. *Physiological Reviews, 69,* 605-670.

Boszormenyi, Z. (1960). Creative urge as an after effect of model psychoses. *Confinia Psychiatrica, 3,* 117-126.

Boutin, R. (1979). Psychoactive drugs: Effective use of low doses. *Psychosomatics, 20,* 403-405, 409.

Bowden, C. (1992). Psychopharmacological treatment of panic disorder. *Bulletin of the Menninger Clinic, 56,* A29-41.

Bower, B. (1989). Alcoholism's elusive genes. *Science News, 134,* 74-79.

Boyd, J. (1986). Use of mental health services for the treatment of panic disorder. *American Journal of Psychiatry, 143,* 1569-1574.

Bracken, M., Eskenazi, B., Sachse, K., et al. (1990). Association of cocaine use with sperm concentration, motility, and morphology. *Fertility and Sterility, 53,* 315-322.

Bradstock, M., Marks, J., Forman, M., Gentry, E., Hogelin, G., Binkin, N., & Trowbridge, F. (1987). Drinking-driving and health lifestyle in the United States: Behavioral risk factors surveys. *Journal of Studies on Alcohol, 48,* 147-152.

Brady, J. (1967). Frigidity. *Medical Aspects of Human Sexuality, 1,* 42-48.

Brandon, T., Tiffany, S., & Baker, T. (1986). The process of smoking relapse. In F. Tims & C. Leukefeld (Eds.), *Relapse and recovery in drug abuse.* NIDA Research Monograph 72.

Brecher, E. (1972). *Licit and illicit drugs.* Boston: Little, Brown.

Brecher, M., Wang, B., Wong, H., & Morgan, J. (1988). Phencyclidine and violence: Clinical and legal issues. *Journal of Clinical Psychopharmacology, 8,* 397-401.

Breggin, P. (1983). *Psychiatric drugs: Hazards to the brain.* New York: Springer.

Brehm, M., & Back, K. (1968). Self-image and attitudes toward drugs. *Journal of Personality, 36,* 299-314.

Bremer, J. (1959). *Asexualization: A follow-up study of 244 cases.* New York: Macmillan.

Brent, R., & Beckman, D. (1990). Environmental teratogens. *Bulletin of the New York Academy of Medicine, 66,* 123-163.

Brien, J., Clarke, D., Richardson, B., & Patrick, J. (1985). Disposition of ethanol in maternal blood, fetal blood, and amniotic fluid of third trimester pregnant ewes. *American Journal of Obstetrics and Gynecology, 152,* 583-590.

Broad, W., & Wade, N. (1982). *Betrayers of the truth.* New York: Simon & Schuster.

Broadhurst, P. (1977). Pharmacogenetics. In L. Iverson, S. Iverson, & S. Snyder (Eds.), *Handbook of psychopharmacology, Vol. 7.* New York: Plenum.

Brody, S. (1990). Violence associated with acute cocaine use in patients admitted to a medical emergency department. In M. De la Rosa, E. Lambert, & B. Gropper (Eds.), *Drugs and violence: Causes, correlates, and consequences.* NIDA Research Monograph 103.

Brookhuis, K., Volkerts, E., & O'Hanlon, J. (1990). Repeated dose effects of lormetazepam and flurazepam upon driving performance. *European Journal of Clinical Pharmacology, 39,* 83-87.

Broverman, D., Klaiber, E., Kobayashi, Y., & Vogel, W. (1968). Roles of activation and inhibition in sex differences in cognitive abilities. *Psychological Reviews, 75,* 23-50.

Brower, K., Blow, F., & Beresford, T. (1989). Treatment implications of chemical dependency models: An integrative approach. *Journal of Substance Abuse Treatment, 6,* 147-157.

Browman, C., Gordon, G., Tepas, D., & Walsh, J. (1977). Reported sleep and drug use of workers: A preliminary report. *Sleep Research, 6,* 111.

Brown, G., & Silverman, L. (1974). The retail price of heroin: Estimation and applications. *Journal of the American Statistical Association, 69,* 595-606.

Brown, T., Chapman, P., Kairiss, E., & Keenan, C. (1988). Long-term potentiation. *Science, 242,* 724-728.

Brown, W., & Harrison, W. (1992). Are patients who are intolerant to one SSRI intolerant to another? *Psychopharmacology Bulletin, 28,* 253-256.

Browne, R. (1986). Discriminative stimulus properties of PCP mimetics. *NIDA Research Monograph, 64,* 134-147.

Browne, R., & Fondren, B. (1978). B-endorphin and the narcotic cue. In F. Colpaert & J. Rosecrans (Eds.), *Stimulus properties of drugs: Ten years of progress.* Amsterdam: Elsevier.

Brumback, R., & Weinberg, W. (1990). Pediatric behavioral neurology: An update on the neurologic aspects of depression, hyperactivity, and learning disabilities. *Pediatric Neurology, 8,* 677-703.

Bry, B. (1978). Research design in drug abuse prevention: Review and recommendations. *International Journal of the Addictions, 13,* 1157-1168.

Bry, B. (1983). Empirical foundations of family-based approaches to adolescent substance abuse. In T. Glynn, C. Leukefeld, & J. Ludford (Eds.), *Preventing adolescent drug abuse: Intervention strategies.* NIDA Research Monograph 47.

Bryant, H., Bernton, E., & Holaday, J. (1990). Immunomodulatory effects of chronic morphine treatment: Pharmacologic and mechanistic studies. *Drugs of Abuse: Chemistry, Pharmacology, Immunology, and AIDS.* NIDA Research Monograph 96.

Buckley, W., Yesalis, C., Friedl, K., et al. (1988). Estimated prevalence of anabolic steroid use among male high school seniors. *Journal of the American Medical Association, 260,* 3441-3445.

Buffum, J. (1986). Pharmacosexology update: Prescription drugs and sexual function. *Journal of Psychoactive Drugs, 18,* 97-106.

Buffum, J., & Moser, C. (1986). MDMA and human sexual function. *Journal of Psychoactive Drugs, 18,* 355-359.

Bukoski, W. (1991). *A framework for drug abuse prevention research.* NIDA Research Monograph 107.

Bunn, W., & Giannini, A. (1992). Cardiovascular complications of cocaine abuse. *American Family Physician, 46,* 769-773.

Bureau of Justice Statistics Sourcebook of Criminal Justice Statistics—1991. (1992). Washington, DC: U.S. Department of Justice.

Bureau of Justice Statistics Bulletin. (1992a). Jail inmates 1991. Washington, DC: U.S. Department of Justice, Office of Justice Programs, Bureau of Justice Statistics.

Bureau of Justice Statistics Bulletin. (1992b). Prisoners in 1991. Washington, DC: U.S. Department of Justice, Office of Justice Programs, Bureau of Justice Statistics.

Burger, A. (1982). Approaches to screening compounds for pharmacological activity. In C. Hamner (Ed.), *Drug development.* Boca Raton, FL: CRC Press.

Burke, L., Baum, C., Jolson, H., & Kennedy, D. (1991). Drug utilization in the US: 1989. Eleventh annual review. Washington, DC: Department of Health and Human Services.

Burns, R., & Lerner, S. (1981). The effects of phencyclidine in man: A review. In E. Domino (Ed.), *PCP (phencyclidine): Historical and current perspectives.* Ann Arbor, MI: NPP Books.

Burroughs, W. (1966). Points of distinction between sedative and conscious-ness-expanding drugs. In D. Solomon (Ed.), *The marihuana papers.* New York: Signet.

Bustamente, J., Jordan, A., Vila, M., et al. (1970). State- dependent learning in humans. *Physiology and Behavior, 5,* 793-796.

Butler, N. (1977). Smoking and pregnancy. In *Smoking and health, II* (DHEW Pub. No. NIH 77-1413). Washington, DC: Government Printing Office.

Byrne, R. (1982). *The 637 best things anybody ever said.* New York: Atheneum.

Caan, B., & Goldhaber, M. (1989). Caffeinated beverages and low birthweight: A case-control study. *American Journal of Public Health, 79,* 1299-1300.

Caldecott-Hazard, S., Morgan, D., DeLeon-Jones, F., et al. (1991). Clinical and biochemical aspects of depressive disorders: II. Transmitter/receptor theo-ries. *Synapse, 9,* 251-301.

Camp, J. (1991). Patient-controlled analgesia. *American Family Physician, 44,* 45-50.

Campbell, M., & Spencer, E. (1988). Psychopharmacology in child and adoles-cent psychiatry: A review of the past five years. *Journal of the American Academy of Child and Adolescent Psychiatry, 27,* 269-279.

Caporaso, N., Hayes, R., Dosemeci, M., et al. (1989). Lung cancer risk, occupa-tional exposure, and the debrisoquine metabolic phenotype. *Cancer Research, 49,* 3675-3679.

Carpenter, W., Hanlon, T., Heinrichs, D., Summerfelt, A., Kirkpatrick, B., Levine, J., & Buchanan, R. (1990). Continuous versus targeted medication in schizophrenic outpatients: Outcome results. *American Journal of Psychiatry, 147,* 1138-1148.

Carroll, M., France, C., & Meisch, R. (1979). Food deprivation increases oral and intravenous drug intake in rats. *Science, 205,* 319-321.

Carskadon, M., & Dement, W. (1982). The Multiple Sleep Latency Test: What does it mean? *Sleep, 5,* 67-72.

Carter, D. (1990). An overview of drug-related misconduct of police officers: Drug abuse and narcotic corruption. In R. Weisheit (Ed.), *Drugs, crime and the criminal justice system.* Highland Heights, KY: Anderson Publishing.

Carter, J., Tyson, J., Tolis, G., et al. (1978). Prolactin-secreting tumors and hypo-gonadism in 22 men. *The New England Journal of Medicine, 299,* 847-852.

Cerletti, A., & Rothlin, E. (1955). Role of 5-hydroxytryptamine in mental diseases and its antagonism to lysergic acid derivatives. *Nature, 176,* 785-786.

Cesura, A., & Pletscher, A. (1992). The new generation of monoamine oxidase inhibitors. *Progress in Drug Research, 38,* 171-297.

Chaiken, M., & Johnson, B. (1988). Characteristics of different types of drug-involved offenders. *National Institute of Justice/Issues and Practices* (1990-262-221). Washington, DC: Government Printing Office.

Chairperson, Public Affairs Committee. (1991). Recommendations for isoretinoin use in women of childbearing potential. *Teratology, 44,* 1-6.

Challem, J. (1979). Resistance to orthomolecular medicine—Or why you don't read about megavitamin therapy. *Orthomolecular Psychiatry, 8,* 248-252.

Chambers, C. (1987). Understanding drugs in dangerous combinations. In C. Chambers, J. Inciardi, D. Petersen, et al. (Eds.), *Chemical dependencies.* Athens: Ohio University Press.

Chambers, C., White, O., & Lindquist, J. (1983). Physician attitudes and prescribing practices: A focus on minor tranquilizers. *Journal of Psychoactive Drugs, 15,* 55-59.

Chance, M. (1946). Aggregation as a factor influencing the toxicity of sympathomimetic amines in mice. *Journal of Pharmacology and Experimental Therapeutics, 87,* 214-219.

Chance, M. (1947). Factors influencing the toxicity of sympathomimetic amines in mice. *Journal of Pharmacology and Experimental Therapeutics, 89,* 289-296.

Charen, S., & Perelman, L. (1946). Personality studies of marihuana addicts. *American Journal of Psychiatry, 102,* 674-682.

Charney, D., Woods, S., Krystal, J., & Heninger, G. (1990). Serotonin function and human anxiety disorders. *Annals of the New York Academy of Sciences, 600,* 558-573.

Chasnoff, I. (1988). Drug use in pregnancy: Parameters of risk. *Pediatric Clinics of North America, 35,* 1403-1412.

Chasnoff, I. (1989). Drug use in pregnancy. *New York State Medical Journal, 89,* 255.

Chasnoff, I., Schnoll, S., Burns, W., & Burns, K. (1984). Maternal nonnarcotic substance abuse during pregnancy: Effects on infant development. *Neurobehavioral Toxicology and Teratology, 6,* 277-280.

Cheaper can be better. (1991, March 18). *Time,* p. 70.

Chein, I., & Wilner, D. (1964). *Narcotics, delinquency, and social policy: The road to H.* London: Tavistock.

Cherubin, C. (1967). The medical sequelae of narcotic addiction. *Annals of Internal Medicine, 67,* 23-33.

Chiang, C., & Hawks, R. (1990). *Research findings on smoking of abused substances.* NIDA Research Monograph 99.

Chiang, C., & Rapaka, R. (1987). Pharmacokinetics and disposition of cannabinoids. In R. Rapaka & A. Makriyannis (Eds.), *Structure-activity relationships of the cannabinoids.* NIDA Research Monograph 79.

Childress, A., McLellan, T., Ehrman, R., & O'Brien, C. (1988). Classically conditioned responses in opioid and cocaine dependence: A role in relapse? In B. Ray (Ed.), *Learning factors in substance abuse.* NIDA Research Monograph 84.

Chiou, G. (1991). Systemic delivery of polypeptide drugs through ocular route. *Annual Review of Pharmacology and Toxicology, 31,* 457-467.

Chopin, P., & Briley, M. (1992). Effects of four non-cholinergic cognitive enhancers in comparison with tacrine and galanthamine on scopolamine-induced amnesia in rats. *Psychopharmacology, 106,* 26-30.

Chopra, R., & Chopra, G. (1939). The present position of hemp drug addiction in India. *Indian Medical Research Memoirs, 31,* 1-119.

Chouinard, G. (1986). Rebound anxiety: Incidence and relationship to subjective cognitive impairment. *Journal of Clinical Psychiatry Monograph Series, 4,* 12-16.

Chouinard, G., Annable, L., & Ross-Chouinard, A. (1986). Supersensitivity psychosis and tardive dyskinesia: A survey in schizophrenic outpatients. *Psychopharmacology Bulletin, 22,* 891-896.

Chouinard, G., Annable, L., Ross-Chouinard, A., & Oliver, M. (1983). Piracetam in elderly psychiatric patients with mild diffuse cerebral impairment. *Psychopharmacology, 81,* 100-106.

Chouinard, G., & Jones, B. (1980). Neuroleptic-induced supersensitivity psychosis: Clinical and pharmacologic characteristics. *American Journal of Psychiatry, 137,* 16-21.

Christensen, L., & Burrows, R. (1990). Dietary treatment of depression. *Behavior Therapy, 21,* 183-193.

Christensen, L., Nielsen, L., & Nielsen, S. (1990). Traffic accidents and drivers suspected for drug influence. *Forensic Science International, 45,* 273-280.

Church, M., & Johnson, L. (1979). Mood and performance of poor sleepers during repeated use of flurazepam. *Psychopharmacology, 61,* 309-316.

Ciotola, P., & Peterson, J. (1976). Personality characteristics of alcoholics and drug addicts in a merged treatment program. *Journal of Studies on Alcohol, 37*, 1229-1235.

Ciraulo, D., Alderson, L., Chapron, D., et al. (1982). Imipramine disposition in alcoholics. *Journal of Clinical Psychopharmacology, 2*, 2-7.

Clark, D., & Agras, W. (1991). The assessment and treatment of performance anxiety in musicians. *American Journal of Psychiatry, 148*, 598-605.

Clark, J., Smith, E., & Davidson, J. (1984). Enhancement of sexual motivation in male rats by yohimbine. *Science, 225*, 847-849.

Clegg, D. (1971). Teratology. *Annual Review of Pharmacology, 11*, 409-424.

Clincke, G., Tritsmans, L., Idzikowski, C., et al. (1988). The effect of R 58735 on memory functions in healthy elderly volunteers. *Psychopharmacology, 94*, 52-57.

Coccaro, E. (1989). Central serotonin and impulsive aggression. *British Journal of Psychiatry, 155*, 52-62.

Cohen, H. (1972). Multiple drug use considered in the light of the stepping-stone hypothesis. *International Journal of Addiction, 7*, 27-55.

Cohen, J., & Cohen, M. (1980). *Dictionary of modern quotations.* New York: Penguin.

Cohen, M., Marinello, M., & Back, N. (1967). Chromosomal damage in human leukocytes induced by lysergic acid diethylamide. *Science, 155*, 1417-1419.

Cohen, S. (1968). Pot, acid, and speed. *Medical Science, 19*, 30-35.

Cohen, S. (1969). *The drug dilemma.* New York: McGraw-Hill.

Cohen, S., Lichtenstein, E., Prochaska, J., et al. (1989). Debunking myths about self-quitting: Evidence from 10 prospective studies of persons who attempt to quit smoking by themselves. *American Psychologist, 44*, 1355-1365.

Cohen, S., Tyrrell, D., & Smith, A. (1991). Psychological stress and susceptibility to the common cold. *The New England Journal of Medicine, 325*, 606-612.

Cole, J., & Chiarello, R. (1990). The benzodiazepines as drugs of abuse. *Journal of Psychiatric Research, 24*, 135-144.

Coleman, R., Roffwarg, H., Kennedy, S., et al. (1982). Sleep-wake disorders based on a polysomnographic diagnosis: A national cooperative study. *Journal of the American Medical Association, 247*, 997-1003.

Coles, C., Smith, I., Lancaster, J., & Falek, A. (1987). Persistence over the first month of neurobehavioral alterations in infants exposed to alcohol prenatally. *Infant Behavior and Development, 10*, 23-37.

Coleston, D., & Hindmarch, I. (1991). Effects of nootropics on information processing. In Psychopharmacology, neuropsychology and psychiatry [Special issue]. *Pharmacopsychoecologia, 4,* 57-59.

Collins, J. (1990). Summary thoughts about drugs and violence. In M. De la Rosa, E. Lambert, & B. Gropper (Eds.), *Drugs and violence: Causes, correlates, and consequences.* NIDA Research Monograph 103.

Colsher, P., & Wallace, R. (1989). Is modest alcohol consumption better than none at all? An epidemiologic assessment. *Annual Review of Public Health, 10,* 203-219.

Committee on Problems of Drug Dependence. (1984). *Testing drugs for physical dependence potential and abuse liability.* NIDA Research Monograph 52.

Comptroller General of the United States. (1981). *Report to the Congress: Stronger crackdown needed on clandestine laboratories manufacturing dangerous drugs.* Washington, DC: U.S. General Accounting Office.

Connell, P. (1958). *Amphetamine psychosis.* London: Chapman & Hall.

Consensus Development Panel. (1985). Mood disorders: Pharmacological prevention of occurrence. *American Journal of Psychiatry, 142,* 469-476.

Cook, L., & Davidson, A. (1968). Effects of yeast RNA and other pharmacological agents on acquisition, retention and performance in animals. In D. Efron (Ed.), *Psychopharmacology: A review of progress* (U.S. Pub. No. 183). Washington, DC: Government Printing Office.

Cook, L., Davidson, A., Davis, D., et al. (1963). Ribonucleic acid: Effect on conditioned behavior in rats. *Science, 141,* 268-269.

Cook, P., Petersen, R., & Moore, D. (1990). *Alcohol, tobacco, and other drugs may harm the unborn* (DHHS Pub. No. [ADM] 90-1711). Washington, DC: U.S. Department of Health and Human Services.

Cooper, J., Bloom, F., & Roth, R. (1991). *The biochemical basis of neuropharmacology.* New York: Oxford University Press.

Cooper, M. (1990). *The business of drugs.* Washington, DC: Congressional Quarterly Inc.

Cotton, N. (1979). The familial incidence of alcoholism. A review. *Quarterly Journal of Studies on Alcohol, 40,* 89-116.

Cotton, P. (1991). Public pressure ends "bundled" drug program, but how much cost will drop remains unclear. *Journal of the American Medical Association, 265,* 837-838.

Cotts, C. (1992, March 9). Hard sell in the drug war. *The Nation,* pp. 300-302.

Counseling to prevent household and environmental injuries. (1990). *American Family Physician, 42,* 135-142.

Cousins, N. (1977, October 1). The mysterious placebo. *Saturday Review,* pp. 9-16.

Coyle, J., Price, D., & DeLong, M. (1983). Alzheimer's disease: A disorder of cortical cholinergic innervation. *Science, 219,* 1184-1190.

Crane, G. (1973). Clinical psychopharmacology in its 20th year. *Science, 181,* 124-128.

Creese, I., Burt, D., & Snyder, S. (1978). Biochemical actions of neuroleptic drugs: Focus on the dopamine receptor. In L. Iversen, S. Iversen, & S. Snyder (Eds.), *Handbook of psychopharmacology.* New York: Plenum.

Crenshaw, T. (1986). *Pharmacological enhancement of sexual function.* Paper presented at meeting of the Society for Sex Therapy and Research, Philadelphia.

Crider, R., & Rouse, B. (Eds.). (1988). *Epidemiology of inhalant abuse: An update.* NIDA Research Monograph 85.

Cromwell, P., Abadie, R., Stephens, J., & Kyle, M. (1989). Hair mineral analysis: Biochemical imbalances and violent criminal behavior. *Psychological Reports, 64,* 259-266.

Crow, T., Ferrier, I., & Johnstone, E. (1986). The 2 syndrome concept and neuroendocrinology of schizophrenia. *Psychiatric Clinics of North America, 9,* 99-113.

Crowe, L., & George, W. (1989). Alcohol and human sexuality: Review and integration. *Psychological Bulletin, 105,* 374-386.

Crowley, T. J. (1988). Learning and unlearning drug abuse in the real world: Clinical treatment and public policy. In B. A. Ray (Ed.), *Learning factors in substance abuse.* NIDA Research Monograph 84.

Curran, H., Sakulsriprong, M., & Lader, M. (1988). Antidepressants and human memory: An investigation of four drugs with different sedative and anticholinergic profiles. *Psychopharmacology, 95,* 520-527.

Cutler, N., Sramek, J., Murphy, M., & Nash, R. (1992). Implications of the study population in the early evaluation of anticholinesterase inhibitors for Alzheimer's disease. *Annals of Pharmacotherapy, 26,* 1118-1122.

Dackis, C., & Gold, M. (1985). New concepts in cocaine addiction. The dopamine depletion hypothesis. *Neuroscience and Biobehavioral Reviews, 9,* 469-477.

Dackis, C., Gold, M., Sweeney, D., et al. (1987). Single-dose bromocriptine reverses cocaine craving. *Psychiatric Research Reports, 20,* 261-264.

Daigle, R., Clark, H., & Landry, M. (1988). A primer on neurotransmitters and cocaine. *Journal of Psychoactive Drugs, 20,* 283-295.

Darley, C., Tinklenberg, J., Roth, W., & Atkinson, R. (1974). The nature of storage deficits and state-dependent retrieval under marijuana. *Psychopharmacologia, 37,* 139-149.

Daughton, D., Heatley, S., Prendergast, J., et al. (1991). Effect of transdermal nicotine delivery as an adjunct to low-intervention smoking cessation therapy. A randomized, placebo-controlled, double-blind study. *Archives of Internal Medicine, 151,* 749-752.

Davidson, J., Camargo, C., & Smith, E. (1979). Effects of androgen on sexual behavior in hypogonadal men. *Journal of Clinical Endocrinology and Metabolism, 48,* 955-958.

Davis, D. (1964). The psychological analysis of aggressive behavior. In W. Etkin (Ed.), *Social behavior and organization among vertebrates.* Chicago: University of Chicago Press.

Davis, H., & Squire, L. (1984). Protein synthesis and memory. A review. *Psychological Bulletin, 96,* 518-559.

Davis, K., Mohs, R., Davis, B., et al. (1983). Oral physostigmine in Alzheimer's disease. *Psychopharmacology Bulletin, 19,* 451-453.

Davis, M. (1990). Animal models of anxiety based on classical conditioning: The conditioned emotional response (CER) and the fear-potentiated startle effect. *Pharmacology and Therapeutics, 47,* 147-165.

Davis, R. (1987). Current trends in cigarette advertising and marketing. *The New England Journal of Medicine, 316,* 725-732.

Davis, W. (1985). *The serpent and the rainbow.* New York: Warner Books.

Dawson, E., Moore, T., & McGanity, W. (1972). Relationship of lithium metabolism to mental hospital admission and homicide. *Diseases of the Nervous System, 33,* 546-556.

Decker, M., & McGaugh, J. (1991). The role of interactions between the cholinergic system and other neuromodulatory systems in learning and memory. *Synapse, 7,* 151-168.

DeFreitas, B., & Schwartz, G. (1979). Effects of caffeine in chronic psychiatric patients. *American Journal of Psychiatry, 132,* 951-953.

DeLeo, D., & Magni, G. (1983). Sexual side effects of antidepressant drugs. *Psychosomatics, 24,* 1076-1082.

De Leon, G. (1988). The therapeutic community and behavioral science. In B. Ray (Ed.), *Learning factors in substance abuse*. NIDA Research Monograph 84.

De Leon, G., & Wexler, H. (1973). Heroin addiction: Its relation to sexual behavior and sexual experience. *Journal of Abnormal Psychology, 81*, 36-38.

Delgado, P., Charney, D., & Price, L. (1990). Serotonin function and the mechanism of antidepressant action: Reversal of antidepressant-induced remission by rapid depletion of plasma tryptophan. *Archives of General Psychiatry, 47*, 411-418.

Dembo, R., & LaGrand, L. (1978). A research model for comprehensive health service oriented understanding of drug use. *Journal of Drug Issues, 3*, 355-371.

Dement, W. (1972). *Some must watch while some must sleep*. Stanford, CA: Stanford Alumni Association.

Dement, W. (1983). Rational basis for the use of sleeping pills. *Pharmacology, 27*, 3-38.

Dement, W., Carskadon, M., Guilleminault, C., & Zarlone, V. (1976). Narcolepsy: Diagnosis and treatment. *Primary Care: Clinics in Office Practice, 3*, 609-623.

Dement, W., Seidel, W., Cohen, S., et al. (1991). Effects of alprazolam, buspirone and diazepam on daytime sedation and performance. *Drug Investigations, 3*, 148-156.

Demoss, B. (1992). [Letter to the editor]. *American Family Physician, 46*, 668.

Deutsch, J. (1971). The cholinergic synapse and the site of memory. *Science, 174*, 788-794.

Deutsch, J. (1983). The cholinergic synapse and the site of memory. In J. Deutsch (Ed.), *The physiological basis of memory*. New York: Academic Press.

Dewan, M., & Koss, M. (1989). The clinical impact of the side effects of psychotropic drugs. In S. Fisher & R. Greenberg (Eds.), *The limits of biological treatments for psychological distress*. Hillsdale, NJ: Lawrence Erlbaum.

Dewey, W. (1986). Cannabinoid pharmacology. *Pharmacological Reviews, 38*, 151-178.

Dewhurst, W. (1970). The blood-brain barrier and other membrane phenomena in psychopharmacology. In W. Clark & J. del Guidice (Eds.), *Principles of psychopharmacology*. New York: Academic Press.

Dews, P. (1955). Studies on behavior. I. Differential sensitivity to pentobarbital of pecking performance in pigeons depending on the schedule of reward. *Journal of Pharmacology and Experimental Therapeutics, 113*, 393-401.

Diagnostic Classification Steering Committee. (1990). *International classification of sleep disorders: Diagnostic and coding manual.* Rochester, MN: American Sleep Disorders Association.

Dimascio, A. (1963). Drug effects on competitive paired associate learning: Relationship to and implications for the Taylor manifest anxiety scale. *Journal of Psychology, 56,* 89-97.

Dimond, S., & Brouwers, E. (1976). Improvement of human memory through the use of drugs. *Psychopharmacology, 49,* 307-309.

Dishotsky, N., Loughman, W., Mogar, R., et al. (1971). LSD and genetic damage. *Science, 172,* 431-440.

Ditman, K., Hayman, M., & Whittlesey, J. (1962). Nature and frequency of claims following LSD. *Journal of Nervous and Mental Disease, 134,* 346-352.

Ditman, K., Moss, T., Forgy, E., et al. (1969). Dimensions of LSD, methylphenidate and chlordiazepoxide experiences. *Psychopharmacologia, 14,* 1-11.

Ditman, K., Moss, T., Forgy, E., et al. (1972). Dimensions of the LSD, methylphenidate, and chlordiazepoxide experiences. In D. Matheson & M. Davison (Eds.), *The behavioral effects of drugs.* New York: Holt, Rinehart & Winston.

Dixon, L., Haas, G., Weiden, P., et al. (1991). Drug abuse in schizophrenic patients: Clinical correlates and reasons for use. *American Journal of Psychiatry, 148,* 224-230.

Doering, C., Kraemer, H., Keith, H., Brodie, H., & Hamburg, D. (1975). A cycle of plasma testosterone in the human male. *Journal of Clinical Endocrinology and Metabolism, 40,* 492-500.

Dohan, F. (1979). Schizophrenia: Are some food derived polypeptides pathogenic? Coeliac disease as a model. In G. Hemmings & W. Hemmings (Eds.), *The biological basis of schizophrenia.* Lancaster, England: MTP Press.

Dole, V. (1988). Implications of methadone maintenance for theories of narcotic addiction. *Journal of the American Medical Association, 260,* 3025-3029.

Domenighetti, G., Tomamichel, M., Gutzwiller, F., et al. (1991). Psychoactive drug use among medical doctors is higher than in the general population. *Social Science and Medicine, 33,* 269-274.

Domer, F. (1971). *Animal experiments in pharmacological analysis.* Springfield, IL: Charles C Thomas.

Donahoe, R. (1990). Drug abuse and AIDS: Causes for the connection. In *Drugs of Abuse: Chemistry, Pharmacology, Immunology, and AIDS.* NIDA Research Monograph 96.

Dorner, G. (1988). Neuroendocrine response to estrogen and brain differentiation in heterosexuals, homosexuals, and transsexuals. *Archives of Sexual Behavior, 17,* 57-75.

Dorow, R., & Duka, T. (1986). Anxiety: Its generation by drugs and their withdrawal. In G. Biggio & E. Costa (Eds.), *GABAergic transmission and anxiety.* New York: Raven.

Douglass, F., & Khavari, K. (1978). The drug use index: A measure of the extent of polydrug use. *International Journal of Addictions, 13,* 981-993.

Drachman, D., & Sahakian, G. (1979). Effects of cholinergic agents on human learning and memory. In J. Barbeau, J. Growdon, & R. Wurtman (Eds.), *Nutrition and the brain.* New York: Raven.

Drake, D., & Uhlman, M. (1993, May 2). Wonder drugs, windfall profits. *This World Magazine.*

Drucker-Colin, R., & Spanis, C. (1976). Is there a sleep transmitter? *Progress in Neurobiology, 6,* 1-22.

The drug revolution. (1970, February). *Playboy,* pp. 53-74.

Dryfoos, J. (1990). *Adolescents at risk.* New York: Oxford University Press.

Duke, P., & Turan, K. (1987). *Call me Anna: The autobiography of Patty Duke.* Toronto: Bantam.

Duncker, K. (1945). On problem solving. *Psychological Monographs,* p. 58.

Dundee, J., Gamble, J., & Assaf, R. (1974). Plasma diazepam levels following intramuscular injection by nurses and doctors. *Lancet, 1,* 1461.

Duvall, H., Locke, B., & Brill, L. (1963). Followup study of narcotic drug addicts five years after hospitalization. *Public Health Report, 78,* 185-193.

Earle, C., Keogh, E., Wisniewski, Z., et al. (1990). Prostaglandin E1 therapy for impotence, comparison with papaverine. *Journal of Urology, 143,* 57-59.

Egger, J., Carter, C., Graham, P., et al. (1985). Controlled trial of oligoantigenic treatment in the hyperkinetic syndrome. *Lancet, 1,* 540-545.

Ehrhardt, A. (1984). Gender differences: A biosocial perspective. In *Nebraska Symposium on Motivation, 1984.* Omaha: University of Nebraska Medical Center.

Ehrhardt, A., & Meyer-Bahlburg, H. (1979). Prenatal sex hormones and the developing brain: Effects on psychosexual differentiation and cognitive function. *Annual Review of Medicine, 30,* 417-430.

Eichelman, B. (1986). The biology and somatic experimental treatment of aggressive disorders. In H. Brodie & P. Berger (Eds.), *The American handbook of psychiatry, Vol. VIII.* New York: Basic Books.

Eichelman, B. (1987). Neurochemical bases of aggressive behavior. *Psychiatric Annals, 17,* 371-374.

Eichelman, B. (1990). Neurochemical and psychopharmacologic aspects of aggressive behavior. *Annual Review of Medicine, 41,* 149-158.

Eichlseder, W. (1985). Ten years experience with 1,000 hyperactive children in a private practice. *American Academy of Pediatrics, 76,* 176-184.

Eidson, M., Philen, R., Sewell, C., et al. (1990). L-tryptophan and eosinophilia-myalgia syndrome in New Mexico. *Lancet, 335,* 645-648.

Eiseman, B., Lam, R., & Rush, B. (1964). Surgery on the narcotic addict. *Annals of Surgery, 159,* 748-757.

El-Guebaly, N. (1990). Substance abuse and mental disorders: The dual diagnoses concept. *Canadian Journal of Psychiatry, 35,* 261-267.

Elkashef, A., Ruskin, P., Bacher, N., & Barrett, D. (1990). Vitamin E in the treatment of tardive dyskinesia. *American Journal of Psychiatry, 147,* 505-506.

Ellinwood, E. (1973). Amphetamine and stimulant drugs. In *Second report of the National Commission on Marijuana and Drug Abuse, Vol. I.* Washington, DC: Government Printing Office.

Ellis, A. (1991, July 21). [Editorial]. *Oakland Tribune.*

Ellison, J. (Ed.). (1989). *The psychotherapist's guide to pharmacotherapy.* Chicago: Year Book.

Ellor, J., & Kurz, D. (1982). Misuse and abuse of prescription and nonprescription drugs by the elderly. *Nursing Clinics of North America, 17,* 319-330.

Elofson, G., & Elofson, S. (1990). Steroids claimed our son's life. *Physician and Sports Medicine, 18,* 15-16.

Emsinger, M., Kellam, S., & Rubin, B. (1983). School and family origins of delinquency. In K. Van Dusen & S. Mednick (Eds.), *Perspective studies of crime and delinquency.* Boston: Kluwer-Nijhoff.

Engelhardt, D. (1974). Pharmacologic basis for use of psychotropic drugs. *New York State Journal of Medicine, 74,* 360-366.

Ennaceur, A., Cavoy, A., Costa, J., & Delacour, J. (1989). A new one-trial test for neurobiological studies of memory in rats: II. Effects of piracetam and pramiracetam. *Behavioural Brain Research, 33,* 197-207.

Erickson, P., & Watson, V. (1990). Women, illicit drugs, and crime. In L. Kozlowski et al. (Eds.), *Alcohol and drug problems, Vol. 10.* New York: Plenum.

Erulkar, S. (1989). Chemically mediated synaptic transmission: An overview. In C. Siegel, B. Agranoff, R. Albers, & P. Molinoff (Eds.), *Basic neurochemistry.* New York: Raven.

Esecover, H., Malitz, S., & Wilkens, B. (1961). Clinical profiles of paid normal subjects volunteering for hallucinogenic drug studies. *American Journal of Psychiatry, 117,* 910-915.

Everett, G. (1975). Amyl nitrite ("poppers") as an aphrodisiac. In M. Sandler & G. Gessa (Eds.), *Sexual behavior: Pharmacology and biochemistry.* New York: Raven.

Everitt, D., Avorn, J., & Baker, M. (1990). Clinical decision-making in the evaluation and treatment of insomnia. *American Journal of Medicine, 89,* 357-262.

Executive Office of the President, Office of National Drug Control Policy. (1992). *National drug control strategy: Budget summary.* Washington, DC: Executive Office of the President.

Eysenck, H. (1963). *Experiments with drugs.* Oxford: Pergamon.

Eysenck, H. (1977). *Personality and motivation of cigarette smokers.* Paper presented at Internationales Symposium, Hamburg, Germany.

Eysenck, H. (1983). Drugs as research tools in psychology: Experiments with drugs in personality research. *Neuropsychobiology, 10,* 29-43.

Fagan, J. (1989). The social organization of drug use and drug dealing among urban gangs. *Criminology, 27,* 633-669.

Fagan, J., & Chin, K. (1990). Violence as regulation and social control in the distribution of crack. In M. De la Rosa, E. Lambert, & B. Gropper (Eds.), *Drugs and violence: Causes, correlates, and consequences.* NIDA Research Monograph 103.

Falcone, D., & Loder, K. (1984). A modified lateral eye-movement measure, the right hemisphere and creativity. *Perceptual and Motor Skills, 58,* 823-830.

Falk, J. (1983). Drug dependence: Myth or motive? *Pharmacology, Biochemistry, and Behavior, 19,* 385-391.

Falk, J. (in press). Oral cocaine as a reinforcer: Acquisition conditions and importance of stimulus control. *Behavioral Pharmacology.*

Falk, J., & Tang, M. (1988). What schedule-induced polydipsia can tell us about alcoholism. *Alcoholism: Clinical and Experimental Research, 12,* 577-584.

FASE Reports. (1989). *Drug rehabilitation: A new perspective, Vol. 8.*

Fava, M., Anderson, K., & Rosenbaum, J. (1990). "Anger attacks": Possible variants of panic and major depressive disorders. *American Journal of Psychiatry, 147,* 867-870.

Fayen, M., Goldman, M., Moulthrop, M., & Luchins, D. (1988). Differential memory function with dopaminergic versus anticholinergic treatment of drug-induced extrapyramidal symptoms. *American Journal of Psychiatry, 145,* 483-486.

FDA Consumer. (1990). *New drug development in the United States* (DHHS Pub. No. 90-3168). Washington, DC: U.S. Department of Health and Human Services.

FDA Consumer. (1990, November 24-27). Testing drugs in older people. *FDA Consumer.*

FDA Talk Paper. (1991, October 18). *Antidepressants update.*

Fejer, D., Smart, R., Whitehead, P., & LaForest, L. (1971). Sources of information about drugs among high school students. *Public Opinion Quarterly, 35,* 235-241.

Fell, J. (1987). *Alcohol involvement rates in fatal crashes: A focus on young drivers and female drivers.* Proceedings of the 31st Annual Conference of the American Association for Automotive Medicine, New Orleans.

Ferguson, H. (1966). Effect of red cedar chip bedding on hexobarbital and pentobarbital sleep time. *Journal of Pharmaceutical Sciences, 55,* 1142-1143.

Fingarette, H. (1988). *Heavy drinking: The myth of alcoholism as a disease.* Berkeley: University of California Press.

Fischer, R., Hill, R., & Warshay, D. (1969). Effects of the psychodysleptic drug psilocybin on visual perception. Changes in brightness preference. *Experientia, 25,* 166-168.

Fischer, R., & Scheib, J. (1971). Creative performance and the hallucinogenic drug-induced creative experience. *Confinia Psychiatrica, 14,* 174-202.

Fischman, M., Foltin, R., Nestadt, G., & Pearlson, G. (1990). Effects of desipramine maintenance on cocaine self-administration by humans. *Journal of Pharmacology and Experimental Therapeutics, 253,* 760-770.

Fish, B., & Bruhnsen, K. (1979). The impact of legal sanctions on illicit drug selling. *Drug Forum, 7,* 239-258.

Fisher, C., Kahn, E., Edwards, A., & Davis, D. (1973). A psychophysiological study of nightmares and night terrors. *Journal of Nervous and Mental Disease, 157,* 75-98.

Fisher, S., et al. (1964). Drug-set interaction: The effect of expectations on drug response in outpatients. *Neuropsychopharmacology, 3,* 149-156.

Fisher, S., & Greenberg, R. (Eds.). (1989a). *The limits of biological treatments for psychological distress.* Hillsdale, NJ: Lawrence Erlbaum.

Fisher, S., & Greenberg, R. (1989b). Rethinking claims of biological psychiatry. In S. Fisher & R. Greenberg (Eds.), *The limits of biological treatments for psychological distress.* Hillsdale, NJ: Lawrence Erlbaum.

Fitten, L., Perryman, K., Hanna, J., & Menon, M. (1990). Effect of BMY 21502 on acquisition of shape discrimination and memory retention in monkey. *Pharmacology, Biochemistry, and Behavior, 35,* 553-556.

Flanagan, T., & Maguire, K. (Eds.), (1990). *Sourcebook of criminal justice statistics-1989.* Washington, DC: U.S. Department of Justice.

Foltin, R., & Fischman, M. (1989a). Effects of the combination of cocaine and marijuana on the task-elicited physiological response. *NIDA Research Monograph, 95,* 359-360.

Foltin, R., & Fischman, M. (1989b). Ethanol and cocaine interactions in humans: Cardiovascular consequences. *Pharmacology, Biochemistry, and Behavior, 31,* 877-883.

Foltin, R., McEntee, M., Capriotti, R., et al. (1988). Effect of cocaine on the task-elicited physiological response. *Pharmacology, Biochemistry, and Behavior, 31,* 387-391.

Fontaine, R., & Chouinard, G. (1986). An open clinical trial of fluoxetine in the treatment of obsessive-compulsive disorder. *Journal of Clinical Psychopharmacology, 6,* 98-101.

Ford, D., & Kamerow, D. (1989). Epidemiologic study of sleep disturbances and psychiatric disorders. An opportunity for prevention? *Journal of the American Medical Association, 262,* 1479-1484.

Fort, J., & Cory, C. (1975). *American drugstore.* Boston: Little, Brown.

Foulds, G. (1963). The design of experiments in psychiatry. In P. Sainsbury & N. Kreitman (Eds.), *Methods of psychiatric research.* London: Oxford University Press.

Fox, C., Ismail, A., Love, D., et al. (1972). Studies on the relationship between plasma testosterone levels and human sexual activity. *Journal of Endocrinology, 52,* 51-58.

Fox, K., Abendschein, D., & Lahcen, R. (1977). Effects of benzodiazepines during gestation and infancy on Y-maze performance of mice. *Pharmacological Research Communications, 9,* 325-338.

Fox, R. (1967). Disulfiram (Antabuse) as an adjunct in the treatment of alcoholism. In R. Fox (Ed.), *Alcoholism.* New York: Springer.

Fram, D., & Stone, N. (1986). Clinical observations in the treatment of adolescent and young adult PCP abusers. In D. Clouet (Ed.), *Phencyclidine: An update.* NIDA Research Monograph 64.

Franks, S., Jacobs, H., Martin, N., & Nabarro, J. (1978). Hyperprolactinemia and impotence. *Clinical Endocrinology, 8,* 277-287.

Freedman, A. (1976). In Sadock, B., Kaplan, H., & Freedman, A. (Eds.), *The sexual experience.* Baltimore, MD: Williams & Wilkins.

Freestone, D. (1969). Formulation and therapeutic efficacy of drugs used in clinical trials. *Lancet, 2,* 98-99.

French, E. (1988). Effects of acute and chronic administration of phencyclidine on A10 dopaminergic mesolimbic system: Electrophysiological and behavioral correlates. *Neuropharmacology, 27,* 791-798.

Fresle, D. (1992, March-April). How many drugs do we really need? *World Health,* p. 9.

Frezza, M., di Padova, C., Pozzato, G., et al. (1990). High blood alcohol levels in women. *The New England Journal of Medicine, 322,* 95-99.

Fried, P. (1982). Marijuana use by pregnant women and effects on offspring: An update. *Neurobehavioral Toxicology and Teratology, 4,* 451-454.

Fried, P. (1985). Postnatal consequences of maternal marijuana use. In T. Pinkert (Ed.), *Current research on the consequences of maternal drug abuse.* NIDA Research Monograph 59.

Friedel, R. (1983). Clinical predictors of treatment response: An update. In J. Davis & J. Maas (Eds.), *The affective disorders.* Washington, DC: American Psychiatric Press.

Friedler, G., & Cochin, J. (1967). Altered post-natal growth pattern of offspring of female rats chronically treated with morphine prior to mating. *Pharmacologist, 9,* 230.

Frierson, R., Wey, J., & Tabler, J. (1991). Psychostimulants for depression in the medically ill. *American Family Physician, 43,* 163-168.

Frykholm, B. (1979). Termination of the drug career: An interview study of 58 ex-addicts. *Acta Psychiatrica Scandinavica, 59,* 370-380.

Fuller, R., Branchey, L., Brightwell, D., et al. (1986). Disulfiram treatment of alcoholism: A Veterans Administration cooperative study. *Journal of the American Medical Association, 256,* 1449-1455.

Funfgeld, E. (1989). A natural and broad spectrum nootropic substance for treatment of SDAT—The Gingko biloba extract. *Progress in Clinical and Biological Research, 317,* 1247-1260.

Gable, R. (1993). Toward a comparative overview of dependence potential and acute toxicity of psychoactive substances used nonmedically. *American Journal of Drug and Alcohol Abuse, 19,* 263-281.

Gadow, K. (1986). *Children on medication, Vol. II.* San Diego, CA: College Hills Press.

Gaillard, J. (1989a). Benzodiazepines and GABA-ergic transmission. In M. Kryger, T. Roth, & W. Dement (Eds.), *Principles and practice of sleep medicine.* Philadelphia: J. B. Saunders.

Gaillard, J. (1989b). Neurotransmission and receptor pharmacology. In M. Kryger, T. Roth, & W. Dement (Eds.), *Principles and practice of sleep medicine.* Philadelphia: J. B. Saunders.

Gaillard, J., Nicholson, A., & Pascoe, P. (1989). Neurotransmitter systems. In M. Kryger, T. Roth, & W. Dement (Eds.), *Principles and practice of sleep medicine.* Philadelphia: J. B. Saunders.

Gainotti, G., Nocentini, U., & Sena, E. (1989). Can the pattern of neuropsychological improvement obtained with cholinergic drugs be used to infer a cholinergic mechanism in other nootropic drugs? *Progress in Neuro-pharmacology, & Biological Psychiatry, 13,* S47-S59.

Gallagher, W. (1986, August). The looming menace of designer drugs. *Discover,* pp. 24-35.

Gardner, C. (1989). Interpretation of behavioral effects of benzodiazepine receptor ligands. *Drugs Future, 14,* 51-67.

Garfield, E. (1979, July 30). *Current Contents,* p. 11.

Gartrell, N. (1986). Increased libido in women receiving trazodone. *American Journal of Psychiatry, 143,* 781-782.

Garza-Trevino, E., Hollister, L., Overall, J., et al. (1989). Efficacy of combinations of intramuscular antipsychotics and sedative-hypnotics for control of psychotic agitation. *American Journal of Psychiatry, 146,* 1598-1561.

Gauron, E., & Rowley, V. (1969). Effects on offspring behavior of mother's early chronic drug experience. *Psychopharmacology, 16,* 5-15.

Gay, G., Newmeyer, J., Elion, R., et al. (1975). Drug-sex practice in the Haight-Ashbury or "the sensuous hippie." In M. Sandler & G. Gessa (Eds.), *Sexual behavior: Pharmacology and biochemistry*. New York: Raven.

Gay, G., & Sheppard, C. (1973). Sex crazed dope fiends—Myth or reality. *Drug Forum, 2*, 125-140.

Gebhard, P. (1965). Situational factors affecting human sexual behavior. In F. Beach (Ed.), *Sex and behavior*. New York: John Wiley.

Gelenberg, A., & Mandel, M. (1977). Catatonic reactions to high-potency neuroleptic drugs. *Archives of General Psychiatry, 34*, 947-950.

Gerard, D., Saenger, G., & Wile, R. (1952). The abstinent alcoholic. *Archives of General Psychiatry, 6*, 83-95.

Geschwind, N., & Galaburda, A. (1987). *Cerebral lateralization*. Cambridge: MIT Press.

Gessa, G., Paglietti, E., & Pellegrini-Quarantotti, B. (1979). Induction of copulatory behaviour in sexually inactive rats by naloxone. *Science, 204*, 203-205.

Gibbons, D., & Connelly, J. (Eds.). (1970). *Selected readings in psychology*. St. Louis: C. V. Mosby.

Gilbert, J., Light, R., & Mosteller, F. (1975). Assessing social innovations: An empirical basis for policy. In C. Bennett & A. Lumsdaine (Eds.), *Evaluation and experiment*. New York: Academic Press.

Gilchrist, L., Gillmore, M., & Lohr, M. (1990). Drug use among pregnant adolescents. *Journal of Consulting Clinical Psychology, 58*, 402-407.

Ginsberg, A. (1966). First manifesto to end the bringdown. In D. Solomon (Ed.), *The marihuana papers*. New York: Signet.

Gitlin, T. (1990). *The psychotherapist's guide to psychopharmacology*. New York: Maxwell Macmillan.

Giurgea, C. (1973). The "nootropic" approach to the pharmacology of the integrative activity of the brain. *Conditional Reflex, 8*, 108-115.

Giurgea, C. (1982). The nootropic concept and its prospective implications. *Drug Development Research, 2*, 441-446.

Glantz, M., Petersen, D., & Whittington, F. (Eds.). (1983). *Drugs and the elderly*. Washington, DC: NIDA.

Glassman, A. (1993). Cigarette smoking: Implications for psychiatric illness. *American Journal of Psychiatry, 150*, 546-553.

Glassman, A., & Perel, J. (1973). The clinical pharmacology of imipramine. *Archives of General Psychiatry, 28,* 649-653.

Godfrey, P., Toone, B., Carney, M., et al. (1990). Enhancement of recovery from psychiatric illness by methylfolate. *Lancet, 336,* 392-395.

Goelet, P., Castellucci, V., Schacher, S., & Kandel, E. (1986). The long and the short of long-term memory—A molecular framework. *Nature, 322,* 419-422.

Goetzl, F. (1953). *A note on the possible usefulness of wine in the management of anorexia.* Oakland, CA: Permanente Foundation.

Gold, M. (1987). *The good news about depression: Cures and treatments in the new age of psychiatry.* New York: Villard Books.

Gold, P. (1991). An integrated memory regulation system: From blood to brain. In R. Frederickson, J. McGaugh, & D. Felten (Eds.), *Peripheral signaling of the brain.* New York: Hogrefe & Huber.

Gold, P. (1992). Modulation of memory processing: Enhancement of memory in rodents and humans. In L. Squire & N. Butters (Eds.), *Neuropsychology of Memory.* New York: Guilford.

Gold, P., & Stone, W. (1988). Neuroendocrine effects on memory in aged-rodents and humans. *Neurobiology of Aging, 9,* 709-717.

Goldberg, S., & Schuster, C. (1967). Conditioned suppression by a stimulus associated with nalorphine in morphine-dependent monkeys. *Journal of Experimental Analysis of Behavior, 10,* 235-242.

Goldstein, A., Kaizer, S., & Whitby, O. (1969). Psychotropic effects of caffeine in man: IV. Quantitative and qualitative differences associated with habituation to coffee. *Clinical Pharmacology and Therapeutics, 10,* 489-497.

Goldstein, A., & Kalant, H. (1990). Drug policy: Striking the right balance. *Science, 249,* 1513-1521.

Goldstein, H. (1987). Cognitive development in low attentive, hyperactive and aggressive 6 through 11 year-old children. *American Academy of Child and Adolescent Psychiatry, 26,* 214-218.

Goldstein, P. (1985). The drugs-violence nexus: A tripartite conceptual framework. *Journal of Drug Issues, 15,* 493-506.

Golub, M., Eisele, J., & Anderson, J. (1986). Maternal-fetal distribution of morphine and alfentanil in near-term sheep and rhesus monkeys. *Developmental Pharmacology and Therapeutics, 9,* 12-22.

Gong, H., Fligiel, S., Tashkin, D., & Barbers, R. (1987). Tracheobronchial changes in habitual, heavy smokers of marijuana with and without tobacco. *American Review of Respiratory Diseases, 136,* 142-149.

Goode, E. (1970). *The marijuana smokers.* New York: Basic Books.

Goode, E. (1972a). *Drugs in American society.* New York: Knopf.

Goode, E. (1972b). Drug use and sexual activity on a college campus. *American Journal of Psychiatry, 128,* 1272-1276.

Goodstadt, M. (1980). Drug education—A turn on or a turn off? *Journal of Drug Education, 10,* 89-99.

Goodstadt, M. (1981). Planning and evaluation of alcohol education programmes. *Journal of Alcohol and Drug Education, 26,* 1-10.

Goodwin, D. (1971). Blackouts and alcohol induced memory dysfunction. In N. Mello & J. Mendelson (Eds.), *Recent advances in studies of alcoholism* (NIMH Pub. No. [HSM] 71-9045). Washington, DC: Government Printing Office.

Goodwin, D. (1985). Alcoholism and genetics: The sins of the fathers. *Archives of General Psychiatry, 42,* 171-174.

Goodwin, D., Johnson, J., Maher, C., et al. (1969). Why people do not drink: A study of teetotalers. *Comprehensive Psychiatry, 10,* 209-214.

Gorelick, D., Wilkins, J., & Wong, C. (1986). Diagnosis and treatment of chronic phencyclidine (PCP) abuse. In D. Clouet (Ed), *Phencyclidine: An update.* NIDA Research Monograph 64.

Gottschalk, L., Aronow, W., & Prakash, R. (1977). Effect of marijuana and placebo-marijuana smoking on psychological state and on psychophysiological cardiovascular functioning in anginal patients. *Biological Psychiatry, 12,* 255-266.

Gray, B. (1975). *Human subjects in medical experimentation.* New York: John Wiley.

Gray, J. (1978, July). Anxiety. *Human Nature,* pp. 38-45.

Green, J., Kim, K., & Bowman, K. (1976). Ocular effects of delta-9-tetrahydrocannabinol. In S. Cohen & R. Stillman (Eds.), *The therapeutic potential of marihuana.* New York: Plenum.

Greenberg, R., & Fisher, S. (1989). Examining antidepressant effectiveness: Findings, ambiguities, and some vexing puzzles. In S. Fisher & R. Greenberg (Eds.), *The limits of biological treatments for psychological distress.* Hillsdale, NJ: Lawrence Erlbaum.

Greenberg, S. (1981). Alcohol and crime: A methodological critique of the literature. In J. Collins (Ed.), *Drinking and crime. Perspectives on the relationships between alcohol consumption and criminal behavior.* New York: Guilford.

Greenblatt, D., Harmatz, J., Engelhardt, N., & Shader, R. (1989). Pharmacokinetic determinants of dynamic differences among three benzodiazepines. *Archives of General Psychiatry, 46,* 326-332.

Greenblatt, D., & Shader, R. (1974). *Benzodiazepines in clinical practice.* New York: Raven.

Greenstein, R., Evans, B., McLellan, T., et al. (1983). Predictors of favorable outcome following naltrexone treatment. *Drug and Alcohol Dependence, 12,* 173-180.

Greer, G., & Tolbert, R. (1986). Subjective reports of the effects of MDMA in a clinical setting. *Journal of Psychoactive Drugs, 18,* 319-327.

Greer, G., & Tolbert, R. (1990). The therapeutic use of MDMA. In S. Peroutka (Ed.), *Ecstasy.* New York: Kluver.

Griffin, K. (1991). The unbearable darkness of being. *Health, 5,* 63-67.

Griffiths, R., Bigelow, G., & Liebson, I. (1986). Human coffee drinking: Reinforcing and physical dependence producing effects of caffeine. *Journal of Pharmacology and Experimental Therapeutics, 239,* 416-425.

Griffiths, R., Stitzer, M., Corker, K., et al. (1977). Drug-produced changes in human social behavior: Facilitation by d-amphetamine. *Pharmacology, Biochemistry, and Behavior, 7,* 365-372.

Grinspoon, L., & Bakalar, J. (1986). Can drugs be used to enhance the psychotherapeutic process? *American Journal of Psychotherapy, 40,* 393-404.

Grinspoon, L., & Bakalar, J. (1993). *Marihuana, the forbidden medicine.* New Haven, CT: Yale University Press.

Grinspoon, L., Ewalt, J., & Shader, R. (1972). *Schizophrenia: Pharmacotherapy and psychotherapy.* Baltimore, MD: Williams & Wilkins.

Grossarth-Maticek, R., & Eysenck, H. (1991a). Coca-Cola, cancers, and coronaries: Personality and stress as mediating factors. *Psychological Reports, 68,* 1083-1087.

Grossarth-Maticek, R., & Eysenck, H. (1991b). Coffee-drinking and personality as factors in the genesis of cancer and coronary heart disease. *Neuropsychobiology, 23,* 153-159.

Grossman, S. (1960). Eating and drinking elicited by direct adrenergic or cholinergic stimulation of hypothalamus. *Science, 132,* 301-302.

Grunt, J., & Young, W. (1952). Differential reactivity of individuals and the response of the male guinea pig to testosterone propionate. *Endocrinology, 52,* 237-248.

Guttman, D. (1977). *A survey of drug-taking behavior of the elderly.* Washington, DC: NIDA.

Haddad, L. (1992). Managing tricyclic antidepressant overdose. *American Family Physician, 46,* 153-159.

Haffner, M. (1991). Orphan products: Origins, progress, and prospects. *Annual Review of Pharmacology and Toxicology, 31,* 603-620.

Halberg, F. (1960). The 24-hour scale: A time dimension of adaptive functional organization. *Perspectives in Biology and Medicine, 3,* 491-527.

Hale, P., Hannah, P., Sandler, M., & Bridges, P. (1989). Tyramine conjugation test for prediction of treatment response in depressed patients. *Lancet, 1,* 234-236.

Halikas, J., Weller, R., & Morse, C. (1982). Effects of regular marijuana use on sexual performance. *Journal of Psychoactive Drugs, 14,* 59-70.

Hall, G. (1980). The pharmacology of tobacco smoking in relation to schizophrenia. In G. Hemmings (Ed.), *Biochemistry of schizophrenia and addiction.* Lancaster, England: MTP Press.

Hall, J., Nelson, R., & Edlin, A. (1967). Effect of temperature on convulsive liability of pentylene tetrazol, strychnine sulfate, and thebaine hydrochloride. *Journal of Pharmaceutical Sciences, 56,* 298-299.

Hall, S., Rugg, D., Tunstall, C., & Jones, R. (1984). Preventing relapse by behavioral skills training. *Journal of Consulting Psychology, 52,* 372-382.

Hall, S., Wasserman, D., & Havassy, B. (1991). Relapse prevention. In R. Pickens, C. Leukefeld, & C. Schuster (Eds.), *Improving drug abuse treatment.* NIDA Research Monograph 106.

Haller, E. & Binder, R. (1990). Clozapine and seizures. *American Journal of Psychiatry, 147,* 1069-1071.

Haller, M. (1989). Bootlegging: The business and politics of violence. In T. Gurr (Ed.), *Violence in America, Vol. 1.* Newbury Park, CA: Sage.

Halperin, S. (1989). Analysis of statistical procedures and designs commonly used in drug research studies. In S. Fisher & R. Greenberg (Eds.), *The limits of biological treatments for psychological distress.* Hillsdale, NJ: Lawrence Erlbaum.

Hanneman, G. (1972). *Dissemination of drug related information*. Storrs: University of Connecticut Community Research Program.

Hans, S. (1989). Developmental consequences of prenatal exposure to methadone. *Annals of the New York Academy of Science, 562*, 195-207.

Hans, S. (1991). Following drug-exposed infants into middle childhood: Challenges to researchers. In M. Kilbey & K. Asghar (Eds.), *Methodological issues in controlled studies on effects of prenatal exposure to drug abuse*. NIDA Research Monograph 114.

Hansen, K., Malloy, T., Gordon, O., et al. (1984-1985). Nitrous oxide and cognitive set: Implications of an altered state of consciousness for creative problem solving. *Imagination, Cognition, and Personality, 4*, 2-24.

Hansen, M., Paredes, J., Koczapski, A., et al. (1987). The relationship between neuroleptic dosage and cognitive functioning in chronic schizophrenic patients. *Clinical and Investigative Medicine, 10: 368-371.*

Harding, C., Zubin, J., & Strauss, J. (1987). Chronicity in schizophrenia: Fact, partial fact, or artifact? *Hospital and Community Psychiatry, 38*, 477-486.

Hare, E., & Willcox, D. (1967). Do psychiatric inpatients take their pills? *British Journal of Psychiatry, 113*, 1435-1439.

Haring, C., Fleischhacker, W., Schett, P., Humpel, C., et al. (1990). Influence of patient-related variables on clozapine plasma levels. *American Journal of Psychiatry, 147*, 1471-1475.

Harlap, S., & Davies, A. (1974). Infant admissions to hospital and maternal smoking. *Lancet, 1*, 529-532.

Harman, W., McKim, R., Mogar, R., et al. (1966). Psychedelic agents in creative problem-solving: A pilot study. *Psychological Reports, 19*, 211-227.

Harruff, R., Francisco, J., Elkins, S., et al. (1988). Cocaine and homicide in Memphis and Shelby County: An epidemic of violence. *Journal of Forensic Science, 33*, 1231-1237.

Hartmann, E., & Cravens, J. (1973). The effects of long-term administration of psychotropic drugs on human sleep: V. The effects of chloral hydrate. *Psychopharmacology, 33*, 219-232.

Hartmann, E., & Greenwald, D. (1984). Tryptophan and human sleep: An analysis of 43 studies. In H. Schlossberger, W. Kochen, B. Linden, & H. Steinhart (Eds.), *Progress in tryptophan and serotonin research*. New York: Walter de Gruyter.

Hattie, J. (1980). Should creativity tests be administered under testlike conditions? An empirical study of three alternative conditions. *Journal of Educational Psychology, 72*, 87-98.

Hauser, P., Zametkin, A., Martinez, P., et al. (1993). Attention deficit-hyperactivity disorder in people with generalized resistance to thyroid hormone. *The New England Journal of Medicine, 328*, 997-1001.

Hawkins, J., Catalano, R., Gillmore, M., & Wells, E. (1989). Skills training for drug abusers: Generalization, maintenance, and effects on drug use. *Journal of Consulting Clinical Psychology, 57*, 559-563.

Hawkins, J., Lishner, D., Jenson, J., & Catalano, R. (1987). Delinquents and drugs: What the evidence suggests about prevention and treatment programming. In B. Brown & A. Mills (Eds.), *Youth at high risk for substance abuse.* Rockville, MD: NIDA.

Hawkins, L., White, M., & Morris, L. (1982, October 13). Smoking, stress and nurses. *Nursing Mirror*, pp. 18-22.

Hayter, A. (1968). *Opium and the romantic imagination.* Berkeley: University of California Press.

Heath and Public Policy Committee, American College of Physicians. (1988). Improving education in therapeutics. *Annals of Internal Medicine, 108*, 145-147.

Hearn, W., Flynn, D., Hime, G., et al. (1991). Cocaethylene: A unique cocaine metabolite displays high affinity for the dopamine transporter. *Journal of Neurochemistry, 56*, 698-701.

Helwig, F. (1940). Beverage alcohol and heart disease. *Journal of the Missouri Medical Association, 37*, 204-206.

Helzer, J. (1985). Specification of predictors of narcotic use versus addiction. In L. Robins (Ed.), *Studying drug abuse.* New Brunswick, NJ: Rutgers University Press.

Hendin, H., Haas, A., Singer, P., et al. (1987). *Living high: Daily marijuana use among adults.* New York: Human Sciences Press.

Henningfield, J., & Goldberg, S. (1983). Control of behavior by intravenous nicotine injections in human subjects. *Pharmacology, Biochemistry, and Behavior, 19*, 1021-1026.

Herbst, A., Scully, R., & Robboy, S. (1975). Effects of maternal DES ingestion on the female genital tract. *Hospital Practice, 10*, 51- 57.

Hernandez-Avila, M., Colditz, G., Stampfer, M., et al. (1991). Caffeine, moderate alcohol intake, and risk of fracture of the hip and forearm in middle-aged women. *American Journal of Clinical Nutrition, 54,* 157-163.

Hernandez-Peon, R. (1965). Central neuro-humoral transmission in sleep and wakefulness. *Progress in Brain Research, 18,* 96-117.

Herning, R., Glover, B., Koeppl, B., et al. (1990). Cognitive deficits in abstaining cocaine abusers. In J. Spencer & J. Boren (Eds.), *Residual effects of abused drugs on behavior.* NIDA Research Monograph 101.

Hersey, P. (1931). Emotional cycles of man. *Journal of Mental Science, 77,* 151-169.

Hertig, A. (1967). The overall problem in man. In K. Benirschke (Ed.), *Comparative aspects of reproductive failure.* Berlin: Springer-Verlag.

High Times Encyclopedia of Recreational Drugs. (1978). New York: Stonehill.

Higley, J., Hasert, M., Suomi, S., & Linnoila, M. (1991). Nonhuman primate model of alcohol abuse: Effects of early experience, personality, and stress on alcohol consumption. *Proceeding of the National Academy of Science, 88,* 7261-7265.

Hill, L., Nunn, A., & Fox, W. (1976). Matching quality of agents employed in "double-blind" controlled clinical trials. *Lancet, 1,* 352-356.

Hiller, S. (1991). A better way to make the medicine go down. *Science, 253,* 1095-1096.

Hilton, M. (1987). Drinking patterns and drinking problems in 1984: Results from a general population survey. *Alcoholism, 11,* 167-175.

Hilts, P. (1989, December 4). A guardian of U.S. health is failing under pressure. *The New York Times.*

Hingson, R., Alpert, J., Day, N., et al. (1982). Effects of maternal drinking and marijuana use on fetal growth and development. *Pediatrics, 70,* 539-546.

Hingson, R., & Howland, J. (1987). Alcohol as a risk factor for injury or death resulting from accidental falls: A review of the literature. *Journal of Studies on Alcohol, 48,* 212-219.

Hingson, R., Zuckerman, B., Amaro, H., et al. (1986). Maternal marijuana use and neonatal outcome. Uncertainty posed by self-reports. *American Journal of Public Health, 76,* 667-669.

Hinshaw, S. (1987). On the distinction between attentional deficits/hyperactivity and conduct problems/aggression in child psychopathology. *Psychological Bulletin, 101,* 443-463.

Hirsch, C. (1972). The dermatopathology of narcotic addiction. *Human Pathology, 3,* 45.

Hoff, A., Shukla, S., Helms, P., et al. (1990). The effects of nortriptyline on cognition in elderly depressed patients. *Journal of Clinical Psychopharmacology, 10,* 231-232.

Hoffeld, D., McNew, J., & Webster, R. (1968). Effect of tranquilizing drugs during pregnancy on activity of offspring. *Nature, 218,* 357-358.

Hogarty, G. (1976). Drug discontinuation among long-term, successfully maintained schizophrenic outpatients. *Diseases of the Nervous System, 37,* 494-500.

Hollister, L. (1986). Health aspects of cannabis. *Pharmacological Reviews, 38,* 1-20.

Hollister, L. (1988). Marijuana and immunity. *Journal of Psychoactive Drugs, 20,* 3-8.

Hollon, S., & Beck, A. (1987). Psychotherapy and drug therapy: Comparisons and combinations. In S. Garfield & A. Bergin (Eds.), *Handbook of psychotherapy and behavior change.* New York: John Wiley.

Hommer, D., Skolnick, P., & Paul, S. (1987). The benzodiazepine/GABA receptor complex and anxiety. In H. Meltzer (Ed.), *Pharmacology: The third generation of progress.* New York: Raven.

Honkanen, R., Ertama, L., Linnoila, M., et al. (1980). Role of drugs in traffic accidents. *British Medical Journal, 281,* 1309-1312.

Houston Chronicle. (1992, March 29).

Howard, J., Beckwith, L., & Rodning, C. (1990). Adaptive behavior in recovering female phencyclidine/polysubstance abusers. In J. Spencer & J. Boren (Eds.), *Residual effects of abused drugs on behavior.* NIDA Research Monograph 101.

Howard, J., Kropenske, V., & Tyler, R. (1986). The long-term effects on neurodevelopment in infants exposed prenatally to PCP. In D. Clouet (Ed.), *Phencyclidine: An update.* NIDA Research Monograph 64.

Howland, J., & Hingson, R. (1987). Alcohol as a risk factor for injuries or death due to fires and burns: Review of the literature. *Public Health Report, 102,* 475-483.

Hu, T., Swisher, J., McDonnell, N., & Stein, J. (1982). *Cost-effectiveness evaluations: A drug abuse prevention alternatives program* (Research Reports for Prevention Branch of NIDA). Rockville, MD: NIDA.

Hubbard, R., & Marsden, M. (1986). Relapse to use of heroin, cocaine, and other drugs in the first year after treatment. In F. Tims & C. Leukefeld (Eds.), *Relapse and recovery in drug abuse.* NIDA Research Monograph 72.

Hubbard, R., Marsden, M., Rachal, J., et al. (1989). *Drug abuse treatment: A national study of effectiveness*. Chapel Hill: University of North Carolina Press.

Hughes, J., Hatsukami, D., Mitchell, J., & Dahlgren, L. (1986). Prevalence of smoking among psychiatric outpatients. *American Journal of Psychiatry, 143,* 993-997.

Hughes, J., & Pierattini, R. (1992). An introduction to pharmacotherapy for mental disorders. In J. Grabowski & G. Vandenbos (Eds.), *Psychopharmacology: Basic mechanisms and applied interventions: Master lecturers in psychology.* Washington, DC: American Psychiatric Association.

Hughes, J., Stewart, M., & Barraclough, B. (1985). Why teetotallers abstain. *British Journal of Psychiatry, 146,* 204-208.

Hume, R., O'Donnell, K., Stanger, C., et al. (1989). In utero cocaine exposure: Observations of fetal behavioral state may predict neonatal outcome. *American Journal of Obstetrics and Gynecology, 161,* 685-690.

Hunt, H. (1956). Some effects of drugs on classical (type S) conditioning. *Annals of the New York Academy of Science, 65,* 258-267.

Hutchings, D., Brake, S., & Morgan, B. (1989). Animal studies of prenatal delta-9-tetrahydrocannabinol: Female embryolethality and effects on somatic and brain growth. *Annals of the New York Academy of Science, 562,* 133-144.

Huxley, A. (1963). *The doors of perception and heaven and hell.* New York: Harper & Row.

Hyyppa, M., Falck, S., & Rinne, U. (1975). Is L-dopa an aphrodisiac in patients with Parkinson's disease? In M. Sandler & G. Gessa (Eds.), *Sexual behavior: Pharmacology and biochemistry.* New York: Raven.

If at first you do succeed. (1991). [Editorial]. *Lancet, 337,* 650-651.

Inciardi, J. (1990). The crack-violence connection within a population of hardcore adolescent offenders. In M. De la Rosa, E. Lambert, & B. Gropper (Eds.), *Drugs and violence: Causes, correlates, and consequences.* NIDA Research Monograph 103.

Indian Hemp Drugs Commission. (1969). *Report of the Indian Hemp Drugs Commission.* Silver Springs, MD: Thomas Jefferson Publishing. [Original work published 1893-1894]

Innes, I., & Nickerson, M. (1965). Drugs acting on postganglionic adrenergic nerve endings and structures innervated by them (sympathomimetic drugs). In L. Goodman & A. Gilman (Eds.), *The pharmacological basis of therapeutics.* New York: Macmillan.

Institute of Medicine. (1990). *Treating drug problems*. Washington, DC: National Academy Press.

Irwin, P. (1985). Greater brain response of left-handers to drugs. *Neuropsychopharmacology, 23*, 61-67.

Irwin, S. (1966). Considerations for the pre-clinical evaluation of new psychiatric drugs: A case study with phenothiazine-like tranquilizers. *Psychopharmacology, 9*, 259-287.

Is there gender bias in drug testing? (1991, April 9-13). *FDA Consumer.*

Itil, T. (1976). Discrimination between some hypnotic and anxiolytic drugs by computer-analyzed sleep. In R. Williams & I. Karacan (Eds.), *Pharmacology of sleep*. New York: John Wiley.

Itil, T., Menon, G., Bozak, M., & Songar, A. (1982). The effects of oxiracetam (ISF-2522) in patients with organic brain syndrome. *Drug Development Research, 2*, 447-461.

Izumi, K. (1970). LSD and architectural design. In B. Aronson & H. Osmond (Eds.), *Psychedelics*. Garden City, NY: Doubleday.

Jacobs, B. (1987). How hallucinogenic drugs work. *American Scientist, 75*, 386-392.

Jacobson, B., Nyberg, K., Gronbladh, L., et al. (1990). Opiate addiction in adult offspring through possible imprinting after obstetric treatment. *British Medical Journal, 301*, 1067-1070.

Jaffe, J. (1965). Narcotic analgesics. In L. Goodman & A. Gilman (Eds.), *The pharmacological basis of therapeutics*. New York: Macmillan.

Jaffe, J. (1984). Evaluating drug abuse treatment: A comment on the state of the art. In F. Tims & J. Ludford (Eds.), *Drug abuse treatment evaluation: Strategies, progress, and prospects*. NIDA Research Monograph 51.

Jaffe, J. (1990). Drug addiction and drug abuse. In A. Gilman, T. Rall, A. Nies, & P. Taylor (Eds.), *The pharmacological basis of therapeutics*. Elmsford, NY: Pergamon.

James, I. (1976). Prescribing for the elderly: Why it's best to keep it simple. *Modern Geriatrics, 6*, 25-28.

Janiger, O., & De Rios, M. (1989). LSD and creativity. *Journal of Psychoactive Drugs, 21*, 129-134.

Jarvik, M. (1965). Drugs used in the treatment of psychiatric disorders. In L. Goodman & A. Gilman (Eds.), *The pharmacological basis of therapeutics*. New York: Macmillan.

Jarvik, M. (1991). Beneficial effects of nicotine. *British Journal of Addiction, 86,* 571-575.

Jarvik, M., Flinn, D., & West, L. (1976). Psychopharmacological treatment of schizophrenia. In L. West & D. Flinn (Eds.), *Treatment of schizophrenia.* New York: Grune & Stratton.

Jarvik, M., & Henningfield, J. (1988). Pharmacological treatment of tobacco dependence. *Pharmacology, Biochemistry, and Behavior, 30,* 379-394.

Jenike, M., Hyman, S., Baer, L., et al. (1990). A controlled trial of fluvoxamine in obsessive-compulsive disorder: Implications for a serotonergic theory. *American Journal of Psychiatry, 147,* 1209-1215.

Joffe, J. (1979). Influence of drug exposure of the father on perinatal outcome. *Clinics in Perinatology, 6,* 21-36.

Joffe, J., Peruzovic, M., & Milkovic, K. (1990). Progeny of male rats treated with methadone: Physiological and behavioural effects. *Mutation Research, 229,* 201-211.

Johanson, C., & Balster, R. (1978). A summary of the results of a drug self-administration study using substitution procedures in rhesus monkeys. *Bulletin on Narcotics, 30,* 43-54.

Johanson, C., Balster, R., & Bonese, K. (1976). Self-administration of psychomotor stimulant drugs; the effects of unlimited access. *Pharmacology, Biochemistry, and Behavior, 4,* 45-51.

Johnsgaard, K. (1989). *The exercise prescription for depression and anxiety.* New York: Plenum.

Johnson, B., Goldstein, P., Preble, E., et al. (1985). *Taking care of business: The economics of crime by heroin abusers.* Lexington, MA: Lexington Books.

Johnson, G. (1969). LSD in the treatment of alcoholism. *American Journal of Psychiatry, 126,* 481-487.

Johnston, L., & O'Malley, P. (1986). Why do the nation's students use drugs and alcohol? Self-reported reasons from nine national surveys. *Journal of Drug Issues, 16,* 29-66.

Johnstone, E., & Meersch, W. (1973). Acetylator status and response to phenelzine in depressed patients. *Lancet, 1,* 567-570.

Jones, B. (1973). Memory impairment on the ascending and descending limbs of the blood alcohol curve. *Journal of Abnormal Psychology, 82,* 24-32.

Jones, B., & Jones, M. (1976). Alcohol effects in women during the menstrual cycle. *Annals of the New York Academy of Science, 273,* 576-587.

Jones, B., & Vega, A. (1971). Cognitive performance measured on the ascending and descending limb of the blood alcohol curve. *Psychopharmacology, 23,* 99-114.

Jones, K., & Smith, D. (1973). Recognition of the fetal alcohol syndrome in early infancy. *Lancet, 2,* 999-1001.

Jones, R. (1983). Cannabis tolerance and dependence. In K. Fehr & H. Kalant (Eds.), *Cannabis and health hazards.* Toronto: Addiction Research Foundation.

Jones, R. (1990). The pharmacology of cocaine smoking in humans. *NIDA Research Monograph, 99,* 30-41.

Jones, R. (1992). Alternative strategies. In *Cocaine: Scientific and social dimensions.* Ciba Foundation Symposium 166. New York: John Wiley.

Joyce, P., & Paykel, E. (1989). Predictors of drug response in depression. *Archives of General Psychiatry, 46,* 89-99.

Julien, R. (1992). *A primer of drug action.* New York: Freeman.

Jurich, A., & Polson, C. (1984). Reasons for drug use: Comparison of drug users and abusers. *Psychological Reports, 55,* 371-378.

Just what the patient ordered. (1990, May 28). *Time,* p. 42.

Kahn, A. (1991). Menstrual cycle important factor when prescribing psychotropic drugs. *Psychiatric News,* p. 24.

Kahn, D. (1990). Current trends in short-term therapeutic approaches to panic disorder. *International Journal of Short-Term Psychotherapy, 5,* 211-245.

Kahn, J., Stevenson, E., Topol, P., & Klein, D. (1986). Agitated depression, alprazolam, and panic anxiety. *American Journal of Psychiatry, 143,* 1172-1173.

Kalat, J. (1992). *Biological psychology.* Belmont, CA: Wadsworth.

Kales, A., Manfredi, R., Vgontzas, A., et al. (1991). Rebound insomnia after only brief and intermittent use of rapidly eliminated benzodiazepines. *Clinical Pharmacology and Therapeutics, 49,* 468-476.

Kales, J., Tan, T., Swearingen, C., & Kales, A. (1971). Are over-the-counter sleep medications effective? All-night EEG studies. *Current Therapeutic Research, 13,* 143-151.

Kalinowsky, L. (1958). Appraisal of the "tranquilizers" and their influence on other somatic treatments in psychiatry. *American Journal of Psychiatry, 115,* 294-300.

Kalow, W. (1967). Pharmacogenetics and the predictability of drug responses. In G. Wolstenholme & R. Porter (Eds.), *Drug response in man*. Boston: Little, Brown.

Kamb, M., Murphy, J., Jones, J., et al. (1992). Eosinophilia-myalgia syndrome in L-tryptophan-exposed patients. *Journal of the American Medical Association, 267*, 77-82.

Kandel, D. (Ed.). (1978). *Longitudinal research on drug use: Empirical findings and methodological issues*. Washington, DC: Hemisphere.

Kandel, D. (1982). Epidemiological and psychosocial perspectives on adolescent drug use. *Journal of the American Academy of Clinical Psychiatry, 21*, 328-347.

Kane, J. (1987). Treatment of schizophrenia. *Schizophrenia Bulletin, 13*, 133-157.

Kane, J., & Lieberman, J. (1984). The efficacy of amoxapine, maprotiline and trazodone in comparison to imipramine and amitriptyline: A review of the literature. *Psychopharmacology Bulletin, 20*, 240-249.

Kaplan, J., Manuck, S., & Shively, C. (1991). The effects of fat and cholesterol on social behavior in monkeys. *Psychosomatic Medicine, 53*, 634-642.

Karno, M., Golding, J., Sorenson, S., & Burnam, M. (1988). The epidemiology of obsessive-compulsive disorder in five US communities. *Archives of General Psychiatry, 45*, 1094-1099.

Karon, B. (1989). Psychotherapy versus medication for schizophrenia: Empirical comparisons. In S. Fisher & R. Greenberg (Eds.), *The limits of biological treatments for psychological distress*. Hillsdale, NJ: Lawrence Erlbaum.

Katz, J., & Halstead, W. (1950). Protein organization and mental function. *Comparative Psychological Monographs, 20*, 1-38.

Katz, R., DeVeaugh-Geiss, J., & Landau, P. (1990). Clomipramine in obsessive-compulsive disorder. *Biological Psychiatry, 28*, 401-414.

Kaufman, E., & McNaul, J. (1992). Recent developments in understanding and treating drug abuse and dependence. *Hospital and Community Psychiatry, 43*, 223-236.

Kay, D. (1975a). Human sleep and EEG through a cycle of methadone dependence. *Electroencephalography and Clinical Neurophysiology, 38*, 35-43.

Kay, D. (1975b). Human sleep during chronic morphine intoxication. *Psychopharmacology, 44*, 117-124.

Kay, D. (1979). Opioid effects on computer-derived sleep and EEG parameters in nondependent human addicts. *Sleep, 2*, 175-191.

Keith, J., & Rudy, J. (1990). Why NMDA-receptor-dependent long-term potentiation may not be a mechanism of learning and memory: Reappraisal of the NMDA-receptor blockade strategy. *Psychobiology, 18,* 251-257.

Kellam, S., & Brown, H. (1982). *Social adaptational and psychological antecedents to adolescent psychopathology ten years later.* Baltimore, MD: Johns Hopkins University Press.

Kellog, C., & Guillet, R. (1988). Developmental effects of neuroactive drugs. In D. Scarpelli & G. Migaki (Eds.), *Transplacental effects on fetal health.* New York: Alan R. Liss.

Kelly, J. (1990, December 20). Senator: Survey "wildly off the mark." *USA Today.*

Kelly, J., & Cavanaugh, J. (1982). Treatment of the sexually dangerous patient. In J. Masserman (Ed.), *Current psychiatric therapies, Vol. 21.* New York: Grune & Stratton.

Kendler, K., Heath, A., Neale, M., et al. (1992). A population-based twin study of alcoholism in women. *Journal of the American Medical Association, 268,* 1877-1882.

Kennard, D., & Wilson, S. (1979). The modification of personality disturbance in a therapeutic community for drug abusers. *British Journal of Medical Psychology, 52,* 215-221.

Kerekjarto, M. (1968). The influence of experimenter's sex on drug effects in normal subjects. In K. Rickels (Ed.), *Non-specific factors in drug therapy.* Springfield, IL: Charles C Thomas.

Kessler, D. (1991). Drug promotion and scientific exchange. The role of the clinical investigator. *The New England Journal of Medicine, 325,* 201-203.

Khanna, J. (1989). The nature of alcohol tolerance: The role of neurotransmitters. *Proceedings of the Indo-US Symposium on Alcohol and Drug Abuse* (NIMHANS Pub. No. 20). Washington, DC: Government Printing Office.

Khanna, J., Le, A., Kalant, H., & LeBlanc, A. (1979). Cross-tolerance between ethanol and morphine with respect to their hypothermic effects. *European Journal of Pharmacology, 59,* 145-149.

Khantzian, E. (1985). The self-medication hypothesis of addictive disorders: Focus on heroin and cocaine dependence. *American Journal of Psychiatry, 142,* 1259-1264.

Khatena, J. (1977). Creative imagination and what we can do to stimulate it. *Gifted Child Quarterly, 21,* 87-96.

Kim, H., Delva, N., & Lawson, J. (1990). Prophylactic medication for unipolar depressive illness: The place of lithium carbonate in combination with antidepressant medication. *Canadian Journal of Psychiatry, 35,* 107-114.

King, D., & Mandell, M. (1978). *A double-blind study of allergic cerebral-viscerosomatic malfunctions evoked by provocative sublingual challenges with allergenic extracts.* Paper presented at 12th Advanced Seminar of Clinical Ecology, Key Biscayne, FL.

Kinsley, M. (1990, April 4). TRB: Regrets only. *New Republic,* p. 49.

Klamt, R. (1973). Homicide and LSD. *Journal of the American Medical Association, 224,* 246.

Klatsky, A., Armstrong, M., & Friedman, G. (1992). Alcohol and mortality. *Annals of Internal Medicine, 117,* 646-654.

Klatsky, A., Armstrong, M., & Friedman, G. (1993). Coffee, tea, and mortality. *Annals of Epidemiology, 3,* 375-381.

Kleiman, M., & Doblin, R. (1991). Marijuana as antiemetic medicine: A survey of oncologists' experiences and attitudes. *Journal of Clinical Oncology, 9,* 1314-1319.

Kleinman, D., & Cohen, L. (1991). The decontextualization of mental illness: The portrayal of work in psychiatric drug advertisements. *Social Science and Medicine, 32,* 867-874.

Kleinman, P., Lukoff, I., & Kail, B. (1977). The magic fix: A critical analysis of methadone maintenance treatment. *Social Problems, 25,* 208-214.

Kleitman, N. (1963). *Sleep and wakefulness.* Chicago: University of Chicago Press.

Klepfisz, A., & Racy, J. (1973). Homicide and LSD. *Journal of the American Medical Association, 223,* 429-430.

Klerman, G. (1970). Clinical efficacy and actions of anti-psychotics. In A. DiMascio & R. Shrader (Eds.), *Clinical handbook of psychopharmacology.* New York: Science House.

Klerman, G. (1986). The National Institute of Mental Health Epidemiologic Catchment Area (NIMH-ECA) program. Background, preliminary findings and implications. *Social Psychiatry, 21,* 159-166.

Klerman, G., Ballenger, J., Burrows, G., et al. (1989). In reply. *Archives of General Psychiatry, 46,* 670-672.

Kline, N. (1959). The challenge of the psychopharmaceuticals. *American Philosophical Society, 103,* 455-462.

Kline, N., & Cooper, T. (1975). Evaluation of lithium therapy in alcoholism. In J. Sinclair & K. Kiianmaa (Eds.), *The effects of centrally active drugs on voluntary alcohol consumption.* Helsinki: Kauppakirjapaino.

Klonoff, H. (1974). Marijuana and driving in real-life situations. *Science, 186,* 317-324.

Knupfer, G. (1987). Drinking for health: The daily light drinker myth. *British Journal of Addiction, 82,* 547-555.

Koff, W. (1974). Marijuana and sexual activity. *Journal of Sex Research, 10,* 194-204.

Kohler, W. (1969). *The task of gestalt psychology.* Princeton, NJ: Princeton University Press.

Kohn, A. (1986). *False prophets.* New York: Basil Blackwell.

Kolansky, H., & Moore, W. (1971). Effects of marihuana on adolescents and young adults. *Journal of the American Medical Association, 216,* 486-492.

Kolata, G. (cited in *Oakland Tribune,* 1991, from *New York Times* article) "Fast track AIDS drug OK by FDA seen as milestone."

Kolb, L. (1962). *Drug addiction: A medical problem.* Springfield, IL: Charles C Thomas.

Kolodny, R., Master, W., Johnson, V., & Biggs, M. (1979). Drugs and sex. In *Textbook of human sexuality for nurses.* Boston: Little, Brown.

Kopelman, M. (1987). Amnesia: Organic and psychogenic. *British Journal of Psychiatry, 150,* 428-442.

Koranyi, E. (1980). Somatic illness in psychiatric patients. *Psychosomatics, 21,* 887-891.

Koren, G., Graham, K., Shear, H., & Einarson, T. (1989). Bias against the null hypothesis: The reproductive hazards of cocaine. *Lancet, 2,* 1440-1442.

Kornetsky, C. (1959). The effects of dextroamphetamine on behavioural deficits produced by sleep loss in humans. *Journal of Pharmacology and Experimental Therapeutics, 127,* 46-50.

Kornetsky, C. (1960). Alterations in psychomotor functions and individual differences in responses produced by psychoactive drugs. In L. Uhr & J. Miller (Eds.), *Drugs and behavior.* New York: John Wiley.

Korngold, M. (1963). LSD and the creative experience. *Psychoanalitic Review, 50,* 682-685.

Koster, A., & Garde, K. (1993). Sexual desire and menopausal development. A prospective study of Danish women born in 1936. *Maturitas, 16,* 49-60.

Kotin, J., Wilbert, D., Verburg, D., et al. (1976). Thioridazine and sexual dysfunction. *American Journal of Psychiatry, 133,* 82-85.

Kramlinger, K., & Post, R. (1989). The addition of lithium carbamazepine. Antidepressant efficacy in treatment-resistant depression. *Archives of General Psychiatry, 46,* 794-800.

Kreek, M. (1990). Immune function in heroin addicts and former heroin addicts in treatment: Pre- and post-AIDS epidemic. In *Drugs of abuse: Chemistry, pharmacology, immunology, and AIDS.* NIDA Research Monograph 96.

Kreek, M. (1991). Using methadone effectively: Achieving goals by application of laboratory, clinical, and evaluation research and by development of innovative programs. In R. Pickens, C. Leukefeld, & C. Schuster (Eds.), *Improving drug abuse treatment.* NIDA Research Monograph 106.

Kripke, D., Simons, R., Garfinkel, L., & Hammond, E. (1979). Short and long sleep and sleeping pills: Is increased mortality associated? *Archives of General Psychiatry, 36,* 103-116.

Krippner, S. (1968). The psychedelic artist. In R. Masters & J. Houston (Eds.), *Psychedelic art.* New York: Grove.

Krippner, S. (1985). Psychedelic drugs and creativity. *Journal of Psychoactive Drugs, 17,* 235-245.

Kristein, M. (1983). How much can business expect to profit from smoking cessation. *Preventive Medicine, 12,* 358-381.

Kuhar, M., Ritz, M., & Boja, J. (1991). The dopamine hypothesis of the reinforcing properties of cocaine. *Trends in Neuroscience, 14,* 299-302.

Kumpfer, K. (1987). *Prevention services for children of substance-abusing parents* (NIDA final technical report, R18DA02758-101/02). Rockville, MD: NIDA.

Kupfer, D., & Spiker, D. (1981). Refractory depression: Prediction of nonresponse by clinical indicators. *Journal of Clinical Psychiatry, 42,* 302-312.

Kupfer, D., Spiker, D., Coble, P., et al. (1978). Amitriptyline and EEG sleep in depressed patients: I. Drug effect. *Sleep, 1,* 149-159.

Kurata, J., Elashoff, J., Nogawa, A., & Haile, B. (1986). Sex and smoking differences in duodenal ulcer mortality. *American Journal of Public Health, 76,* 700-702.

Kushner, M., Sher, K., & Beitman, B. (1990). The relation between alcohol problems and the anxiety disorders. *American Journal of Psychiatry, 147,* 685-695.

Kutner, S., & Brown, S. (1972). History of depression as a risk factor for depression with oral contraceptives and discontinuance. *Journal of Nervous and Mental Diseases, 155,* 163-169.

LaBarre, W. (1975). Anthropological perspectives on hallucination and hallucinogens. In R. Siegel & L. West (Eds.), *Hallucinations: Behavior, experience and theory.* New York: John Wiley.

LaCroix, A., Mead, L., Liang, K., et al. (1986). Coffee consumption and the incidence of coronary heart disease. *The New England Journal of Medicine, 315,* 977-982.

Ladewig, D. (1983). Abuse of benzodiazepine in western European society—incidence and prevalence, motives, drug acquisition. *Pharmacopsychiatria, 16,* 103-106.

Lake, C., Rosenberg, D., & Quirk, R. (1990). Phenylpropanolamine and caffeine use among diet center clients. *International Journal of Obesity, 14,* 575-582.

Langevin, R., Ben-Aron, M., Coulthard, R., et al. (1985). The effect of alcohol on penile erection. In R. Langevin (Ed.), *Erotic preference, gender identity, and aggression in men.* Hillsdale, NJ: Lawrence Erlbaum.

Langevin, T. (1991). The role of implanted systems in the control of temporal drug delivery. In W. Hrushesky, R. Langer, & F. Theeuwes (Eds.), *Temporal control of drug delivery.* New York: New York Academy of Sciences.

Lasagna, L. (1972). Research, regulation and development of new pharmaceuticals: Past, present, and future. *American Journal of Medical Science, 263,* 8-18, 66-78.

Lasagna, L., & von Felsinger, J. (1954). The volunteer subject in research. *Science, 120,* 359-361.

Lashley, K. (1917). The effect of strychnine and caffeine upon rate of learning. *Psychobiology, 1,* 141-170.

Laties, V. (1961). Modification of affect, social behavior and performance by sleep deprivation and drugs. *Journal of Psychiatric Research, 1,* 12-25.

Leake, C., & Silverman, M. (1966). *Alcoholic beverages in clinical medicine.* Cleveland, OH: World.

Leary, T. (1968). *The politics of ecstasy.* New York: Putnam.

Leathwood, P. (1989). Nutritional modulation of neurotransmitter metabolism. In J. Kinney & P. Borum (Eds.), *Perspectives in clinical nutrition.* Baltimore, MD: Urban & Schwarzenberg.

Leavitt, F. (1991). *Research methods for behavioral scientists.* Madison, WI: William C. Brown.

Lee, C., & Chiang, N. (1985). Appendix—Maternal-fetal transfer of abused substances: Pharmacokinetic and pharmacodynamic data. In C. Lee & N. Chiang (Eds.), *Prenatal drug exposure: Kinetics and dynamics.* NIDA Research Monograph 60.

Lefton, L. (1991). *Psychology.* Needham Heights, MA: Allyn & Bacon.

Lehmann, H. (1970). The philosophy of long-acting medication in psychiatry. *Diseases of the Nervous System, 31,* 7-9.

Lehmann, H. (1966). Individual differences in response to pharmacotherapy. In J. Wittenborn & P. May (Eds.), *Prediction of response to pharmacotherapy.* Springfield, IL: Charles C Thomas.

Lemere, F. (1966). The danger of amphetamine dependency. *American Journal of Psychiatry, 123,* 569-572.

Leon, G. (1991). Retention in drug-free therapeutic communities. In R. Pickens, C. Leukefeld, & C. Schuster (Eds.), *Improving drug abuse treatment.* NIDA Research Monograph 106.

Leonhard, B. (1992). *Fundamentals of psychopharmacology.* West Sussex: John Wiley.

Lerner, S., & Burns, R. (1978). Phencyclidine use among youth: History, epidemiology, and acute and chronic intoxication. In R. Petersen & R. Stillman (Eds.), *Phencyclidine PCP abuse: An appraisal.* NIDA Research Monograph 21.

Lerner, S., & Burns, R. (1986). Legal issues associated with PCP abuse—The role of the forensic expert. In D. Clouet (Ed), *Phencyclidine: An update.* NIDA Research Monograph 64.

Lesar, T., Briceland, L., Delcoure, K., et al. (1990). Medication prescribing errors in a teaching hospital. *Journal of the American Medical Association, 263,* 2329-2334.

Lesko, L., Stotland, N., & Segraves, R. (1982). Three cases of female anorgasmia associated with MAOIs. *American Journal of Psychiatry, 139,* 1353-1354.

Leslie, A. (1954). Ethics and practice of placebo therapy. *American Journal of Medicine, 16,* 854-862.

Leukefeld, D., & Bukoski, W. (1991). *Drug abuse prevention intervention research: Methodological issues.* NIDA Research Monograph Series 107.

Levin, R. (1987). Principles of drug disposition and therapy in neonates, infants, and children. In A. Rudolph & J. Hoffman (Eds.), *Pediatrics*. Norwalk, CT: Appleton & Lange.

Levy, G. (1992). Publication bias: Its implications for clinical pharmacology. *Clinical Pharmacology and Therapeutics, 52,* 115-119.

Lewy, A., Sack, R., Singer, C., et al. (1988). Winter depression and the phase-shift hypothesis for bright light's therapeutic effects: History, theory, and experimental evidence. *Journal of Biological Rythms, 3,* 121-134.

Lieberman, H., Wurtman, R., Emde, G., et al. (1987). The effects of low doses of caffeine on human performance and mood. *Psychopharmacology, 92,* 308-312.

Lifschitz, M., & Wilson, G. (1991). Patterns of growth and development in narcotic-exposed children. In M. Kilbey & K. Asghar (Eds.), *Methodological issues in controlled studies on effects of prenatal exposure to drug abuse*. NIDA Research Monograph 114.

Lijinsky, W. (1977). *Identification of toxic substances as carcinogens by testing in animals*. Proceedings of the Second Annual Toxic Substances Control Conference, Washington, DC.

Lin, K., Poland, R., Nuccio, I., et al. (1989). A longitudinal assessment of haloperidol doses and serum concentrations in Asian and Caucasian schizophrenic patients. *American Journal of Psychiatry, 146,* 1307-1311.

Lindenbaum, J., Mellow, M., Blackstone, M., et al. (1971). Variation in biologic availability of digoxin from four preparations. *The New England Journal of Medicine, 285,* 1344-1347.

Lindqvist, P. (1991). Homicides committed by abusers of alcohol and illicit drugs. *British Journal of Addiction, 86,* 321-326.

Links, P., Boyle, M., & Offord, D. (1989). The prevalence of emotional disorder in children. *Journal of Nervous and Mental Disease, 177,* 85-91.

Linnoila, M., Erwin, C., & Logue, P. (1980). Efficacy and side effects of flurazepam and a combination of amobarbital and secobarbital on insomniac patients. *Journal of Clinical Pharmacology, 20,* 117-122.

Lipman, R. (1989). Pharmacotherapy of the anxiety disorders. In S. Fisher & R. Greenberg (Eds.), *The limits of biological treatments for psychological distress*. Hillsdale, NJ: Lawrence Erlbaum.

Lipman, R., Park, L., & Rickels, K. (1966). Paradoxical influence of a therapeutic side effect interpretation. *Archives of General Psychiatry, 15,* 462-474.

Lipscomb, W. (1976). Quoted in *Psychiatric News*, April 1976, p. 1.

Lipton, M., & Burnett, G. (1979). Pharmacological treatment of schizophrenia. In L. Bellak (Ed.), *Disorders of the schizophrenic syndrome.* New York: Basic Books.

Lockwood, A. (1989). Medical problems of musicians. *The New England Journal of Medicine, 320,* 221-226.

Logan, J. (1978). *Movie stars, real people, and me.* New York: Delacorte.

Lolli, G. (1962). Role of wine in treatment of obesity. *New York Journal of Medicine, 62,* 3438-3443.

Lomberg, J. (1983). The tripping eye. In L. Grinspoon & J. Bakalar (Eds.), *Psychedelic reflections.* New York: Human Sciences Press.

Longo, V., & de Carolis, A. (1968). Anticholinergic hallucinogens: Laboratory results versus clinical trials. In P. Bradley & M. Fink (Eds.), *Anticholinergic drugs and brain functions in animals and man.* Amsterdam: Elsevier.

Lorenzo, A., Fernandez, C., & Roth, L. (1965). Physiologically induced alteration of sulfate penetration into brain. *Archives of Neurology, 12,* 128-132.

Lost tribes, lost knowledge. (1991, September 23). *Time,* pp. 46-56.

Louria, D. (1968). *The drug scene.* New York: McGraw-Hill.

Lowe, G. (1981). State-dependent recall decrements with moderate doses of alcohol. *Current Psychological Research, 1,* 3-8.

Lowe, G. (1988). State-dependent retrieval effects with social drugs. In M. Gruneberg, P. Morris, & R. Sykes (Eds.), *Practical aspects of memory: Current research and issues.* New York: John Wiley.

Lowinger, P. (1975). Speaking in film *Do no harm.* Health Education Media Inc.

Luchins, A. (1946). Classroom experiments on mental set. *American Journal of Psychology, 59,* 295-298.

Ludwig, A. (1990). Alcohol input and creative output. *British Journal of Addiction, 85,* 953-963.

Lue, T. (1988). Impotence: New concepts regarding therapy. In M. Resnick (Ed.), *Current trends in urology, Vol. 4.* Baltimore, MD: Williams & Wilkins.

Lutwak-Mann, C. (1964). Observations of progeny of thalidomide-treated male rabbits. *British Medical Journal, 1,* 1090-1091.

Lyons, T., & French, J. (1991). Modafinil: The unique properties of a new stimulant. *Aviation, Space, & Environmental Medicine, 62,* 432-435.

MacFarlane, C., Reynolds, W., & Rosencrantz, D. (1983). Yohimbine an alternative treatment for erectile dysfunction. *Weekly Urology Clinic Letter,* p. 27.

Maddux, J., & Desmond, D. (1982). Residence relocation inhibits opioid dependence. *Archives of General Psychiatry, 39,* 1313-1317.

Madrid, Y., Feigenbaum, L., Brem, H., & Langer, R. (1991). New directions in the delivery of drugs and other substances to the central nervous system. In J. August, M. Anders, & F. Murad (Eds.), *Advances in pharmacology, Vol. 22.* New York: Academic Press.

Magura, S., Goldsmith, D., Casriel, C., et al. (1987). The validity of methadone clients' self-reported drug use. *International Journal of Addictions, 22,* 727-749.

Malcolm, R., Currey, H., Mitchell, M., & Keil, J. (1986). Silver acetate gum as a deterrent to smoking. *Chest, 90,* 107-111.

Mandell, A., Spooner, C., & Brunet, D. (1969). Whither the "sleep transmitter"? *Biological Psychiatry, 1,* 13-30.

Mann, K., Abbott, E., Gray, J., et al. (1982). Sexual dysfunction with B-blocker therapy: More common than we think? *Sexuality and Disability, 5,* 67-77.

Mann, R., Smart, R., Anglin, L., & Adlaf, E. (1991). Reductions in cirrhosis deaths in the United States: Associations with per capita consumption and AA membership. *Journal of Studies on Alcohol, 52,* 361-365.

Manning, C., Hall, J., & Gold, P. (1990). Glucose effects on memory and other neuropsychological tests in elderly humans. *Psychology and Science, 1,* 307-311.

Manning, C., Parsons, M., & Gold, P. (1992). Anterograde and retrograde enhancement of 24-hour memory by glucose in elderly humans. *Behavioral Neural Biology, 58,* 125-130.

Marder, S. (1979). Predicting drug-free improvement in schizophrenic psychosis. *Archives of General Psychiatry, 36,* 1080-1085.

Margraf, J., Ehlers, A., Roth, W., et al. (1991). How "blind" are double-blind studies? *Journal of Consulting Clinical Psychology, 59,* 184-187.

Marholin, D., & Phillips, D. (1976). Methodological issues in psychopharmacological research: Chlorpromaxine—A case in point. *American Journal of Orthopsychiatry, 46,* 477-495.

Marks, I., De Albuquerque, A., Cottraux, J., et al. (1989). The "efficacy" of alprazolam in panic disorder and agoraphobia: A critique of recent reports. *Archives of General Psychiatry, 46,* 668-670.

Marlatt, G., & Gordon, J. (1980). Determinants of relapse: Implication for the maintenance of behavior change. In P. Davidson & S. Davidson (Eds.), *Behavioral medicine: Changing lifestyles.* New York: Bruner/Mazel.

Marlatt, A., & Rohsenow, D. (1981). The think-drink effect. *Psychology Today, 93,* pp. 60-69.

Martin, B., Dewey, W., & Harris, L. (1984). Pharmacological activity of delta-9-THC metabolites and analogs of CBD, delta-8-THC and delta-9-THC. In S. Agurell, W. Dewey, & R. Willette (Eds.), *The cannabinoids: Chemical, pharmacologic and therapeutic aspects.* New York: Academic Press.

Martin, M., & Edmonds, L. (1991). Use of birth defects monitoring programs for assessing the effects of maternal substance abuse on pregnancy outcomes. In M. Kilbey & K. Asghar (Eds.), *Methodological issues in controlled studies on effects of prenatal exposure to drug abuse.* NIDA Research Monograph 114.

Martin, M., Owen, C., & Morisha, J. (1987). An overview of neurotransmitters and neuroreceptors. In R. Hales & S. Yudofsky (Eds.), *Textbook of psychiatry.* Washington, DC: American Psychiatric Press.

Martin, T., & Bracken, M. (1987). The association between low birth weight and caffeine consumption during pregnancy. *American Journal of Epidemiology, 126,* 813-821.

Martindale, C., Hines, D., Mitchell, L., & Covell, E. (1984). EEG alpha asymmetry and creativity. *Personality and Individual Differences, 5,* 77-86.

Martinez, J. (1986). Memory: Drugs and hormones. In J. Martinez & R. Kesner (Eds.), *Learning and memory.* New York: Academic Press.

Martinez, J., Schulteis, G., & Weinberger, S. (1991). How to increase and decrease the strength of memory traces: The effects of drugs and hormones. In J. Martinez & R. Kesner (Eds.), *Learning and memory.* New York: Academic Press.

Martinez, J., Vasquez, B., Rigter, H., et al. (1980). Attenuation of amphetamine-induced enhancement of learning by adrenal demedullation. *Brain Research, 195,* 433-443.

Mason, J., Langenbach, R., Shelby, M., et al. (1990). Ability of short-term tests to predict carcinogenesis in rodents. *Annual Review of Pharmacology, 30,* 149-168.

Mason, A., Nerviano, V., & DeBurger, R. (1977). Patterns of antipsychotic drug use in four southeastern state hospitals. *Diseases of the Nervous System, 38,* 541-545.

Masters, R., & Houston, J. (1968). *Psychedelic art.* New York: Grove.

Masters, W., & Johnson, V. (1970). *Human sexual inadequacy.* Boston: Little, Brown.

Mathis, J. (1970). Sexual aspects of heroin addiction. *Medical Aspects of Human Sex, 4,* 98-109.

Maugh, T. (1977). Drinkers rejoice: A little wine may kill your virus. *Science, 196,* 1074.

Maugh, T. (1978). Chemical carcinogens: The scientific basis for regulation. *Science, 201,* 1200-1205.

May, P. (1968). *Treatment of schizophrenia.* New York: Science House.

Mayfield, D., McLeod, G., & Hall, P. (1974). The CAGE questionnaire: Validation of a new alcoholism screening instrument. *American Journal of Psychiatry, 131,* 1121-1123.

McBride, W., Murphy, J., Lumeng, L., & Li, T. (1988). Effects of Ro 15-4513, fluoxetine and desipramine on the intake of ethanol, water and food by the alcohol-preferring (P) and -nonpreferring (NP) lines of rats. *Pharmacology, Biochemistry, and Behavior, 30,* 1045-1050.

McCarron, M., Schulze, B., Thompson, G., et al. (1981). Acute phencyclidine intoxication: Incidence of clinical findings in 1,000 cases. *Annals of Emergency Medicine, 10,* 237-242.

McCarthy, T. (1974). Chemical incompatibility of parenteral drug admixtures. *South African Medical Journal, 48,* 1951-1953.

McCoy, N., & Davidson, J. (1985). A longitudinal study of the effects of menopause on sexuality. *Maturitas, 7,* 203-211.

McCoy, N., Cutler, W., & Davidson, J. (1985). Relationships among sexual behavior, hot flashes, and hormone levels in perimenopausal women. *Archives of Sexual Behavior, 14,* 385-394.

McGaugh, J. (1973). Drug facilitation of learning and memory. *Annual Review of Psychopharmacology, 13,* 229-241.

McGlothlin, W., Cohen, S., & McGlothlin, M. (1969). Long-lasting effects of LSD on normals. In J. Cole & J. Wittenborn (Eds.), *Drug abuse.* Springfield, IL: Charles C Thomas.

McGowan, J., Altman, R., & Kanto, W. (1988). Neonatal withdrawal symptoms after chronic maternal ingestion of caffeine. *Southern Medicine, 81,* 1092-1094.

McGuiness, D. (1989). Attention deficit disorder: The emperor's clothes, animal "pharm," and other fiction. In S. Fisher & R. Greenberg (Eds.), *The limits of biological treatments for psychological distress.* Hillsdale, NJ: Lawrence Erlbaum.

McGuire, W. (1985). Attitudes and attitude change. In G. Lindzey & E. Aronson (Eds.), *Handbook of social psychology, Vol. 2.* New York: Random House.

McIntosh, T., Vallano, M., & Barfield, R. (1980). Effects of morphine, B-endorphin and naloxone on catecholamine levels and sexual behavior in male rats. *Pharmacology, Biochemistry, and Behavior, 13,* 435-441.

McKirnan, D., & Johnson, T. (1986). Alcohol and drug use among "street" adolescents. *Addictive Behaviors, 11,* 201-205.

McLellan, A., Woody, G., & O'Brien, C. (1979). Development of psychiatric disorders in drug abusers. *The New England Journal of Medicine, 301,* 1310-1314.

McLellan, T., & Alterman, A. (1991). Patient treatment matching: A conceptual and methodological review with suggestions for future research. In R. Pickens, C. Leukefeld, & C. Schuster (Eds.), *Improving drug abuse treatment.* NIDA Research Monograph 106.

McWilliams, S., & Tuttle, R. (1973). Long-term psychological effects of LSD. *Psychological Bulletin, 79,* 341-351.

Mehta, K., Sorofman, B., & Rowland, C. (1989). Prescription drug advertising trends: A study of oral hypoglycemics. *Social Science and Medicine, 29,* 853-857.

Melander, A. (1978). Influence of food on the bioavailability of drugs. *Clinical Pharmacokinetics, 3,* 337-351.

Mellinger, G., Balter, M., & Uhlenhuth, E. (1984). Prevalence and correlates of the long-term regular use of anxiolytics. *Journal of the American Medical Association, 251,* 375-379.

Mellinger, G., Balter, M., & Uhlenhuth, E. (1985). Insomnia and its treatment. Prevalence and correlates. *Archives of General Psychiatry, 42,* 225-232.

Mello, N. (1975). A semantic aspect of alcoholism. In H. Cappell & A. LeBlanc (Eds.), *Biological and behavioural approaches to drug dependence.* Toronto: Addiction Research Foundation.

Mello, N. (1992). Behavioral strategies for the evaluation of new pharmacotherapies for drug abuse treatment. In L. Harris (Ed.), *Problems of drug dependence 1991.* NIDA Research Monograph 119.

Mello, N., Mendelson, J., Bree, M., & Lukas, S. (1989). Buprenorphine suppresses cocaine self-administration in rhesus monkeys. *NIDA Research Monograph, 95,* 333-334.

Mendels, J. (1974). Biological aspects of affective illness. In S. Arieti & E. Brody (Eds.), *American handbook of psychiatry.* New York: Basic Books.

Merry, J. (1966). The "loss of control" myth. *Lancet, 1,* 1257-1258.

Meyer, P. (1975). *Medical experimentation on prisoners: Some economic considerations.* Washington, DC: Correctional Economics Center of the American Bar Association.

Miczek, K. (1973). Effects of scopolamine, amphetamine and chlordiazepoxide on punishment. *Psychopharmacology, 28,* 373-389.

Miczek, K., & Tidey, J. (1989). Amphetamines: Aggressive and social behavior. In K. Asghar & E. Souza (Eds.), *Pharmacology and toxicology of amphetamine and related designer drugs.* NIDA Research Monograph 94.

Millenson, J., & Leslie, J. (1974). The conditioned emotional response (CER) as a baseline for the study of anti-anxiety drugs. *Neuropharmacology, 13,* 1-9.

Miller, B. (1990). The interrelationships between alcohol and drugs and family violence. In M. De la Rosa, E. Lambert, & B. Gropper (Eds.), *Drugs and violence: Causes, correlates, and consequences.* NIDA Research Monograph 103.

Miller, L., & Branconnier, R. (1983). Cannabis: Effects on memory and the cholinergic limbic system. *Psychological Bulletin, 93,* 441-456.

Miracle drugs or media drugs. (1992, March). *Consumer Reports,* pp. 142-146.

Mirin, S., Weiss, R., Griffin, M., & Michael, J. (1991). Psychopathology in drug abusers and their families. *Comprehensive Psychiatry, 32,* 36-51.

Mitchell, P., & Redman, J. (1992). Effects of caffeine, time of day and user history on study-related performance. *Psychopharmacology, 109,* 121-126.

Mitic, W., McGuire, D., & Neumann, B. (1985). Perceived stress and adolescents' cigarette use. *Psychological Reports, 57,* 1043-1048.

Mitler, M., & Hajdukovic, R. (1991). Relative efficacy of drugs for the treatment of sleepiness in narcolepsy. *Sleep, 14,* 218-220.

Moglia, A., Corsico, R., Zandrini, C., et al. (1986). Activity of oxiracetam in patients with OBS: A neuropsychological study. *Clinical Neuropharmacology, 9,* S73-S78.

Mohler, H. (1992). GABAergic synaptic transmission. Regulation by drug. *Arzneimittel-Forschung, 42,* 211-214.

Mondadori, C., Ducret, T., & Borkowski, J. (1991). How long does "memory consolidation" take? New compounds can improve retention performance, even if administered up to 24 hours after the learning experience. *Brain Research, 555,* 107-111.

Mondadori, C., & Etienne, P. (1990). Nootropic effects of ACE inhibitors in mice. *Psychopharmacology, 100,* 301-307.

Money, J. (1970). Use of an androgen-depleting hormone in the treatment of male sex offenders. *Journal of Sex Research, 6,* 165-172.

Monnier, M., Dudler, L., Gachter, R., et al. (1977). The delta sleep-inducing peptide (DSIP). Comparative properties of the original and synthetic nonapeptide. *Experientia, 33,* 548-552.

Monti, J. (1987). Disturbances of sleep and wakefulness associated with the use of antihypertensive agents. *Life Sciences, 41,* 1979-1988.

Monti, P., Brown, W., & Corriveau, D. (1977). Testosterone and components of aggressive and sexual behavior in man. *American Journal of Psychiatry, 134,* 692-694.

Moore, R., Bone, L., Geller, G., et al. (1989). Prevalence, detection, and treatment of alcoholism in hospitalized patients. *Journal of the American Medical Association, 261,* 403-407.

Moore, J. (1990). Gangs, drugs, and violence. In M. De la Rosa, E. Lambert, & B. Gropper (Eds.), *Drugs and violence: Causes, correlates, and consequences.* NIDA Research Monograph 103.

Morales, A., Surridge, D., Marshall, P., & Fenemore, J. (1982). Nonhormonal pharmacological treatment of organic impotence. *Journal of Urology, 128,* 45-47.

Morgan, K. (1990). Hypnotics in the elderly: What cause for concern? *Drugs, 40,* 688-696.

Morris, R., Anderson, E., Lynch, G., & Baudry, M. (1986). Selective impairment of learning and blockade of long-term potentiation by an N-methyl-D-aspartate receptor antagonist, AP5. *Nature, 319,* 774-776.

Moskowitz, J. (1989). The primary prevention of alcohol problems: A critical review of the research literature. *Journal of Studies on Alcohol, 50,* 54-88.

Muldoon, M., Kaplan, J., Manuck, S., & Mann, J. (1992). Effects of a low-fat diet on brain serotonergic responsivity in cynomolgus monkeys. *Biological Psychiatry, 31,* 53-56.

Muldoon, M., Manuck, S., & Matthews, K. (1990). Lowering cholesterol concentrations and mortality: A quantitative review of primary prevention trials. *British Medical Journal, 301,* 309-314.

Murphy, D. (1990). Neuropsychiatric disorders and the multiple human brain serotonin receptor subtypes and subsystems. *Neuropsychopharmacology, 3,* 457-471.

Murray, E. (1989). Measurement issues in the evaluation of psychopharmacological therapy. In S. Fisher & R. Greenberg (Eds.), *The limits of biological treatments for psychological distress.* Hillsdale, NJ: Lawrence Erlbaum.

Muzet, A., Johnson, L., & Spinweber, C. (1982). Benzodiazepines increase heart rate during sleep. *Sleep, 5,* 256-261.

Myers, J., Weissman, M., Tischler, G., et al. (1984). Six-month prevalence of psychiatric disorders in three communities. *Archives of General Psychiatry, 41,* 959-967.

Myers, M. (1988). Effects of caffeine on blood pressure. *Archives of Internal Medicine, 148,* 1189-1193.

Myers, T. (1986). An analysis of context and alcohol and consumption in a group of criminal events. *Alcohol, 21,* 389-395.

Nadelmann, E. (1988). The case for legalization. *The Public Interest, 2,* 3-31.

Naranjo, C., Sellers, E., Sullivan, J., et al. (1987). The serotonin uptake inhibitor citalopram attenuates ethanol intake. *Clinical Pharmacology and Therapeutics, 41,* 266-274.

Naranjo, C., Sellers, E., Roach, C., et al. (1984). Zimelidine-induced variations in alcohol intake by nondepressed heavy drinkers. *Clinical Pharmacology and Therapeutics, 35,* 374-381.

National Cancer Institute. (1991). *Clearing the air* (NIH Publication No. 91-1647). Washington, DC: Government Printing Office.

National Commission on the Causes and Prevention of Violence. (1970). *Crimes of violence.* Washington, DC: Government Printing Office.

National Household Survey on Drug Abuse: 1988. (1990). DHHS Pub. No. (ADM) 90-1681. Washington, DC: Government Printing Office.

Nau, H. (1986). Species differences in pharmacokinetics and drug teratogenesis. *Environmental Health Perspectives, 70,* 113-129.

Neill, D., & Grossman, S. (1970). Behavioral effects of lesions or cholinergic blockade of the dorsal and ventral caudate of rats. *Journal of Comparative and Physiological Psychology, 71,* 311-317.

Nelson, J., Phillips, R., & Goldstein, L. (1977). Interhemispheric EEG laterality relationships following psychoactive agents and during operant performance in rabbits. In S. Harnad, R. Doty, L. Goldstein et al. (Eds.), *Lateralization in the nervous system*. New York: Academic Press.

Newcomb, M., Chou, C., Bentler, P., & Huba, G. (1988). Cognitive motivations for drug use among adolescents: Longitudinal tests of gender differences and predictors of change in drug use. *Journal of Counseling Psychology, 35*, 426-438.

Newman, R., Weingartner, H., Smallberg, S., & Calne, D. (1984). Effortful and automatic memory processes: Effects of dopamine. *Neurology, 34*, 805-807.

Newman, T., Browner, W., & Hulley, S. (1992). Childhood cholesterol screening: Contraindicated. *Journal of the American Medical Association, 267*, 100-101.

Ney, T., Gale, A., & Morris, H. (1989). *Smoking and human behavior*. New York: John Wiley.

Nicholson, A. (1989). Hypnotics: Clinical pharmacology and therapeutics. In M. Kryger, T. Roth, & W. Dement (Eds.), *Principles and practice of sleep medicine*. Philadelphia: J. B. Saunders.

Nicholson, A., Bradley, C., & Pascoe, P. (1989). Medications: Effect on sleep and wakefulness. In M. Kryger, T. Roth, & W. Dement (Eds.), *Principles and practice of sleep medicine*. Philadelphia: J. B. Saunders.

Nicholson, C. (1990). Pharmacology of nootropics and metabolically active compounds in relation to their use in dementia. *Psychopharmacology, 101*, 147-159.

NIDA. (1974). *Methadone: The drug and its therapeutic uses in the treatment of addiction* (Rep. Ser. 31, No. 1). Washington, DC: U.S. Department of Health and Human Services.

NIDA. (1981). *Prevention planning workbook* (DHHS Pub. No. [ADM] 81-1062). Washington, DC: U.S. Department of Health and Human Services.

NIDA. (1991). *National Household Survey on Drug Abuse: Highlights 1988*. Washington, DC: U.S. Department of Health and Human Services.

Niebergall, P., Sugita, E., & Schnaare, R. (1974). Potential dangers of common drug dosing regimens. *American Journal of Hospital Pharmacy, 31*, 53-58.

Nieforth, K. (1971). Psychotomimetic phenethylamines. *Journal of Pharmacological Science, 60*, 655-665.

Nino-Murcia, G., & Dement, W. (1987). Psychophysiological and pharmacological aspects of somnambulism and night terrors in children. In H.

Meltzer (Ed.), *Psychopharmacology: The third generation of progress.* New York: Raven.

Nisbett, R., & Schachter, S. (1966). Cognitive manipulation of pain. *Journal of Experimental and Social Psychology, 2,* 227-236.

Noback, C., & Demarest, R. (1972). *The nervous system: Introduction and review.* New York: McGraw-Hill.

Noback, C., & Demarest, R. (1986). *The nervous system* (3rd ed.). New York: McGraw-Hill.

Noel, P. (1973). *Traditional animal screening tests. Meeting on pharmacological models to assess toxicity and side effects of fertility regulating agents.* Geneva, September 17-20.

Nube, J. (1991). Beta-blockers: Effects on performing musicians. *Medical Problems of Performing Artists, 6,* 61-67.

Nyberg, K., Allebeck, P., Eklund, G., & Jacobson, B. (1992). Socio-economic versus obstetric risk factors for drug addiction in offspring. *British Journal of Addiction, 87,* 1669-1676.

Oakland Tribune. (1984, November 24).

Oakland Tribune. (1993, February 8).

Oakland Tribune. (1993, February 26).

O'Brien, C. (1976). Experimental analysis of conditioning factors in human narcotic addiction. *Pharmacological Reviews, 27,* 533-543.

O'Brien, C. (1987). Treatment research. In *Drug abuse and drug abuse research, Second triennial report to Congress* (DHHS Pub. No. [ADM] 87-1486). Washington, DC: Government Printing Office.

O'Brien, C., Childress, A., Arndt, I., et al. (1988). Pharmacological and behavioral treatments of cocaine dependence: Controlled studies. *Journal of Clinical Psychiatry, 49,* 17-22.

O'Brien, C., McLellan, T., Alterman, A., & Childress, A. (1992). Psychotherapy for cocaine dependence. In *Cocaine: Scientific and social dimensions.* Ciba Foundation Symposium 166. New York: John Wiley.

O'Brien, C., & Ternes, J. (1977). Conditioning as a cause of relapse in narcotic addiction. In E. Gottheil, A. McLellan, K. Druley, & A. Alterman (Eds.), *Addiction research and treatment: Converging trends.* Elmsford, NY: Pergamon.

O'Brien, C., Testa, T., O'Brien, T., et al. (1977). Conditioned narcotic withdrawal in humans. *Science, 195,* 1000-1002.

O'Donnell, J. (1968). Social factors and follow-up studies in opioid addiction. *Research Publications Association for Research in Nervous and Mental Disease, 46,* 333-346.

Oei, T., Singer, G., & Jefferys, D. (1980). The interaction of a fixed time food delivery schedule and body weight on self-administration of narcotic analgesics. *Psychopharmacology, 67,* 171-176.

Office of Substance Abuse Prevention. (1989). *Stopping alcohol and other drug use before it starts: The future of prevention* (DHHS Pub. No. [ADM] 89-1645). Washington, DC: U.S. Department of Health and Human Services.

Ohta, T., Ando, K., Iwata, T., et al. (1991). Treatment of persistent sleep-wake schedule disorders in adolescents with methylcobalamin (Vitamin B_{12}). *Sleep, 14,* 414-418.

Okamoto, M., Boisse, N., Rosenberg, H., & Rosen, R. (1978). Characteristics of functional tolerance during barbiturate physical dependence production. *Journal of Pharmacology and Experimental Therapeutics, 207,* 906-915.

Okawa, M., Mishima, K., Hishikawa, Y., & Takahashi, K. (1991). Vitamin B_{12} treatment for sleep-wake rhythm disorder. In G. Racagni et al. (Eds.), *Biological psychiatry, Vol. 1.* New York: Elsevier.

Okawa, M., Mishima, K., Nanami, T., et al. (1990). Vitamin B_{12} treatment for sleep-wake rhythm disorders. *Sleep, 13,* 15-23.

Okuyama, S., & Aihara, H. (1988). Action of nootropic drugs on transcallosal responses in rats. *Neuropharmacology, 27,* 67-72.

Oldendorf, W. (1978). The blood-brain barrier. In L. Bito, H. Davson, & J. Fenstermacher (Eds.), *The ocular and cerebrospinal fluids.* New York: Academic Press.

Onken, L. (1991). Using psychotherapy effectively in drug abuse treatment. In R. Pickens, C. Leukefeld, & C. Schuster (Eds.), *Improving drug abuse treatment.* NIDA Research Monograph 106.

Oral contraceptives in the '80s. (1982). *Population Reports,* series A, no. 6.

Ordy, J., Samorajski, T., Collins, R., et al. (1966). Prenatal chlorpromazine effects on liver, survival and behavior of mice offspring. *Journal of Pharmacology and Experimental Therapeutics, 151,* 110-125.

Orlowski, J., & Wateska, L. (1992). The effects of pharmaceutical firm enticements on physician prescribing patterns. There's no such thing as a free lunch. *Chest, 102,* 270-273.

Osborne, D. (1983). Cognitive effects of passive smoking. *Ergonomics, 26,* 1163-1172.

Oscar-Berman, M. (1990). Learning and memory deficits in detoxified alcoholics. In J. Spencer & J. Boren (Eds.), *Residual effects of abused drugs on behavior.* NIDA Research Monograph 101.

Ostrowski, J. (1990, July 12). Has the time come to legalize drugs? *USA Today,* pp. 27-30.

Oswald, I. (1968). Drugs and sleep. *Pharmacological Reviews, 20,* 273-303.

Overton, D. (1973). State-dependent learning produced by addicting drugs. In S. Fisher & A. Freedman (Eds.), *Opiate addiction: Origins and treatment.* New York: John Wiley.

Overton, D. (1974). Experimental methods for the study of state-dependent learning. *Federation Proceedings, 33,* 1800-1813.

Owicki, J., & Parce, J. (1990). Bioassays with a microphysiometer. *Nature, 344,* 271-272.

PADS: A look at prescription drug abuse. *Ohio State Medical Journal, 82,* 33-38.

Pahnke, W., & Richards, W. (1969). Implications of LSD and experimental mysticism. In C. Tart (Ed.), *Altered states of consciousness.* New York: John Wiley.

Painting under LSD. (1969, December 5). *Time,* p. 88.

Pam, A. (1990). A critique of the scientific status of biological psychiatry. *Acta Psychiatrica Scandinavica, 82,* 1-35.

Pappenheimer, J. (1979). "Nature's soft nurse": A sleep-promoting factor isolated from brain. *Johns Hopkins Medical Journal, 145,* 49-56.

Pappenheimer, J., Fencl, V., Karnovsky, M., et al. (1974). Peptides in cerebrospinal fluid and their relation to sleep and activity. *Research Publications Association for Research in Nervous and Mental Disease, 53,* 201-208.

Pappenheimer, J., Miller, T., & Goodrich, C. (1967). Sleep-promoting effects of cerebrospinal fluid from sleep-deprived goats. *Proceedings of the National Academy of Science of the United States, 58,* 513-517.

Parade Magazine. (1980, May 25). p. 17.

Parker, S., Zuckerman, B., Bauchner, H., et al. (1990). Jitteriness in full-term neonates: Prevalence and correlates. *Pediatrics, 85,* 17-23.

Parnes, S., & Meadow, A. (1959). Effects of "brain-storming" instructions on creative problem-solving by trained and untrained subjects. *Journal of Educational Psychology, 50,* 171-176.

Parr, D. (1976). Sexual aspects of drug abuse in narcotic addicts. *British Journal of Addiction, 71,* 261-268.

Parsons, M., & Gold, P. (1992). Glucose enhancement of memory in elderly humans: An inverted-U dose-response curve. *Neurobiology of Aging, 13,* 401-404.

Parsons, O. (1987). Neuropsychological consequences of alcohol abuse: Many questions—some answers. In O. Parsons, N. Butters, & P. Nathan (Eds.), *Neuropsychology of alcoholism: Implications for diagnosis and treatment.* New York: Guilford.

Pato, M., Zohar-Kadouch, R., Zohar, J., & Murphy, D. (1988). Return of symptoms after discontinuation of clomipramine in patients with obsessive-compulsive disorder. *American Journal of Psychiatry, 145,* 1521-1525.

Paton, W. (1960). The principles of drug action. *Proceedings of the Royal Society of Medicine, 53,* 815-820.

Peachey, J., & Annis, H. (1984). Pharmacologic treatment of chronic alcoholism. *Psychiatric Clinics of North America, 7,* 745-756.

Pearl, R. (1926). *Alcohol and longevity.* New York: Knopf.

Pepeu, G., & Spignoli, G. (1989). Nootropic drugs and brain cholinergic mechanisms. *Progress in Neuro-pharmacology, & Biological Psychiatry, 13,* S77-S88.

Perez-Reyes, Mario. (1990). Marijuana smoking: Factors that influence the bioavailability of tetrahydrocannabinol. *NIDA Research Monograph, 99,* 42-62.

Peroutka, S., & Snyder, S. (1980). Relationship of neuroleptic drug effects as brain dopamine, serotonin, alpha-adrenergic, and histamine receptors to clinical potency. *American Journal of Psychiatry, 137,* 1518-1522.

Peters, R., & McGee, R. (1982). Cigarette smoking and state dependent memory. *Psychopharmacology, 76,* 232-235.

Petrie, K., Conaglen, J., Thompson, L., & Chamberlain, K. (1989). Effect of melatonin on jet lag after long haul flights. *British Medical Journal, 298,* 705-707.

Pfeiffer, C. (1987). *Nutrition and mental illness.* Rochester, VT: Healing Arts Press.

Piazza, P., Deminiere, J., LeMoal, M., & Simon, H. (1989). Factors that predict individual vulnerability to amphetamine self-administration. *Science, 245,* 1511-1514.

Pickens, R., & Heston, L. (1981). Personality factors in human drug self-administration. In T. Thompson & C. Johanson (Eds.), *Behavioral pharmacology of human drug dependence.* NIDA Research Monograph 37.

Pickens, R., & Svikis, D. (1988). *Genetic vulnerability to drug abuse.* NIDA Research Monograph 89.

Pierce, D., & West, J. (1986a). Alcohol-induced microencephaly during the third trimester equivalent: Relationship to dose and blood alcohol concentration. *Alcohol, 3,* 185-191.

Pierce, D., & West, J. (1986b). Blood alcohol concentration: A critical factor for producing fetal alcohol effects. *Alcohol, 3,* 269-272.

Pihl, R., Peterson, J., & Finn, P. (1990). Inherited predisposition to alcoholism: Characteristics of sons of male alcoholics. *Journal of Abnormal Psychology, 99,* 291-301.

Pillai, R., & Watson, R. (1990). In vitro immunotoxicology and immunopharmacology: Studies on drugs of abuse. *Toxicology Letters, 53,* 269-283.

Pirke, K., Kockott, G., & Dittmar, F. (1974). Psychosexual stimulation and plasma testosterone in man. *Archives of Sexual Behavior, 3,* 577-584.

Placidi, G., Lenzi, A., & Lazzerini, F. (1986). The comparative efficacy and safety of carbamazepine versus lithium: A randomized double-blind 3-year trial in 83 patients. *Journal of Clinical Psychiatry, 47,* 490-494.

Plante, T., & Rodin, J. (1990). Physical fitness and enhanced psychological health. *Current Psychology, 9,* 3-24.

Platt, M., Anand, K., & Aynsley-Green, A. (1989). The ontogeny of the metabolic and endocrine stress response in the human fetus, neonate and child. *Intensive Care Medicine, 15,* S44-S45.

Pliner, P., & Cappell, H. (1974). Modification of affective consequences of alcohol. *Journal of Abnormal Psychology, 83,* 418-425.

Plumridge, R. (1983). A review of factors influencing drug prescribing. *Australian Journal of Hospital Pharmacy, 13,* 16.

Poklis, A., Maginn, D., & Barr, J. (1987). Drug findings in "driving under the influence of drugs" cases: A problem of illicit drug use. *Drug and Alcohol Dependence, 20,* 57-62.

Polich, J., Armor, D., & Braiker, H. (1979). *The course of alcoholism: Four years after treatment.* Santa Monica, CA: Rand Corporation.

Pope, H., Ionescu-Pioggia, M., Aizley, H., & Varma, D. (1990). Drug use and life style among college undergraduates in 1989: A comparison with 1969 and 1978. *American Journal of Psychiatry, 147,* 998-1001.

Pope, H., & Katz, D. (1988). Affective and psychotic symptoms associated with anabolic steroid use. *American Journal of Psychiatry, 145,* 487-490.

Porchet, H., Benowitz, N., & Sheiner, L. (1988). Pharmacodynamic model of tolerance: Application to nicotine. *Journal of Pharmacology and Experimental Therapeutics, 244,* 231-236.

Porter, I. (1966). The genetics of drug susceptibility. *Diseases of the Nervous System, 27,* 25-36.

Post, R., Kramlinger, K., Altshuler, L., et al. (1990). Treatment of rapid cycling bipolar illness. *Psychopharmacology Bulletin, 26,* 37-47.

Prakash, R., & Aronow, W. (1976). Effects of marijuana in coronary heart disease. Reply. *Clinical Pharmacology and Therapeutics, 19,* 94, 95.

Prange, A., Garbutt, J., & Loosen, P. (1987). The hypothalamic-pituitary-thyroid axis in affective disorders. In H. Meltzer (Ed.), *Psychopharmacology: The third generation of progress.* New York: Raven.

Prentice, R. (1979). Patterns of psychoactive drug use among the elderly. In *The aging process and psychoactive drug use.* NIDA Service Research Monograph Series.

Preskorn, S., & Burke, M. (1992). Somatic therapy for major depressive disorder: Selection of an antidepressant. *Journal of Clinical Psychiatry, 53,* 5-18.

Price, L., Charney, D., Delgado, P., & Heninger, G. (1990). Lithium and serotonin function: Implications for the serotonin hypothesis of depression. *Psychopharmacology, 100,* 3-12.

Price, L., Charney, D., & Heninger, G. (1985). Efficacy of lithium-tranylcypromine treatment in refractory depression. *American Journal of Psychiatry, 142,* 619-623.

Prien, R., & Kupfer, D. (1986). Continuation drug therapy for major depressive episodes: How long should it be maintained? *American Journal of Psychiatry, 143,* 18-23.

Pryor, G. (1990). Persisting neurotoxic consequences of solvent abuse: A developing animal model for toluene-induced neurotoxicity. In J. Spencer & J.

Boren (Eds.), *Residual effects of abused drugs on behavior.* NIDA Research Monograph 101.

Puccio, E., McPhillips, J., Barrett-Connor, E., & Ganiats, T. (1990). Clustering of atherogenic behaviors in coffee drinkers. *American Journal of Public Health, 80,* 1310-1313.

Pushing drugs to doctors. (1992, February). *Consumer Reports,* pp. 87-94.

Quadagno, D., Briscoe, R., & Quadagno, J. (1977). Effect of perinatal hormones on selected nonsexual behavior patterns: A critical assessment of the non-human and human literature. *Psychological Bulletin, 84,* 62-80.

Quadbeck, G. (1962). Effects of phenothiazine derivatives on blood brain barrier system. *Psychopharmacology Service Center Bulletin, 2,* 83- 84.

Quitkin, F., Stewart, J., McGrath, P., et al. (1988). Phenelzine versus imipramine in the treatment of probable atypical depression: Defining syndrome boundaries of selective MAOI responders. *American Journal of Psychiatry, 145,* 306-311.

Rabkin, J., Markowitz, J., Stewart, J., et al. (1986). How blind is blind? Assessment of patient and doctor medication guesses in a placebo-controlled trial of imipramine and phenelzine. *Psychiatric Research, 19,* 75-86.

Rabkin, J., Stewart, J., McGrath, P., et al. (1987). Baseline characteristics of 10-day placebo washout responders in antidepressant trials. *Psychiatric Research, 21,* 9-22.

Rafaelson, O. (1973). Cannabis and alcohol: Effects on simulated car driving. *Science, 179,* 920-923.

Rai, G., Shovlin, C., & Wesnes, K. (1991). A double-blind, placebo controlled study of Gingko biloba extract ("tanakan") in elderly outpatients with mild to moderate memory impairment. *Current Medical Research and Opinion, 12,* 350-355.

Randrup, A., & Munkvad, I. (1967). Stereotyped activities produced by amphetamine in several animal species and man. *Psychopharmcology, 11,* 300-310.

Rang, H., & Dale, M. (1987). *Pharmacology.* Edinburgh: Churchill Livingstone.

Rapaka, R., & Hawks, R. (Eds.). (1993). *Medications development: Drug discovery, databases, and computer-aided drug design.* NIDA Monograph 134.

Rastogi, S., & McMillan, D. (1984). The effects of cimetidine on schedule-controlled responding and locomotor activity in rats. *Pharmacology, Biochemistry, and Behavior, 20,* 63-67.

Reardon, G., Rifkin, A., Schwartz, A., et al. (1989). Changing patterns of neuroleptic dosage over a decade. *American Journal of Psychiatry, 146*, 726-729.

Regier, D., Boyd, J., Burke, B., et al. (1988). One-month prevalence of mental disorders in the U.S.—Based on five epidemiologic catchment area sites. *Archives of General Psychiatry, 45*, 977-986.

Reid, K., Surridge, D., Morales, A., et al. (1987). Double-blind trial of yohimbine in treatment of psychogenic impotence. *Lancet, 2*, 421-423.

Reimann, H. (1967). Caffeinism. A cause of long continued low-grade fever. *Journal of the American Medical Association, 202*, 1105-1106.

Reinberg, A. (1991). Concepts of circadian chronopharmacology. In W. Hrushesky, R. Langer, & F. Theeuwes (Eds.), *Temporal control of drug delivery*. New York: New York Academy of Sciences.

Reinberg, A., & Smolensky, M. (1983). *Biological rhythms and medicine*. New York: Springer.

Reuter, P. (1990). Can the borders be sealed? In R. Weisheit (Ed.), *Drugs, crime and the criminal justice system*. Highland Heights, KY: Anderson Publishing.

Reynolds, G. (1983). Increased concentrations and lateral asymmetry of amygdala dopamine in schizophrenia. *Nature, 305*, 527-529.

Ricaurte, G., & McCann, U. (1992). Neurotoxic amphetamine analogues: Effects in monkeys and implications for humans. *Annals of the New York Academy of Sciences, 648*, 371-382.

Richardson, J., Fredrickson, P., & Lin, S. (1990). Narcolepsy update. *Mayo Clinic Proceedings, 65*, 991-998.

Ricjman, A., Jackson, G., & Trigg, H. (1973). Follow-up of methadone maintenance patients hospitalized for abuse of alcohol and barbiturates. *Proceedings of the 5th National Conference on Methadone Treatment*, pp. 1484-1503. Washington, DC: Government Printing Office.

Rickels, K. (Ed.). (1968). *Non-specific factors in drug therapy*. Springfield, IL: Charles C Thomas.

Rickles, K. (1990). Buspirone in clinical practice. *Journal of Clinical Psychiatry, 51*, 51-54.

Rickels, K., Case, G., Downing, R., & Fridman, R. (1986). One-year follow-up of anxious patients treated with diazepam. *Journal of Clinical Psychopharmacology, 6*, 32-36.

Rickels, K., Case, G., Schweizer, E., et al. (1991). Long-term benzodiazepine users 3 years after participation in a discontinuation program. *American Journal of Psychiatry, 148,* 757-761.

Rickels, K., & Schweizer, E. (1990). Clinical overview of serotonin reuptake inhibitors. *Journal of Clinical Psychiatry, 51,* 9-12.

Ritchie, J., Cohen, P., & Dripps, R. (1965). Cocaine, procaine and other synthetic local anesthetics. In L. Goodman & A. Gilman (Eds.), *The pharmacological basis of therapeutics.* New York: Macmillan.

Robbins, T., Jones, G., & Sahakian, B. (1989). Central stimulants, transmitters and attentional disorder: A perspective from animal studies. In T. Sagvolden & T. Archer (Eds.), *Attention deficit disorder.* Hillsdale, NJ: Lawrence Erlbaum.

Robertson, J., Koegel, P., & Ferguson, L. (1989). Alcohol use and abuse among homeless adolescents in Hollywood. *Contemporary Drug Problems, 16,* 415-453.

Robins, L. (1973). *The Vietnam drug user returns.* Washington, DC: Government Printing Office.

Robins, L., Helzer, J., Weissman, M., et al. (1984). Lifetime prevalence of specific psychiatric disorders in three sites. *Archives of General Psychiatry, 41,* 949-958.

Robinson, R., & Zwillich, C. (1989). The effects of drugs on breathing during sleep. In M. Kryger, T. Roth, & W. Dement (Eds.), *Principles and practice of sleep medicine.* Philadelphia: J. B. Saunders.

Roche, A., Lipman, R., Overall, J., & Hung, W. (1979). The effects of stimulant medication on the growth of hyperkinetic children. *Pediatrics, 63,* 847-850.

Rodriguez, E., Aregullin, M., Nishida, T., et al. (1985). Thiaubrine A, a bioactive constituent of Aspilia (Asteracea) consumed by wild chimpanzees. *Experientia, 41,* 419-420.

Roehrich, H., & Gold, M. (1988). 800-COCAINE: Origin, significance, and findings. *Yale Journal of Biological Medicine, 61,* 149-155.

Roffwarg, H., Muzio, J., & Dement, W. (1966). Ontogenetic development of the human sleep-dream cycle. *Science, 152,* 604-619.

Rogers, A., Spencer, M., Stone, B., & Nicholson, A. (1989). The influence of a 1 h nap on performance overnight. *Ergonomics, 32,* 1193-1205.

Roizen, J., & Schneberk, D. (1977). Alcohol and crime. In M. Aarens, T. Cameron, J. Roizen et al. (Eds.), *Alcohol, casualties and crime.* Berkeley: University of California, Social Research Group.

Room, R. (1990). Measuring alcohol consumption in the United States: Methods and rationales. In L. Kozlowski et al. (Eds.), *Alcohol and drug problems, Vol. 10*. New York: Plenum.

Rosenbaum, M., & Murphy, S. (1984, Summer). Always a junkie?: The arduous task of getting off methadone maintenance. *Journal of Drug Issues*, pp. 527-552.

Rosenthal, L., Roehrs, T., Zwyghuizen-Doorenbos, B., et al. (1991). Alerting effects of caffeine after normal and restricted sleep. *Neuropsychopharmacology, 4*, 103-108.

Rosenthal, R., & Rosnow, R. (1969). The volunteer subject. In *Artifacts in behavioral research*. New York: Academic Press.

Rosevear, J. (1967). *Pot: A handbook of marijuana*. New York: University Books.

Rosmarin, P., Applegate, W., & Somes, G. (1990a). Coffee consumption and blood pressure: A randomized, crossover clinical trial. *Journal of General Internal Medicine, 5*, 211-213.

Rosmarin, P., Applegate, W., & Somes, G. (1990b). Coffee consumption and serum lipids: A randomized, crossover clinical trial. *American Journal of Medicine, 88*, 349-356.

Ross, S. (1973). A study of living and residence patterns of former heroin addicts as a result of their participation in a methadone treatment program. In *Proceedings of the Fifth National Conference on Methadone Treatment*. New York: National Association for the Prevention of Addiction to Narcotics.

Rothberg, A., & Lits, B. (1991). Psychosocial support for maternal stress during pregnancy: Effect on birth weight. *American Journal of Obstetrics and Gynecology, 165*, 403-407.

Rothenberg, A. (1990). *Creativity and madness: New findings and old stereotypes*. Baltimore, MD: Johns Hopkins University Press.

Roy, A., Virkkunen, M., & Linnoila, M. (1987). Reduced central serotonin turnover in a subgroup of alcoholics. *Progress in Neuropsychopharmacolgy and Biological Psychiatry, 11*, 173-177.

Rubin, V., & Comitas, L. (1976). *Ganja in Jamaica*. Garden City, NY: Anchor.

Rudd, C., & Brazy, J. (1988). Drugs in the perinatal period: Implications for the preterm infant. *Comprehensive Therapy, 14*, 30-37.

Russell, M. (1971a). Cigarette dependence: I. Nature and classification. *British Medical Journal, 2*, 330-331.

Russell, M. (1971b). Cigarette dependence: II. Doctor's role in management. *British Medical Journal, 2*, 393-395.

Russell, M. (1971c). Cigarette smoking: Natural history of a dependence disorder. *British Journal of Medical Psychology, 44,* 1-16.

Russell, W., & Nathan, P. (1946). Traumatic amnesia. *Brain, 69,* 180-300.

Rylander, G. (1969). Clinical and medico-criminological aspects of addiction to central stimulating drugs. In F. Sjoqvist & M. Tottie (Eds.), *Abuse of central stimulants.* New York: Raven.

Sachs, J., Ungar, J., Waser, P., & Borbely, A. (1976). Factors in cerebrospinal fluid affecting motor activity in the rat. *Neuroscience Letter, 2,* 83-86.

Sackett, D. (1976). The magnitude of compliance and noncompliance. In D. Sackett & R. Haynes (Eds.), *Compliance with therapeutic regimes.* Baltimore, MD: Johns Hopkins University Press.

Sackett, D. (1980). Is there a compliance problem? If so, what do we do about it? In L. Lasagna (Ed.), *Controversies in therapeutics.* Philadelphia: J. B. Saunders.

Safer, R., Allen, D., & Barr, E. (1972). Depression of growth in hyperactive children on stimulant drugs. *The New England Journal of Medicine, 287,* 217-220.

Salzman, C. (1991). The APA task force report on benzodiazepine dependence, toxicity, and abuse. *American Journal of Psychiatry, 148,* 151-152.

Salzman, C., & Shader, R. (1978). Depression in the elderly. II. Possible drug etiologies; differential diagnostic criteria. *Journal of the American Geriatric Society, 26,* 303-308.

San Francisco Chronicle. (1971, March 2).

San Francisco Chronicle. (1971, April 3).

San Francisco Examiner. (1991, November 1).

Sanders, D., Warner, P., Backstrom, T., & Bancroft, J. (1983). Mood, sexuality, hormones and the menstrual cycle. I. Changes in mood and physical state: Description of subjects and method. *Psychosomatic Medicine, 45,* 487-501.

Sansone, M., Castellano, C., Battaglia, M., & Ammassari-Teule, M. (1990). Oxiracetam prevents mecamylamine-induced impairment of active, but not passive, avoidance learning in mice. *Pharmacology, Biochemistry, and Behavior, 36,* 389-392.

Sansone, M., & Oliverio, A. (1989). Avoidance facilitation by nootropics. *Progress in Neuropsychopharmacology and Biological Psychiatry, 13,* S89-S97.

Sassen-Koob, S. (1989). New York City's informal economy. In A. Portes, M. Castells, & L. Benton (Eds.), *The informal economy: Studies in advanced and less developed countries*. Baltimore, MD: Johns Hopkins University Press.

Satin, M., Winsberg, B., Monetti, C., Sverd, J., & Foss, D. (1985). A central population screen for attention deficit disorder with hyperactivity. *American Academy of Child Psychiatry, 24*, 756-764.

Satinoff, E. (1988). Thermal influences on REM sleep. In R. Lydic & J. Biebuyck (Eds.), *Clinical physiology of sleep*. Baltimore, MD: Waverly Press.

Savage, C., et al. (1963). A follow-up note on the psychedelic experience. Cited in *Psychedelic Review, 1*, 18-26.

Schachter, S., Silverstein, B., Kozlowski, L., et al. (1977). Studies of the interaction of psychological and pharmacological determinants of smoking. *Journal of Experimental Psychology, 106*, 3-40.

Schaeffer, J., Andrysiak, T., & Ungerleider, J. (1981). Cognition and long-term use of ganja (cannabis). *Science, 213*, 465-466.

Schapira, K., McClelland, H., Griffiths, M., & Newell, D. (1970). Study on the effects of tablet colour in the treatment of anxiety states. *British Medical Journal, 2*, 446-449.

Schaps, E., DiBartolo, R., Moskowitz, J., et al. (1981). A review of 127 drug abuse prevention evaluations. *Journal of Drug Issues, 11*, 17-43.

Scharf, M., Fletcher, K., & Graham, J. (1988). Comparative amnestic effects of benzodiazepine hypnotic agents. *Journal of Clinical Psychiatry, 49*, 134-137.

Scharf, M., & Sachais, B. (1990). Sleep laboratory evaluation of the effects and efficacy of trazodone in depressed insomniac patients. *Journal of Clinical Psychiatry, 51*, 13-17.

Schectman, G., Byrd, J., & Hoffmann, R. (1991). Ascorbic acid requirements for smokers: Analysis of a population survey. *Journal of Clinical Nutrition, 53*, 1466-1470.

Schenk, S., Horger, B., & Snow, S. (1989-1990). Caffeine preexposure sensitizes rats to the motor activating effects of cocaine. *Behavioral Pharmacology, 1*, 447-451.

Scher, J. (1961). Group structure and narcotic addiction: Notes for a natural history. *International Journal of Group Psychotherapy, 6*, 88-93.

Scher, M., Richardson, G., Coble, P., et al. (1988). The effects of prenatal alcohol and marijuana exposure: Disturbances in neonatal sleep cycling and arousal. *Pediatric Research, 24*, 101-105.

Scheuplein, R., Shoaf, S., & Brown, R. (1990). Role of pharmacokinetics in safety evaluation and regulatory considerations. *Annual Review of Pharmacology and Toxicology, 30,* 197-218.

Schmidt, W., Popham, R., & Israel, Y. (1987). Dose-specific effects of alcohol on the lifespan of mice and the possible relevance to man. *British Journal of Addictions, 82,* 775-788.

Schofield, P., Shivers, B., & Seeburg, P. (1990). The role of receptor subtype diversity in the CNS. *Trends in Neuroscience, 13,* 8-11.

Schou, M. (1979). Artistic productivity and lithium prophylaxis in manic-depressive illness. *British Journal of Psychiatry, 135,* 97-103.

Schou, M. (1986). Lithium treatment: A refresher course. *British Journal of Psychiatry, 149,* 541-547.

Schrag, P. (1978). *Mind control.* New York: Pantheon.

Schrauzer, G., & Shrestha, K. (1990). Lithium in drinking water and the incidences of crimes, suicides, and arrests related to drug addictions. *Biological Trace Element Research, 25,* 105-113.

Schroeder, N., Caffey, E., & Lorei, T. (1977). Antipsychotic drug use: Physician prescribing practices in relation to current recommendations. *Diseases of the Nervous System, 38,* 114-116.

Schuckit, M. (1979). *Drug and alcohol abuse.* New York: Plenum.

Schuckit, M., Hauger, R., Monteiro, M., et al. (1991). Response of three hormones to diazepam challenge in sons of alcoholics and controls. *Alcoholism: Clinical and Experimental Research, 15,* 537-542.

Schultes, R. (1963). The widening panorama in medical botany. *Rhodora, 65,* 97-120.

Schwartz, J. (1987). *Review and evaluation of smoking cessation methods: The United States and Canada, 1978-1985* (NIH Pub. No. 87-2940). Washington, DC: Government Printing Office.

Schwartz, R. (1991). Heavy marijuana use and recent memory impairment. *Psychiatric Annals, 21,* 80-82.

Seeman, P., & Lee, T. (1975). Antipsychotic drugs: Direct correlation between clinical potency and presynaptic action on dopamine neurons. *Science, 188,* 1217-1219.

Segawa, S. (1990). Clinical trials: It's still a man's world. *Nature, 345,* 754.

Segraves, R. (1985). Psychiatric drugs and orgasm in the human female. *Journal of Psychosomatic Obstetrics and Gynecology, 4*, 125-128.

Segraves, R. (1988a). Drugs and desire. In S. Leiblum & R. Rosen (Eds.), *Sexual desire disorders*. New York: Guilford.

Segraves, R. (1988b). Hormones and libido. In S. Leiblum & R. Rosen (Eds.), *Sexual desire disorders*. New York: Guilford.

Segraves, R. (1988c). Psychiatric drugs and inhibited female orgasm. *Journal of Sex and Marital Therapy, 14*, 202-207.

Segraves, R. (1989). Effects of psychotropic drugs on human erection and ejaculation. *Archives of General Psychiatry, 46*, 275-284.

Segraves, R., Bari, M., Segraves, K., & Spirnak, P. (1991). Effect of apomorphine on penile tumescence in men with psychogenic impotence. *Journal of Urology, 145*, 1174-1175.

Seidel, W., Roth, T., Roehrs, T., et al. (1984). Treatment of a 12-hour shift of sleep schedule with benzodiazepines. *Science, 224*, 1262-1264.

Seidel, W., Cohen, S., Wilson, L., & Dement, W. (1985). Effects of alprazolam and diazepam on the daytime sleepiness of non-anxious subjects. *Psychopharmacology, 87*, 194-197.

Sellers, E., Busto, U., & Kaplan, H. (1989). Pharmacokinetic and pharmacodynamic drug interactions: Implications for abuse liability testing. *NIDA Research Monograph, 92*, 287-306.

Sells, S. (1977). Methadone maintenance in perspective. *Journal of Drug Issues, 7*, 13-22.

Senay, E. (1989). Case reports and the assessment of drug abuse liability. In M. Fischman & N. Mello (Eds.), *Testing for abuse liability of drugs in humans*. NIDA Research Monograph 92.

Serafetinides, E. (1965). The significance of the temporal lobes and of hemispheric dominance in the production of LSD-25 symptomatology in man. *Neuropsychology, 3*, 69-79.

Seventh Special Report to U.S. Congress on Alcohol and Health. (1990). Washington, DC: U.S. Department of Health and Human Services.

Shader, R., & Jackson, A. (1975). Approaches to schizophrenia. In R. Shader (Ed.), *Manual of psychiatric therapeutics*. Boston: Little, Brown.

Shagass, C. (1960). Drug thresholds as indicators of personality and affect. In L. Uhr & J. Miller (Eds.), *Drugs and behavior*. New York: John Wiley.

Shapiro, A., & Morris, L. (1978). The placebo effect in medical and psychological therapies. In S. Garfield & H. Bergin (Eds.), *Handbook of psychotherapy and behavior change*. Hawthorne, NY: Aldine de Gruyter.

Sheard, M. (1963). The influence of doctor's attitude on the patient response to antidepressant medication. *Journal of Nervous and Mental Disease, 136*, 555-560.

Shedler, J., & Block, J. (1990). Adolescent drug use and psychological health: A longitudinal inquiry. *American Psychologist, 45*, 612-630.

Shekerjian, D. (1990). *Uncommon genius*. New York: Viking.

Shen, W., & Sata, L. (1990). Inhibited female orgasm resulting from psychotropic drugs: A five-year, updated, clinical review. *Journal of Reproductive Medicine, 35*, 11-14.

Shoaf, S., & Linnoila, M. (1991). Interaction of ethanol and smoking on the pharmacokinetics and pharmacodynamics of psychotropic medications. *Psychopharmacology Bulletin, 27*, 577-609.

Shopsin, B., Friedman, E., & Gershon, S. (1976). Parachlorophenylalanine reversal of tranylcypromine effects in depressed outpatients. *Archives of General Psychiatry, 33*, 811-819.

Shulgin, A. (1983). *Drugs of perception*. Invited address, Psychedelic Conference, Santa Barbara, CA.

Sidney, S. (1990). Evidence of discrepant data regarding trends in marijuana use and supply, 1985-1988. *Journal of Psychoactive Drugs, 22*, 319-324.

Siegel, R. (1977). Hallucinations. *Scientific American, 237*, 132-140.

Siegel, R. (1978a). Phencyclidine and ketamine intoxication: A study of four populations of recreational users. In R. Petersen & R. Stillman (Eds.), *Phencyclidine (PCP) abuse: An appraisal*. NIDA Research Monograph 21.

Siegel, R. (1978b). Phencyclidine, criminal behavior, and the defense of diminished capacity. In R. Petersen & R. Stillman (Eds.), *Phencyclidine (PCP) abuse: An appraisal*. NIDA Research Monograph 21.

Siegel, R. (1982). Cocaine and sexual dysfunction: The curse of mama coca. *Journal of Psychoactive Drugs, 14*, 71-74.

Siegel, R. (1986, March). Jungle revelers. *Omni*, pp. 70-72, 74, 100.

Siegel, R. (1989). *Intoxication: Life in pursuit of artificial paradise*. New York: NAL/E. P. Dutton.

Siegel, S. (1988). Drug anticipation and the treatment of dependence. *NIDA Research Monograph, 84,* 1-24.

Silverman, I. (1982). Women, crime and drugs. *Journal of Drug Issues, 12,* 167-183.

Simcha-Fagan, O., Gersten, J., & Langner, T. (1986). Early precursors and concurrent correlates of patterns of illicit drug use in adolescence. *Journal of Drug Issues, 16,* 7-28.

Simes, R. (1986). Publication bias: The case for an international registry of clinical trials. *Psychopharmacology, 100,* 3-12.

Simon, E., & Hiller, J. (1989). Opiate peptides and opioid receptors. In G. Siegel, B. Agranoff, R. Albers, & P. Molinoff (Eds.), *Basic neurochemistry.* New York: Raven.

Simonds, J., & Kashani, J. (1980). Specific drug use and violence in delinquent boys. *American Journal of Drug and Alcohol Abuse, 7,* 305-322.

Simpson, D., & Sells, S. (1982). Effectiveness of treatment for drug abuse: An overview of the DARP research program. *Advances in Alcohol & Substance Abuse, 2,* 7-29.

Singh, N., & Winton, A. (1989). Behavioral pharmacology. In J. Luiselli (Ed.), *Behavioral medicine and developmental disabilities.* New York: Springer.

Siomopoulos, V. (1981). Violence: The ugly face of amphetamine abuse. *Illinois Medical Journal, 159,* 375-377.

Skolnick, A. (1990). Illicit drugs take still another toll—Death or injury from vehicle-associated trauma. *Journal of the American Medical Association, 263,* 3122-3123.

Slag, M., Morley, J., Elson, M., et al. (1983). Impotence in medical clinic outpatients. *Journal of the American Medical Association, 249,* 1736-1740.

Small, J., Milstein, V., Perez, H., et al. (1972). EEG and neurophysiological studies of lithium in normal volunteers. *Biological Psychiatry, 5,* 65-77.

Smart, R. (1991a). Crack cocaine use: A review of prevalence and adverse effects. *American Journal of Drug and Alcohol Abuse, 17,* 13-26.

Smart, R. (1991b). World trends in alcohol consumption. *World Health Forum, 12,* 99-103.

Smart, R., & Adlaf, E. (1991). Substance use and problems among Toronto street youth. *British Journal of Addictions, 86,* 999-1010.

Smith, A., Traganza, E., & Harrison, G. (1969). Studies on the effectiveness of antidepressant drugs [Special issue]. *Psychopharmacology Bulletin.*

Smith, D., & Vernier, V. (1978). Antidepressants, new drugs, discovery and development. *Drugs and the Pharmaceutical Sciences, 5,* 204.

Smith, D., & Wesson, D. (1978). Cocaine. *Journal of Psychedelic Drugs, 10,* 351-360.

Smith, E., Lee, R., Schnur, S., & Davidson, J. (1987a). Alpha2-adrenoreceptor antagonists and male sexual behavior: I. Mating behavior. *Physiology and Behavior, 41,* 7-14.

Smith, E., Lee, R., Schnur, S., & Davidson, J. (1987b). Alpha2-adrenoreceptor antagonists and male sexual behavior: II. Erectile and ejaculatory reflexes. *Physiology and Behavior, 41,* 15-19.

Smith, L., & Lang, W. (1980). Changes occurring in self administration of nicotine by rats over a 28-day period. *Pharmacology, Biochemistry, and Behavior, 13,* 215-220.

Smith, R. (1979). Study finds sleeping pills overprescribed. *Science, 204,* 287-288.

Smith, S., & Rawlins, M. (1973). *Variability in human drug response.* London: Butterworth.

Smoking-attributable mortality and years of potential life lost—United States, 1988. (1991). *Morbidity and Mortality Weekly Report, 40,* 62-63, 69-71.

Snyder, S. (1971). *Uses of marijuana.* New York: Oxford University Press.

Soderstrom, C., Trifillis, A., Shankar, B., & Clark, W. (1988). Marijuana and alcohol use among 1023 trauma patients: A prospective study. *Archives of Surgery, 123,* 733-737.

Sotsky, S., Glass, D., Shea, M., et al. (1991). Patient predictors of response to psychotherapy and pharmacotherapy: Findings in the NIMH treatment of depression collaborative research program. *American Journal of Psychiatry, 148,* 997-1008.

Sox, H., Margulies, I., & Sox, C. (1981). Psychologically mediated effects of diagnostic tests. *Annals of Internal Medicine, 95,* 680-685.

Spencer, J., & Boren, J. (Eds.), (1990). *Residual effects of abused drugs on behavior.* NIDA Research Monograph 101.

Speroff, L. (1988, March 26). *Androgens in the menopause.* Symposium Proceedings, Atlanta, GA.

Spielberg, S. (1984). Pharmacogenetics. In S. Macleod & I. Raddle (Eds.), *Textbook of pediatric clinical pharmacology.* Littleton, MA: PSG Publishing.

Spotts, J., & Shontz, F. (1991). Drugs and personality: Comparison of drug users, nonusers, and other clinical groups on the 16PF. *International Journal of Addictions, 26,* 1019-1054.

Spunt, B., Goldstein, P., Belluci, P., & Miller, T. (1990a). Drug relationships in violence among methadone maintenance treatment clients. *Advances in Alcohol & Substance Abuse, 9,* 81-99.

Spunt, B., Goldstein, P., Belluci, P., & Miller, T. (1990b). Race/ethnicity and gender differences in the drugs-violence relationship. *Journal of Psychoactive Drugs, 22,* 293-303.

Spunt, B., Tarshish, C., Fendrich, M., et al. (1990, November). *Using correctional data to understand the drugs-homicide nexus: Findings from New York State.* Paper presented at the Annual Meetings of the American Society of Criminology, Baltimore, MD.

Squire, L. (1992). Memory and the hippocampus: A synthesis from findings with rats, monkeys, and humans. *Psychological Review, 99,* 195-231.

Stachnik, T. (1972). The case against criminal penalties for illicit drug use. *American Psychologist, 27,* 637-642.

Stafford, P., & Golightly, B. (1967). *LSD: The problem-solving psychedelic.* New York: Award.

Steele, C., & Josephs, R. (1990). Alcohol myopia: Its prized and dangerous effects. *American Psychologist, 45,* 921-933.

Steenland, K. (1992). Passive smoking and the risk of heart disease. *Journal of the American Medical Association, 267,* 94-99.

Stein, J., Swisher, J., Hu, T., & McDonnell, N. (1984). Cost-effectiveness evaluation of a Channel One program. *Journal of Drug Education, 14,* 251-269.

Stewart, D. (1992). High fiber diet and serum tricyclic antidepressant levels. *Journal of Clinical Psychopharmacology, 12,* 438-440.

Stimson, G. (1977). Do drug advertisements provide therapeutic information? *Journal of Medical Ethics, 3,* 7-13.

Stitzer, M., Bigelow, G., & Gross, J. (1989). Behavioral treatment of drug abuse. In *Treatments of psychiatric disorders: A task force report of the American Psychiatric Association.* Washington, DC: American Psychiatric Association.

Stone, A., Cox, D., Valdimarsdottir, H., et al. (1987). Evidence that secretory IgA antibody is associated with daily mood. *Journal of Personality and Social Personality, 52,* 988-993.

Stone, W., Rudd, R., & Gold, P. (1990). Amphetamine, epinephrine, and glucose enhancement of memory retrieval. *Psychobiology, 18,* 227-230.

Stone, W., Wenk, G., Stone, S., & Gold, P. (1992). Glucose attenuation of paradoxical sleep deficits in old rats. *Behavioral Neural Biology, 57,* 79-86.

Strassman, R. (1984). Adverse reactions to psychedelic drugs: A review of the literature. *Journal of Nervous and Mental Disease, 172,* 577-595.

Straus, H. (1987, June). From crack to ecstasy. *American Health Magazine,* pp. 50-52, 54.

Streissguth, A., Barr, H., Sampson, P., et al. (1986). Attention, distraction and reaction time at age 7 years and prenatal alcohol exposure. *Neurobehavioral Toxicology and Teratology, 8,* 717-725.

Streissguth, A., Treder, R., Barr, H., et al. (1987). Aspirin and acetaminophen use by pregnant women and subsequent child I IQ and attention decrements. *Teratology, 35,* 211-219.

Stripling, J., & Hendricks, C. (1981). Effect of cocaine and lidocaine on the expression of kindled seizures in the rat. *Pharmacology, Biochemistry, and Behavior, 14,* 397-403.

Study shows major role of alcohol in crimes. (1985, November 4). *Oakland Tribune.*

Stuppaeck, C., Barnas, C., Miller, C., et al. (1990). Carbamazepine in the prophyaxis of mood disorders. *Journal of Clinical Psychopharmacology, 10,* 39-42.

Sturup, G. (1979). Castration: The total treatment. In H. Resnick & M. Wolfgang (Eds.), *Sexual behavior: Social and legal aspects.* Boston: Little, Brown.

Subcommittee on Health, Committee on Labor and Public Welfare, U.S. Senate. (1974). *Examination of the pharmaceutical industry.* Washington, DC: Government Printing Office.

Surgeon General's report. (1979). *Smoking and health* (DHEW Pub. No. [PHS] 79-50066). Washington, DC: Government Printing Office.

Sutherland, G., Stapleton, J., Russell, M., et al. (1992). Randomised controlled trial of nasal nicotine spray in smoking cessation. *Lancet, 340,* 324-329.

Sutker, P., & Archer, R. (1979). MMPI characteristics of opiate addicts, alcoholics, and other drug abusers. In C. Newark (Ed.), *MMPI: Clinical and research trends.* New York: Praeger.

Suzdak, P., Glowa, J., Crawley, J., et al. (1986). A selective imidazobenzodiazepine antagonist of ethanol in the rat. *Science, 234,* 1243-1274.

Svarstad, B. (1983). Stress and the use of nonprescription drugs: An epidemiological study. *Research in Community Mental Health, 3,* 233-254.

Svensson, C. (1989). Representation of American blacks in clinical trials of new drugs. *Journal of the American Medical Association, 261,* 263-265.

Swartz, M., Landerman, R., George, L., et al. (1991). Benzodiazepine anti-anxiety agents: prevalence and correlates of use in a Southern community. *American Journal of Public Health, 81,* 592-596.

Swisher, J., & Hu, T (1983). *Alternatives to drug abuse: Some are and some are not.* NIDA Research Monograph 47.

Tang, M., Ahrendsen, K., & Falk, J. (1981). Barbiturate dependence and drug preference. *Pharmacology, Biochemistry, and Behavior, 14,* 405-408.

Tang, M., Brown, C., & Falk, J. (1982). Complete reversal of chronic ethanol polydipsia by schedule withdrawal. *Pharmacology, Biochemistry, and Behavior, 16,* 155-158.

Tart, C. (1971). *On being stoned.* Palo Alto, CA: Science & Behavior.

Tarter, R., Moss, H., Arria, A., & Van Thiel, D. (1990). Hepatic, nutritional, and genetic influences on cognitive process in alcoholics. In J. Spencer & J. Boren (Eds.), *Residual effects of abused drugs on behavior.* NIDA Research Monograph 101.

Taylor, J., & Tinklenberg, J. (1987). Cognitive impairment and benzodiazepines. In H. Meltzer (Ed.), *Psychopharmacology: The third generation of progress.* New York: Raven.

Teboul, E., & Chouinard, G. (1991). A guide to benzodiazepine selection. Part II: Clinical aspects. *Canadian Journal of Psychiatry, 36,* 62-73.

Teicher, M., Glod, C., & Cole, J. (1990). Emergence of intense suicidal preoccupation during fluoxetine treatment. *American Journal of Psychiatry, 147,* 207-210.

Tennant, F., & Groesbeck, C. (1972). Psychiatric effects of hashish. *Archives of General Psychiatry, 27,* 133-136.

Tennant, F., Tarver, A., & Rawson, R. (1984). Clinical evaluation of mecamylamine for withdrawal from nicotine dependence. In L. Harris (Ed.), *Problems in drug dependence 1983.* NIDA Research Monograph 49.

Tennes, K., Avitable, N., Blackard, C., Boyles, C., Hassoun, B., Holmes, L., & Kreye, M. (1985). Marijuana: Prenatal and postnatal exposure in the human. In T. Pinkert (Ed.), *Current research on the consequences of maternal drug abuse.* NIDA Research Monograph 59.

Testing drugs in older people. (1990, November 24-27). *FDA Consumer.*

Teyler, T., & Discenna, P. (1987). Long-term potentiation. *Annual Review of Neuroscience, 10,* 131-161.

Third triennial report to Congress. (1991). *Drug abuse and drug abuse research* (DHHS Pub. No. [ADM]91-1704). Washington, DC: Government Printing Office.

Thompson, J., & Thompson, M. (1986). *Genetics in medicine.* Philadelphia: J. B. Saunders.

Thompson, P. (1991). Antidepressants and memory: A review. *Human Psychopharmacology Clinical and Experimental, 6,* 79-90.

Thompson, R. (1985). *The brain.* New York: Freeman.

Thompson, W., & Olian, S. (1961). Some effects on offspring behavior of maternal adrenalin injection during pregnancy in three inbred mouse strains. *Psychological Reports, 8,* 87-90.

Thomson, R. (1982). Side effects and placebo amplification. *British Journal of Psychiatry, 140,* 64-68.

Ticku, M., & Kulkarnisk, K. (1988). Molecular interactions of ethanol with GABAergic system and potential of Ro15-4513 as an ethanol antagonist. *Pharmacology, Biochemistry, and Behavior, 30,* 501-510.

Tinkleberg, J. (1974). Marijuana and human aggression. In L. Miller (Ed.), *Marijuana: Effects on human behavior.* New York: Academic Press.

Tonini, G., & Montanari, C. (1955). Effects of experimentally induced psychoses on artistic expression. *Confinia Neurologica, 15,* 225-239.

Tonnesen, P., Norregaard, J., Simonsen, K., & Sawe, U. (1991). A double-blind trial of a 16-hour transdermal nicotine patch in smoking cessation. *The New England Journal of Medicine, 325,* 311-315.

Tournier, R. (1979). Alcoholics Anonymous as a treatment and ideology. *Journal of Studies on Alcohol, 40,* 230-239.

Trebach, A. (1987). *The great drug war.* New York: Macmillan.

Trebach, A. (1991, May/June). "Socialist realism" in the service of the drug war. *The Drug Policy Letter.*

Trebach, A., & Zeese, K. (1990). *Drug prohibition and the conscience of nations.* Washington, DC: Drug Policy Foundation.

Trussell, J., & Kost, K. (1987). Contraceptive failure in the United States: A critical review of the literature. *Studies in Family Planning, 18,* 237-283.

Tsoi, W. (1991). Insomnia: Drug treatment. *Annals of the Academy of Medicine, Singapore, 20,* 269-272.

Tueting, P. (1991). Psychophysiological predictors of drug treatment response. *Psychiatric Medicine, 9,* 145-161.

Turner, C. (1966). *General endocrinology.* Philadelphia: J. B. Saunders.

Uhlenhuth, E. (1966). Drug, doctor's verbal attitudes and clinical setting in the symptomatic response to pharmacotherapy. *Psychopharmacology, 9,* 392-418.

Uhlenhuth, E., Canter, A., Neustadt, J., & Payson, H. (1959). The symptomatic relief of anxiety with meprobamate, phenobarbital and placebo. *American Journal of Psychiatry, 115,* 905-910.

Unger, S. (1967). In H. Abramson (Ed.), *The use of LSD in psychotherapy and alcoholism* (p. 366). Indianapolis: Bobbs-Merrill.

Ungerer, J., Harford, R., Brown, F., & Kleber, H. (1976). Sex guilt and preferences for illegal drugs among drug abusers. *Journal of Clinical Psychology, 32,* 891-895.

Uno, H., Lohmiller, L., Thieme, C., et al. (1990). Brain damage induced by prenatal exposure to dexamethasone in fetal rhesus macaques. I. Hippocampus. *Developmental Brain Research, 53,* 157-167.

Update: Eosinophilia-myalgia syndrome associated with the ingestion of L-tryptophan—United States. (1989). *Morbidity and Mortality Weekly Report, 38,* 842-843.

U.S. Department of Health and Human Services. (1982a). *The health consequences of smoking: Cancer: A report of the Surgeon General, 1982* (DHHS Pub. No. [PHS] 82-50179). Washington, DC: U.S. Department of Health and Human Services.

U.S. Department of Health and Human Services. (1982b). *The health consequences of smoking: Cardiovascular disease: A report of the Surgeon General, 1982* (DHHS Pub. No. [PHS] 84-50204). Washington, DC: U.S. Department of Health and Human Services.

U.S. Department of Health and Human Services. (1989). *Reducing the health consequences of smoking: 25 years of progress. A Report of the Surgeon General.* Washington, DC: U.S. Department of Health and Human Services.

U.S. Department of Justice. (1989a). *Drugs of abuse.* Washington, DC: Government Printing Office.

U.S. Department of Justice, Bureau of Justice Statistics. (1989b, July). *Federal criminal cases, 1980-87* (Special Report NCJ-118311). Washington, DC: U.S. Department of Justice.

U.S. General Accounting Office. (1990). *Drug-exposed infants: A generation at risk.* Washington, DC: U.S. General Accounting Office.

U.S. Public Health Service (1980). *The health consequences of smoking for women.* Washington, DC: Government Printing Office.

Van Baar, A. (1990). Development of infants of drug dependent mothers. *Journal of Child Psychology and Psychiatry, 31,* 911-920.

Van Baar, A., Fleury, P., Soepatmi, S., et al. (1989). Neonatal behaviour after drug dependent pregnancy. *Archives of Disease in Children, 64,* 235-240.

Van Baar, A., Fleury, P., & Ultee, C. (1989). Behaviour in first year after drug dependent pregnancy. *Archives of Disease in Children, 64,* 241-245.

Van der Kilk, B. (1988). The trauma spectrum: The interaction of biological and social events in the genesis of the trauma response. *Journal of Traumatic Stress, 1,* 273-290.

Van Kammen, D., Bunney, W., Docherty, J., et al. (1982). d-Amphetamine-induced heterogenous changes in psychotic behavior in schizophrenia. *American Journal of Psychiatry, 139,* 991-997.

Van Putten, T. (1974). Why do schizophrenic patients refuse to take their drugs? *Archives of General Psychiatry, 31,* 67-72.

Van Putten, T., & Mutalipassi, L. (1975). Fluphenazine enanthate induced decompensation. *Psychosomatics, 16,* 37-40.

Vargas, G., Pildes, R., & Vidyasagar, D. (1975). Effect of maternal heroin addiction on 67 liveborn neonates. *Clinical Pediatrics, 14,* 751-757.

Vaughan, F. (1983). Perception and knowledge. In L. Grinspoon & J. Bakalar (Eds.), *Psychedelic reflections.* New York: Human Sciences Press.

Veleber, D., & Templer, D. (1984). Effects of caffeine on anxiety and depression. *Journal of Abnormal Psychology, 93,* 120-122.

Verbrugge, L. (1982). Sex differences in legal drug use. *Journal of Social Issues, 38,* 59-76.

Verghese, C., Kessel, J., & Simpson, G. (1991). Clinical pharmacokinetics of neuroleptics. *Psychopharmacology Bulletin, 27,* 541-564.

Vesell, E. (1979). Pharmacogenetics: Multiple interactions between genes and environment as determinants of drug response. *American Journal of Medicine, 66,* 183-187.

Vesell, E., Lang, C., White, W., et al. (1973). Hepatic drug metabolism in rats: Impairment in a dirty environment. *Science, 179,* 896-897.

Virag, R. (1982). Intracavernous injection of papaverine for erectile failure. [Letter to the Editor]. *Lancet, 2,* 938.

Virag, R., Shoukry, K., Nollet, F., & Greco, E. (1991). Intracavernous self-injection of vasoactive drugs in the treatment of impotence: 8-year experience with 615 cases. *Journal of Urology, 145,* 287-293.

Virkkunen, M. (1987). Metabolic dysfunctions among habitually violent offenders: Reactive hypoglycemia and cholesterol levels. In S. Mednick, T. Moffitt, & S. Stack (Eds.), *The causes of crime.* New York: Cambridge University Press.

Virkkunen, M., DeJong, J., Bartko, J., et al. (1989). Relationship of psychobiological variables to recidivism in violent offenders and impulsive fire setters. *Archives of General Psychiatry, 46,* 600-603.

Vocci, F. (1989). The necessity and utility of abuse liability evaluations in human subjects: The FDA perspective. In M. Fischman & N. Mello (Eds.), *Testing for abuse liability of drugs in humans.* NIDA Research Monograph 92.

Voetglin, W., Broz, W., & O'Hollaren, P. (1941). Conditioned reflex therapy of chronic alcoholics: IV. A preliminary report on the value of reinforcement. *Quarterly Journal of Studies on Alcohol, 2,* 505-511.

Vogel, G., Buffenstein, A., Minter, K., & Hennessey, A. (1990). Drug effects on REM sleep and on endogenous depression. *Neuroscience and Biobehavioral Reviews, 14,* 49-63.

Volgyesi, F. (1954). "School for patients": Hypnosis-therapy and psychoprophylaxis. *British Journal of Medical Hypnosis, 5,* 8-16.

Vom Saal, F., & Bronson, F. (1980). Sexual characteristics of adult female mice are correlated with their blood testosterone levels during prenatal development. *Science, 208,* 597-599.

Vornoff, S. (1941). *From cretin to genius.* New York: Alliance.

Wade, V., Mansfield, P., & McDonald, P. (1989). Drug companies' evidence to justify advertising. *Lancet, 2,* 1261-1264.

Walker, D., & Gold, P. (1991). Effects of the novel NMDA antagonist, NPC 12626, on long-term potentiation, learning and memory. *Brain Research, 549,* 213-221.

Walkup, J. (1991). Increased anticholinergic levels, memory and judgment. *Human Psychopharmacology, 6,* 189-196.

Wallace, J. (1972). Drinkers and abstainers in Norway: A national survey. *Quarterly Journal of Studies on Alcohol, 33,* 129-151.

Walsh, J., Humm, T., Muehlbach, M., et al. (1991). Sedative effects of ethanol at night. *Journal of Studies on Alcohol, 52*, 597-600.

Walsh, J., Muehlbach, M., Humm, T., et al. (1990). Effect of caffeine on physiological sleep tendency and ability to sustain wakefulness at night. *Psychopharmacology, 101*, 271-273.

Walsh, J., Sugerman, J., Muehlbach, M., & Schweitzer, P. (1988). Physiological sleep tendency on a simulated night shift: Adaptation and effects of triazolam. *Sleep, 11*, 251-264.

Ware, J., Brown, F., Moorad, P., et al. (1989). Effects on sleep: A double blind study comparing imipramine to the sedating tricyclic antidepressant trimipramine in depressed insomniac patients. *Sleep, 12*, 537-549.

Ware, J., & Pittard, J. (1990). Increased deep sleep after trazodone use: A double-blind placebo controlled study in healthy young adults. *Journal of Clinical Psychiatry, 51*, 18-22.

Warner, K. (1977). *Possible increases in the understanding of cigarette consumption.* Paper presented at 105th annual meeting of the American Public Health Association, Washington, DC.

Warner, K. (1987). Health and economic implications of a tobacco-free society. *Journal of the American Medical Association, 258*, 2080-2086.

Warner, K., Goldenhar, L., & McLaughlin, C. (1992). Cigarette advertising and magazine coverage of the hazards of smoking. *The New England Journal of Medicine, 326*, 305-309.

The Washington Post. (1991, August 27).

The Washington Post. (1991, September 23).

Wasson, G. (1968). *Soma, divine mushroom of immortality.* New York: Harcourt.

Watzman, N., Barry, H., Kinnard, W., & Buckley, J. (1968). Some conditions under which pentobarbital stimulates spontaneous motor activity of mice. *Journal of Pharmaceutical Sciences, 57*, 1572-1576.

Webb, W. (1978). The sleep of conjoined twins. *Sleep, 1*, 205-211.

Wechsler, H., Grosser, G., & Greenblatt, M. (1965). Research evaluating antidepressant medications on hospitalized mental patients: A survey of published reports during a five-year period. *Journal of Nervous and Mental Disease, 141*, 231-239.

Weil, A., Zinberg, N., & Nelson, J. (1968). Clinical and psychological effects of marihuana in man. *Science, 162*, 1234-1242.

Weingartner, H., Hommer, D., Lister, R., et al. (1992). Selective effects of triazolam on memory. *Psychopharmacology, 106*, 341-345.

Weinshilboum, R. (1984). Human pharmacogenetics. *Federation Proceedings, 43*, 2295-2297.

Weiss, B., & Laties, V. (1962). Enhancement of human performance by caffeine and the amphetamines. *Pharmacological Reviews, 14*, 1-36.

Weiss, J., & Tanner, P. (1981). Twenty questions. *Journal of Operational Psychiatry, 12*, 144-146.

Weiss, R., & Mirin, S. (1986). Subtypes of cocaine abusers. *Psychiatric Clinics of North America, 9*, 491-501.

Weissman, A. (1990). What it takes to validate behavioral toxicology tests: A belated commentary on the collaborative behavioral teratology study. *Neurotoxicology and Teratology, 12*, 497-501.

Weissman, M. (1988). The epidemiology of anxiety disorders. Rates, risks and familial patterns. *Journal of Psychiatric Research* (Suppl. 1), 99-114.

Wender, P. (1988). Attention deficit disorder residual type (ADD-RT) or adult hyperactivity. In J. Tupin, R. Shader, & D. Harnett (Eds.), *Handbook of clinical psychopharmacology*. Northvale, NJ: Jason Aronson.

Werboff, J., & Havlena, J. (1962). Postnatal behavioral effects of tranquilizers administered to the gravid rat. *Experimental Neurology, 6*, 263-269.

Wernicke, W. (1985). The side effect profile and safety of fluoxetine. *Journal of Clinical Psychiatry, 46*, 59-67.

Wesnes, K., & Simpson, P. (1988). Can scopolamine produce a model of the memory deficits seen in aging and dementia? In M. Gruneberg, P. Morris, & R. Sykes (Eds.), *Practical aspects of memory: Current research and issues*. New York: John Wiley.

Wesson, D., & Smith, D. (1985). Cocaine: Treatment perspectives. In N. Kozel & E. Adams (Eds.), *Cocaine use in America: Epidemiologic and clinical perspectives*. NIDA Research Monograph 61.

Wheatley, D. (1968). Effects of doctors' and patients' attitudes and other factors on response to drugs. In K. Rickels (Ed.), *Non-specific factors in drug therapy*. Springfield, IL: Charles C Thomas.

Who profits from drugs? (1989). *Frontline* [PBS TV].

Wieland, W., & Yunger, M. (1970). Sexual effects and side effects of heroin and methadone. In *Proceedings, Third National Conference on Methadone Treatment*. Washington, DC: Government Printing Office.

Wikler, A. (1948). Recent progress in research on the neurophysiologic basis of morphine addiction. *American Journal of Psychiatry, 105,* 329-338.

Wilder, J. (1957). The law of initial value in neurology and psychiatry. Facts and problems. *Journal of Nervous and Mental Disease, 125,* 73-86.

Wilkes, M., Doblin, B., & Shapiro, M. (1992). Pharmaceutical advertisements in leading medical journals: Experts' assessments. *Annals of Internal Medicine, 116,* 912-919.

Willcox, D., Gillan, R., & Hare, E. (1965). Do psychiatric outpatients take their drugs? *British Medical Journal, 2,* 790-792.

Wills, T. (1986). Stress and coping in early adolescence: Relationships to smoking and alcohol use in urban school samples. *Health Psychology, 5,* 503-529.

Wills, T. (1990). Stress and coping factors in the epidemiology of substance use. In L. Kozlowski et al. (Eds.), *Alcohol and drug problems, Vol. 10.* New York: Plenum.

Wilsher, C. (1986). Effects of piracetam on developmental dyslexia. *International Journal of Psychophysiology, 4,* 29-40.

Wilsher, C., Bennett, D., Chase, C., et al. (1987). Piracetam and dyslexia: Effects on reading tests. *Journal of Clinical Pharmacology, 7,* 230-237.

Wilsnack, S., Klassen, A., Schur, B., & Wilsnack, R. (1991). Predicting onset and chronicity of women's problem drinking: A five-year longitudinal analysis. *American Journal of Public Health, 81,* 305- 318.

Wilson, G. (1989). Clinical studies of infants and children exposed prenatally to heroin. *Annals of the New York Academy of Science, 562,* 183-194.

Wilson, G., & Abrams, D. (1977). Effects of alcohol on social anxiety and physiological arousal: Cognitive versus pharmacological processes. *Cognitive Therapeutic Research, 1,* 195-210.

Wilson, G., & Lawson, D. (1976). Expectancies, alcohol, and sexual arousal in male social drinkers. *Journal of Abnormal Psychology, 85,* 587-594.

Winter, E. (1991). Effects of an extract of Gingko biloba on learning and memory in mice. *Pharmacology, Biochemistry and Behavior, 38,* 109-114.

Wish, E. (1986). PCP and crime: Just another illicit drug? In D. Clouet (Ed.), *Phencyclidine: An update.* NIDA Research Monograph 64.

Wolf, S. (1950). Effects of suggestion and conditioning on the action of chemical agents in human subjects—The pharmacology of placebos. *Journal of Clinical Investigation, 29,* 100-109.

Wolf, S. (1962). Placebos: Problems and pitfalls. *Clinical Pharmacology and Therapeutics, 3*, 254-257.

Wolfe, A. (1986). *National roadside breathtesting survey: Procedures and results.* Washington, DC: Insurance Institute for Highway Safety.

Wolkowitz, O., Tinklenberg, J., & Weingartner, H. (1985). A psychopharmacological perspective of cognitive functions. II. Specific pharmacologic agents. *Neuropsychobiology, 14*, 133-156.

Wood, R. (1978). Stimulus properties of inhaled substances. *Environmental Health Perspectives, 26*, 69-76.

Woods, J. (1989). Pharmacokinetics of cocaine: Fetal lamb studies. *Annals of the New York Academy of Science.*

Woody, G., McLellan, T., & O'Brien (1990). Clinical-behavioral observations of the long-term effects of drug abuse. In J. Spencer & J. Boren (Eds.), *Residual effects of abused drugs on behavior.* NIDA Research Monograph 101.

Woody, G., O'Brien, C., & Greenstein, R. (1978). Multimodality treatment of narcotic addiction: An overview. In R. Petersen (Ed.), *The international challenge of drug abuse.* NIDA Research Monograph 19.

Woolf, N., & Butcher, L. (1989). Cholinergic systems: synopsis of anatomy and overview of physiology and pathology. In A.Scheibel & A. Wechsler (Eds.), *The Biological Substrates of Alzheimer's Disease.* New York: Academic.

Worden, A. (1974). Toxicological methods. *Toxicology, 2*, 359-370.

Wright, H. (1980). Violence and PCP abuse. *American Journal of Psychiatry, 137*, 752-753.

Wysowski, D., & Baum, C. (1989). Antipsychotic drug use in the United States, 1976-1985. *Archives of General Psychiatry, 46*, 929-932.

Yanagita, T. (1973). An experimental framework for evaluation of dependence liability of various types of drugs in monkeys. *Bulletin on Narcotics, 25*, 57-64.

Yazigi, R., Odem, R., & Polakoski, K. (1991). Demonstration of specific binding of cocaine to human spermatozoa. *Journal of the American Medical Association, 266*, 1956-1959.

Yeats, E. (1989). Pharmacotherapy from the perspective of family ecology. In J. Ellison (Ed.), *The psychotherapist's guide to pharmacotherapy.* Chicago: Year Book Medical.

Yoken, C., & Berman, J. (1984). Does paying a fee for psychotherapy alter the effectiveness of treatment? *Journal of Consulting Clinical Psychology, 52*, 254-260.

Yolles, S. (1968). *Recent research on LSD, marijuana, and other dangerous drugs* [Statement before Committee on the Judiciary, U.S. Senate].

Yonkers, K., Kando, J., Cole, J., & Blumenthal, S. (1992). Gender differences in pharmacokinetics and pharmacodynamics of psychotropic medication. *American Journal of Psychiatry, 149,* 587-595.

Young, L., Richter, J., Bradley, L., & Anderson, K. (1987). Disorders of the upper gastrointestinal system: An overview. *Annals of Behavioral Medicine, 9,* 7-12.

Zamula, E. (1989, June). Drugs and pregnancy: Often the two don't mix. *FDA Consumer Magazine.*

Zarcone, V. (1973). Marijuana and ethanol: Effects on sleep. *Psychiatric Medicine, 4,* 201-212.

Zarcone, V. (1989). Sleep hygiene. In M. Kryger, T. Roth, & W. Dement (Eds.), *Principles and practice of sleep medicine.* Philadelphia: J. B. Saunders.

Zeese, K. (1989, July/August). Housing: The new battleground in the war on drugs. *The Drug Policy Letter.*

Zegans, L., Pollard, J., & Brown, D. (1967). The effects of LSD-25 on creativity and tolerance to regression. *Archives of General Psychiatry, 16,* 740-749.

Zeichner, A., & Phil, R. (1979). Effects of alcohol and behavior contingencies on human aggression. *Journal of Abnormal Psychology, 88,* 153-160.

Zhou, H., Koshakji, R., Silberstein, D., Wilkinson, G., & Wood, A. (1989). Racial differences in drug response: Altered sensitivity to and clearance of propranolol in men of Chinese descent as compared with American whites. *The New England Journal of Medicine, 320,* 565-570.

Zito, J., Craig, T., Wanderling, J., & Siegel, C. (1987). Pharmaco-epidemiology in 136 hospitalized schizophrenic patients. *American Journal of Psychiatry, 144,* 778-782.

Zito, J., Craig, T., Wanderling, J., Siegel, C., & Green, M. (1988). Pharmacotherapy of the hospitalized young adult schizophrenic patient. *Comprehensive Psychiatry, 29,* 379-386.

Zorc, J., Larson, D., Lyons, J., & Beardsley, R. (1991). Expenditures for psychotropic medications in the United States in 1985. *American Journal of Psychiatry, 148,* 644-647.

Zorgniotti, A., & Lefleur, R. (1985). Auto-injection of the corpus cavernosum with a vasoactive drug combination for vasculogenic impotence. *Journal of Urology, 133,* 39-41.

Zuckerman, B. (1991). Selected methodological issues in investigations of prenatal effects of cocaine: Lessons from the past. In M. Kilbey & K. Asghar (Eds.), *Methodological issues in controlled studies on effects of prenatal exposure to drug abuse.* NIDA Research Monograph 114.

Zuckerman, B., Amaro, H., & Cabral, H. (1989). The validity of self-reported marijuana and cocaine use among pregnant adolescents. *Journal of Pediatrics, 115,* 812-815.

Zuckerman, B., Frank, D., Bauchner, H., et al. (1989). Effects of maternal marijuana and cocaine use on fetal growth: The importance of biological markers. *Pediatric Research, 25,* 79A.

Zuckerman, B., Frank, D., Hingson, R., et al. (1989). Effects of maternal marijuana and cocaine use on fetal growth. *The New England Journal of Medicine, 320,* 762-768.

Zweben, J., & Payte (1990). Methadone maintenance in the treatment of opioid dependence—A current perspective. *Western Journal of Medicine, 152,* 588-599.

Zweben, J., & Sorensen, J. (1988). Misunderstandings about methadone. *Journal of Psychoactive Drugs, 20,* 275-281.

Zwyghuizen-Doorenbos, A., Roehrs, T., Lipschutz, L., et al. (1990). Effects of caffeine on alertness. *Psychopharmacology, 100,* 36-39.

Zwyghuizen-Doorenbos, A., Roehrs, T., Timms, V., & Roth, T. (1990). Individual differences in the sedating effects of ethanol. *Alcoholism, Clinical and Experimental Research, 14,* 400-404.

Drug and Substance Index

EDITOR'S NOTE: Please note that additional information about general classes of drugs as well as certain important drugs can be found in the Subject Index.

Subject Index